Insomniac

The publisher gratefully acknowledges the generous contribution to this book provided by the General Endowment Fund of the University of California Press Foundation.

Insomniac

Gayle Greene

UNIVERSITY OF CALIFORNIA PRESS

Berkeley Los Angeles London

University of California Press, one of the most
distinguished university presses in the United States,
enriches lives around the world by advancing scholarship
in the humanities, social sciences, and natural sciences.
Its activities are supported by the UC Press Foundation
and by philanthropic contributions from individuals and
institutions. For more information, visit www.ucpress
.edu.

University of California Press
Berkeley and Los Angeles, California

University of California Press, Ltd.
London, England

Library of Congress Cataloging-in-Publication Data

Greene, Gayle.
  Insomniac / Gayle Greene.
    p. ; cm.
  Includes bibliographical references and index.
  ISBN 978-0-520-24630-0 (cloth : alk. paper)
    1. Insomnia.   2. Insomnia—Miscellanea.
3. Sleep disorders.   I. Title.
[DNLM: 1. Sleep Initiation and Maintenance Disorders.
2. Personal Narratives.   WM 188 G799i 2008]
RC547.G75   2008
616.8'498—dc22   2007008838

Manufactured in the United States of America
17   16   15   14   13   12   11   10   09   08
10   9   8   7   6   5   4   3   2

To insomniacs of the world . . .

Behold the wreckage
of night, one heck
of a mess: covers . . .
cast off in vast
deserts of insomnia
where trepidations bomb
tranquillity to rubble.

Stephen Cushman,
"Make the Bed"

Contents

Acknowledgments

I want first to thank the insomniacs who shared their stories with me, who took the time and trouble to write me or talk to me about their experiences and ideas: Judy Baxter, Rusty Cady, Edie Cross, Jill Delsigne, Cynthia Greenberg, Naomi Katz, Laura Lockwood, Tiffany Ingersoll, Jenny Warburg, Bill West, Kees Wiese, and Henry Wortis. There are many more I would have named but couldn't reach to ask if they wanted to be named (since changed e-mails leave no forwarding addresses), so I'll say thank you, Arjun, Barbara, Bonnie, Darren, Desiree, Dina, Geoff, Helen, Isabella, Jason, John, Josh, Joseph, Ken, Joan, Leonore, Linda, Nancy, Pat, Rose, Ross, Tanya, Tom, and others I'm sure I'm forgetting or whose names I never knew. (Most preferred to remain anonymous— such is the stigma that attaches to this condition.) Thanks also to the researchers who gave me interviews in person, by telephone, or through e-mail—Daniel Buysse, William Dement, Michael Gershon, Peter Hauri, Michael Irwin, Daniel Kripke, Charles Medawar, Bruce McEwen, Louis Ptacek, Allan Rechtschaffen, Nick Rosenlicht, Martin Scharf, and Michael Young—and heartfelt appreciation to those who hung in there when I kept coming back with questions: Michael Bonnet, Irwin Feinberg, and Emmanuel Mignot.

I am indebted to many people who talked to me at the conferences and whose words helped me get a grasp or an angle on some small part of this vast, sprawling subject: Donna Arand, Sara Arber, Roseanne Armitage, Georgianna Bell, Jed Black, John Brottem, David Dinges, Jenny Hislop, Gregg Jacobs, Leonid Kayumov, Leon Lack, Lynne Lamberg, Karen Moe, Adrian Morrison, Patricia Murphy, Jessica Payne, Tarja Porkka-Heiskanen, Katie Ramos, Tom Scammell, Dan Watenpaugh, Margaret White, and Elizabeth Wyatt. I had the good fortune to know personally or chance to meet several physicians and psychotherapists who gave me insights into what the problem of insomnia looks like to a professional faced with the challenge of treating it: Dr. Peter Barglow, Dr. Anne Coffey, Dr. Steven Freedman, Dr. Richard Levine, Dr. Anne Marshall, Dr. Beth McDougall, Dr. Vicki Ratner, and others who prefer to remain unnamed. I am grateful to Bob Cloud for helping me understand what narcolepsy feels like, and what a travesty it would have been had Xyrem not been approved as a treatment for this condition, as it almost was not; and to Steven Wm. Foukes for sharing with me his considerable knowledge about GHB. Laurel Martin-Harris took me on a memorable tour of Rockefeller Institute and helped me meet researchers there. Filmmaker Alan Berliner helped me see, in his moving autobiographical documentary, *Wide Awake,* and in conversation, how aspects of the condition that eluded my powers of description could be rendered cinematically.

Two writing groups saw this book or parts of it through its various incarnations, and thanks go to Marilyn Fabe, Claire Kahane, Sherry Keith, Wendy Martin, and Margaret Schaefer, with special gratitude to Mardi Louiselle, Kay Trimberger, and Ilene Philipson, who threw themselves into draft after draft with dedication and aplomb. Ilene's contributions as a clinical psychologist who sees insomnia in her practice and as a person who has sometimes experienced it herself were especially illuminating. The readings of Nick Rosenlicht, Richard Lewis, and Laura Hoopes were extremely helpful in keeping me on scientific track. Marcia Cavell and Jill Delsigne also came through with thoughtful, insightful suggestions. Friends from my former days as a Shakespearean, Ann Jones, Carol Neely, and Madelon Sprengnether, made time in their busy lives to read parts or all of the manuscript, bringing to the task the keen critical intelligence and sensibilities of readers steeped in imaginative literature.

Special appreciation to Roberta Johnson, my longtime friend and fellow insomniac: her readings of drafts and our ongoing discussions through the long gestation of this project helped shape it into what it's become. Elizabeth Minnich's comments on chapters she read and our conversations around them inspired me to think about the subject in the broadest terms. A chance meeting with Bill West, who'd been troubleshooting his condition for years, directed my attention, early on, to crucial studies and showed me how a person living with a chronic condition can be so motivated to research that condition that he achieves a command of the scientific literature that would astonish the professionals. I owe a debt of gratitude to Tim Miller, who, though we'd never met, engaged with my chapters with the generosity of an old friend and brought to his readings the eye of a clinical psychologist with long experience helping people deal with sleep, and considerable wisdom as a human being—as well as a keen eye for the flabby sentence.

I'd like also to thank my agent, Jean Naggar, and my editor at University of California Press, Naomi Schneider, for their steadfast, enthusiastic support. Thanks to Scripps College for providing faculty research fellowships that gave me the means to attend the many conferences that I did, and especially to Dean Michael Lamkin and Lisa Sullivan, who encouraged me to apply for a Mellon grant that gave sabbatical support. I am grateful to Julie Lyss for inviting me to air the project at a Humanities Institute event; to Sasha Lilley for inviting me to speak on KPFA Radio; and to the *Women's Review of Books,* which published a piece in their 2003 issue on women aging. These events led to a flood of responses that were brimming with new leads and information. Heartfelt appreciation to student assistants Jaime Willis and Shiyuan Deng for their tireless tracking of sources, to my student Hannah Graves for the author photo (though we had no idea then that it would be an author photo), and to Becky Ballinger for support beyond the secretarial call of duty, not only with this project but with my complicated teaching life. Other friends whose warmth and encouragement kept me going through the long ordeal of this book are Janet Adelman, Kim Beeman, Rich Bowen, David Claus, Rena Fraden, Jed Harris, Wendy Martin, Frances McConnel, Robert Osserman, John Peavoy, Kay Trimberger, Cheryl Walker, Nancy Ware, and Jean Wyatt.

And the book would not have happened if it hadn't been for Robert Jourdain. For his belief in me and the project, his unflagging willingness to talk it through, often in the wee hours of the night, and to read it through yet again, and for much else besides, I owe more than I can say.

CHAPTER 1

Insomnia

The cure for insomnia? Get plenty of sleep.
W. C. Fields

The first thing to go is your sense of humor. Then goes the desire to do the things you used to do, then the desire to do anything at all. Parts of your body ache that you don't even know the names of, and your eyes forget how to focus. Words you once knew aren't there anymore, and there's less and less to say. People you once cared about fall by the way and you let them go, too.

Insomnia is a problem most insomniacs don't want to talk about. In fact, it's a problem many of us don't know *how* to talk about. "Oh, you know, a bad night," I say to a colleague's "What's wrong?" on one of my walking-into-walls days. "Why, Gayle, what do *you* have to lose sleep about? You've got no problems," says my colleague, eyebrows raised. If I'd been up with a bad tooth or a sick child, that's something he would understand. If I just plain can't sleep, that's weird. Anyhow, chronic insomnia is not just "a bad night." *Chronic* (i.e., lasting, constant, continuous) insomnia is a bad night that goes on and on.

Look on the Web, read what insomniacs say on Sleepnet.com and Talkaboutsleep.com, and you'll find stories of lives wrecked by this affliction, marriages ruined, educations abandoned, jobs lost, careers destroyed. *I can't work, I can't date, I can't connect with anyone anymore. I had to drop out of school. I used to be a lawyer; now I'm the walking dead. I was a teacher once; there's no way I could face a classroom now. It's like being punished for something, only I don't know what I did. Does anybody have any advice? Please, please, can somebody tell me what to do?* (Here—and throughout the book—I've italicized the words of insomniacs. Since most of the names I'd attach to insomniacs' quotes would be pseudonyms, I've left names off, except where speakers have told me they're willing to be identified.)

We reach for metaphors, analogies, figures of speech to say what "it's like." *It's like someone opened a tap at the bottom of your body and just tapped out all the blood, and it's just gone, there's nothing left. It's like some vital juice is drained away and what's left is bone on bone. It's like I'm wasting away, slipping away, losin' it. It's like I'm being sucked dry, eaten away, stolen away, swallowed up, coming unglued*—these are the terms I hear. *It's a beast that can pounce on you without warning or cause. It chews you up and spits you out.*

When you have insomnia, you're never really asleep, and you're never really awake, says a character in the film *Fight Club. It's a claustrophobia of crawling through a tunnel of unbroken, undifferentiated time, a nighttime landscape that's neither sleep nor dream,* says an insomniac I interviewed. Says Romanian writer E. M. Cioran,

> Normally someone who goes to bed and sleeps all night almost begins a new life the next day. . . . He has a present, a future, and so on. But for someone who doesn't sleep, from the time of going to bed at night to waking up in the morning, it's all continuous, there's no interruption . . . no suppression of consciousness. . . . So, instead of starting a new life, at 8 in the morning you're like you were at 8 the evening before. The nightmare continues . . . and in the morning that new life doesn't exist. . . .
> When that's stretched out for months and years . . . you do not see what future to look toward, because you don't have any future.

He adds, "And it requires an extraordinary will to not succumb."

"Succumb to what?" asks his interviewer.

"To the temptation of suicide. In my opinion, almost all suicides, about 90%, say, are due to insomnia. I can't prove that, but I'm convinced." Studies corroborate Cioran's suspicion, suggesting that insomnia may well be a risk factor for suicide. It is certainly a risk factor for alcoholism.

Insomnia has been with us as long as we've had language. Ancient Egyptian hieroglyphs record a lament for "three living hells," one of which is "to be in bed and sleep not." The sorrows of Job, in the book of Genesis, include the lament "When shall I arise, and the night be gone? I am full of tossings to and fro unto the dawning of the day." In the Latin epic *Silvae*, a first-century-A.D. insomniac prays to Somnus, the Roman god of sleep, the "gentlest of the gods": "By what crime or error of mine have I deserved that I alone lack thy bounty?" References abound, in the literary texts, diaries, letters, and legal documents of Europe and America of two hundred to five hundred years ago, to "restless" sleep, troubled sleep, broken sleep. The Pharaohs' tombs held urns of sleep-inducing herbs to guard against sleepless nights in the life to come. Remedies are described in ancient Greece and Rome, in medieval and Renaissance Europe and England. They include anointing the soles of the feet with the fat of a dormouse, brushing the teeth with the earwax of a dog, anointing the temples with a mixture of camphor and woman's milk, drinking a potion made from the gall of a castrated boar, and drinking hemlock—which may have induced a longer sleep than intended.

Insomnia may come with the territory of being human, but it has, for a variety of reasons, become the plague of modern times. Surveys indicate that about a third of the American population suffers with it enough to complain about it, and that as many as 10 to 15 percent have it chronically. Incidence is this high in other industrialized countries, the United Kingdom, Europe, Japan. Among the poor, the female, and the elderly, the incidence is much higher—in people over sixty-five, estimates are as high as 60 percent. Since there are no outward and apparent signs for what we have, no wounds, scars, crutches, casts, wheelchairs, this is an invisible epidemic. Insomnia is not seen, and it's certainly not heard, since insomniacs are not speaking out. Sleep researchers estimate that seven out of ten people with sleep problems never even discuss the problem with a professional. "Insomniacs are seen as neurotics who should have more will power," says Stanford researcher Richard Coleman. "Knowing that they'll be granted little sympathy if they mention some of their miserable daytime symptoms . . . or ask for sick leave, insomniacs tend to keep their sleep complaints to themselves. . . . They prefer medication and go on secretly living with insomnia."

Mostly I have been reluctant to complain about insomnia to doctors, an insomniac wrote me. *I'm becoming aware of how much I have internalized the stigma associated with it, the assumption that it's something I'm doing wrong, some emotional problem or bad sleep habits.* From a U.K. insomniac, I hear, *Most people don't want to talk about it because of the way we are regarded, I think.* Some tell me, *You're the first person I've talked to about this. I never talk about it to anyone.* Some don't want to talk about it at all: *you'll just see how neurotic I am.* Several say that it's an issue too private or painful to go into, or that talking about it might make it worse: *I find myself reluctant to talk about it, for fear of invoking it.* From more than one I hear: *I'm not an insomniac, I just can't sleep.*

I understand, nobody wants to wear a badge that says *neurotic.* And yet, by not owning up to it, not naming it, we leave it, well, unnamed—unrecognized, undiagnosed, underresearched, underground, "the great underground ailment of modern society." Insomnia is, as one insomniac called it, *the world's best-kept secret. It's like a dirty little secret we sweep under the carpet, hoping it'll go away.*

But for the chronic insomniac, it doesn't go away.

✳

When it began for me, I can't remember. The truth is, I remember very little of my childhood. What I do remember is the following scene, played at various times throughout my youth, most vividly in my early adolescence: "But I can't sleep!" I'd protest as my parents tried to wrestle me into bed at what they called a *decent* hour, meaning any time before 1 A.M.

"Nonsense," said my father, "of course you can. Everyone knows how to sleep. Why, even animals know how to sleep. Just close your eyes, relax, and you'll get sleepy. It's the most natural thing in the world, sleep." My father was a normal sleeper, and to the normal sleeper, sleep is "the most natural thing in the world."

"But Daddy, I *can't!* I don't know how!"

"Well, you get all wound up. Now if you'd only listen to your mother and go to bed earlier . . ." He knew it was something I was bringing on myself, some obstinacy of mine that I could change, if only I would do something different, *be* something different—if only I would *change my attitude, change my ways.*

My father was a doctor, an old-style family practitioner who carried a black bag and delivered babies at home, one of a heroic, vanished breed. But that didn't mean he knew a thing about sleep. Sleep had no part in the medical school curriculum at Yale in the 1930s when he was there. Sleep has little part in medical curricula today, when doctors get an average of one to two hours' instruction in sleep and sleep disorders. The advice he gave me is a version of the advice I've been hearing ever since: you're stressed out, you're anxious, you're depressed, you have bad habits. These are the things insomniacs are still told. There may be— there often is—truth to such explanations, but they may also be ways of passing the buck back to the sufferer, a thing doctors have been known to do when confronted with problems they don't well understand.

We also hear a lot of cheer-up-it's-not-so-bad advice:

"Don't worry about it—you probably just worry too much."

"You probably just need more exercise—try yogi" (that's not a typo). I do yoga stretches. I swim three times a week and walk on the days I don't swim.

"As you get older, you need less sleep." A myth that's been called into question by recent research: we may get less sleep as we age, but it's not clear that we *need* less sleep.

"You probably sleep more than you think you do—people often do." I run this one by my partner, Bob. "No-o-o-o, I don't think so," he says. Too many of my sleepless nights have become his.

Psychophysiological insomnia is the diagnosis given to garden-variety insomniacs like myself, people who have no egregious psychological or medical problems. It's a sort of catchall term for insomnia that cannot otherwise be explained. The *psycho* suggests that the mind (or psyche) is involved; the *physiological* suggests that the body's there, too, except that nobody—neither the doctors nor the writers of the self-help books that crowd the bookstore shelves nor the researchers themselves—seems much interested in the body's part. No doctor I ever saw showed the slightest curiosity about the cocktail of hormones, estrogen, proges- terone, thyroid, that I ingest daily, though any of these might affect sleep. The *psycho* explanation is so much easier. When 501 physicians were interviewed about how they treated insomnia, "they revealed that they asked an average of 2.5 questions and their questions were most likely to be about psychological problems." Fewer than a quarter "even asked about patients' evening coffee intake."

"Uh, Psychiatry handles that," said my primary caretaker at my HMO when I asked him for a sleep med. I made an appointment with "Psychiatry" (which took six weeks) and talked to a nice man who made sure I wasn't suicidal, referred me to an "antianxiety workbook," and offered me an antidepressant, though I told him that antidepressants make me, well, depressed. "Sure, that's how it works," says a psycho- therapist friend, Ilene, who works with patients referred to her by the HMOs. "The hardcore insomniacs get shunted to us. As though *we* know how to deal with it!" "The patient with a chronic complaint of in- somnia (even though it may have a purely physical etiology) will usually be referred to the psychiatrist," concludes a 1980 survey. Maybe this is why so few insomniacs take their problem to a doctor.

"Sleep in a dark, quiet room," "Make sure you have a comfortable mattress"—these are things I get told. All very true, but what kind of an idiot would I have to be to have lived this long with this problem and not know this? "Go to bed earlier," "Go to bed every night at the same time and get up at the same time," "When you can't sleep, get out of bed and do something else," "Never use the bed to read or work." All very well, but nothing I didn't hear from my father those many years ago—except now there are new names: *sleep hygiene* (a term that makes me feel like I'm not only a bad sleeper, but a dirty sleeper) and *sleep restriction therapy* (restrict time in bed to the hours you sleep consecutively) and *stimulus control therapy* (learn to associate the bed only with sleep) and *cognitive restructuring* (change your way of thinking about the problem) and *cognitive behavioral therapy to deal with maladaptive thought patterns*. A real mouthful, that, but what it all comes down to is—*change your attitude, change your ways.*

Friends and family weigh in with further advice. "Oh, I had insomnia once. I just got up and did something else. I told myself, 'Just cut this out,' and after a week or so, I was fine. If I don't worry about it, it goes away." Everybody's had a bad night now and then, so everybody's an expert, right?

"You're probably not 'getting enough.'" *Sex,* he meant. But for some reason, most of the things that put other people out perk me right up: sex, hot baths, whiskey, meditation, eating carbohydrates at night, eating protein at night, eating nothing at all.

Or, "A little warm milk—puts you right out."

Or, "A shot of whiskey does the trick."

"A hot bath . . ."

"A big plate of pasta . . ."

"Have you tried melatonin?" Yes, I have tried melatonin. I've tried (nearly) everything anyone has ever told me worked for them, and it's taken me some strange ways: lathering myself in sesame oil, brewing a Chinese herbal tea so foul that my dog fled the kitchen when it steeped, concocting a magnesium supplement that hissed and spat like something out of Harry Potter. I've driven across two counties to a guru who claimed to have the secret of sleep. I've tried valerian, kava kava, chamomile, skullcap, passionflower, homeopathic concoctions, l-tryptophan, 5-HTP, GABA, melatonin, Elavil, Zoloft, trazodone, tricyclics, and pills whose names I never knew. I took the talking cure with a psychiatrist and a psychologist, and though the psychologist helped me sort things out, she hadn't a clue why I sleep so badly or what I should do about it. I've tried most of the benzodiazepines—Librium, Valium, Xanax, Dalmane, Klonopin, Restoril, Halcion, and more Ativan than I care to remember or probably can remember, since this drug erodes memory. I've taken the nonbenzodiazepines Ambien and Sonata and, in the bad old days, I dipped into Nembutal, Seconal, and Miltown, as well as over-the-counter products like Sominex, Nytol, Sleep-Eze, and others whose names I've repressed. I've tried acupuncture, biofeedback, meditation, hypnosis, self-hypnosis, relaxation tapes, ayurvedic medicine, adrenal support supplements, blackstrap molasses, wheat germ, bananas by the bunch, licorice root, SAM-e, St. John's wort, yoga positions, and at one point, I was swimming three to four miles a day. I've worn a magnet necklace. And yes, I have tried regularizing and restricting my sleep, cutting out all caffeine and alcohol, doing all those "sleep hygienic" things we're told to do. I thought I'd tried everything there was to try, but when I started talking to insomniacs, I realized I'd missed a few: I have *not* consulted a psychic, hung in a flotation tank, done cranial electrical stimulation, or slept with a cathode ion collector dish by the bed. I have not tried chelation treatment (getting the lead out), colostrom (don't ask), sleeping with my head pointed north or west, or ordeal therapy, unless you call vacuuming the house at 4 A.M., which I used to do, "ordeal therapy."

"If there's any illness for which people offer many remedies," says a character in Anton Chekhov's *The Cherry Orchard*, "you may be sure that particular illness is incurable."

People cannot hear that I am an insomniac without offering some apparently entirely foolproof, it's-always-worked-for-me remedy, and they honestly seem to think, these people, that I must never have tried switching the light on and reading for a bit, or having a hot bath before I go to bed, or a cup of hot milk or counting backwards from a hundred, or one of the hundreds of low-level herbal remedies . . . none of which have any effect on proper, fuck-off insomnia. So says the main character of *Time for Bed,* a novel by British comedian David Baddiel. In one of his stand-up routines, Baddiel asks why, when people hear he's an insomniac, they say, "Really? Cos I fall asleep the second my head hits the pillow": *When I see someone in a wheelchair, I don't say, "Really, cos I can do this . . ."* and he hops around the stage on one leg. Says Bonnie, a San Francisco freelance artist, *If you had a physical disability, there'd be more understanding. When I got sick, it was, like, a blessing. I was in the emergency room. People understand that.*

When people can *see* a problem, they can understand and empathize. But when a condition is invisible—and when it goes on and on for no apparent reason—it calls forth a lot of dumb advice. Friends of mine who live with chronic pain, headache, back pain, arthritis tell me they get this kind of advice, too.

"You probably don't need that much sleep"—this we hear from friends, family, doctors, and even from some sleep researchers. "Insomniacs may be naturally short sleepers who are unaware of their lessened need for sleep," wrote a Stanford researcher in 1993. "Their notion that they need more sleep is an 'erroneous assumption.'" "Worries by such insomniacs about a 'lack of sleep' are unjustified," says British researcher James Horne, who is (as he told me) a good sleeper himself: insomniacs "just need to be reassured that their sleep is sufficient, despite what they believe in this respect." As though I hadn't tried, a million times, to convince myself that it was so, telling myself cheerily, as I looked in the mirror, "Well, maybe today I'll be okay on four hours," never mind those bright red eyes and the blue-black caverns under them. Trust me, if I were a short sleeper, I'd know it by now. I have known such people, been on intimate terms with one or two, men who seemed to suck energy from the air. I'm not one. I'm a person with normal sleep needs, trapped in a body that seems to think I'm someone else.

"Although [insomniacs] may report feeling 'tired' throughout the day," says Horne, "it may not be sleepiness but lethargy and disinterest due to depression." So—I only want more sleep because I'm depressed and trying to avoid my life? With all due respect, this is so ass-backward. The reason I want more sleep is so that I *won't* feel depressed. I need sleep, *not* to avoid my life, but so that I can *live* it.

*

For half a century I've been hearing this kind of useless, well-intended advice from doctors, family, friends. But with each passing year, I find it harder to take—harder to take the advice, harder to take the sleep loss, harder to tolerate the pills I take to minimize the sleep loss. The sad fact about sleeping pills is that they don't make sleep better; they make it worse. And they make *me* worse: they impair memory, balance, coordination, things I'd like to hold on to as I age.

So I set out, in my fifty-eighth year, in search of some explanation why, being of sound mind and reasonably untroubled life, I still can't sleep. I want to know what is known about this beast, what the research is turning up, why there is not much better help for me today than there was half a century ago. I start with the library at the University of California, Berkeley, then I hit interlibrary loan, exhausting the patience of librarians and student assistants. I travel to Seattle, Chicago, Philadelphia, Denver, Washington, Prague, San Diego, Salt Lake City, and Minneapolis, to conferences where scientists, doctors, and sleep professionals gather to exchange the latest in research and clinical findings. I fly around the country to interview researchers. And I talk to insomniacs.

I track down everyone I've ever heard of or known who has insomnia—friends, friends of friends, relatives of friends, acquaintances, colleagues, students. I talk to taxi drivers, bartenders, strangers on planes, in airport lounges, in line at the movies. I place ads in the *New York Review of Books, The Nation,* the *Women's Review of Books,* the *East Bay Guardian,* Craigslist.org. I spend late night hours on the Web, surfing not only the insomnia sites but blogs and newsgroups I click into by chance. Whenever I talk about these issues in public or in print, I'm flooded with responses. I scarf up every story, every tidbit and trifle, however odd or inconsequential it may seem. When asked what my method is, I reply, "Total immersion."

I find out some strange and troubling things. I learn that insomnia is, of all the things that commonly go wrong with people, one of the least well understood. "We do not know the real causes of insomnia, nor do we know whether any treatments, including behavioral and psychological treatments, actually treat these causes," says Daniel Buysse, Department of Psychiatry, University of Pittsburgh School of Medicine. "We do not know . . . the nature of the basic neural mechanisms underlying primary insomnia. Nor do we know the identity of specific neurotransmitters that might be involved, or even whether specific neurotransmitter systems are involved. The genetics of the disorder are also not known," say Gary Richardson and Thomas Roth of the Sleep Disorders and Research Center, Henry Ford Hospital, Detroit. There is little agreement, reported James Walsh in 2006, about "the most basic of questions about the definition, prevalence, pathophysiology, and consequences of and treatments for this disorder (symptom? illness? complaint? syndrome? condition?)." These are some of the most eminent figures in the field saying these things: "We do not know . . . We do not know . . ." When, in June 2005, the National Institutes of Health (NIH) held a "Consensus Conference" on insomnia, researchers found that they were so far from consensus that they dropped the word and renamed it a "State-of-the-Science" conference.

And yet in spite of how little is known, in spite of the vast numbers of people who suffer with insomnia and the enormous toll it takes, the NIH, the source of most biomedical research in this country, spent, in 2005, less than $20 million on insomnia research, most of which went to treatments, therapies, and "management" of insomnia. Pharmaceutical giant Sanofi-Aventis spent *$123 million,* that same year, advertising Ambien.

I learn that not much is known about sleep itself. Sleep science—or *sciences,* I should say, since the subject of sleep spans disciplines—is a new field. It's been around about as long as I've had insomnia. It was born in 1953, in the lab of Nathaniel Kleitman at the University of Chicago, when Eugene Aserinsky, a graduate student, happened to notice, ninety minutes into the sleep of the subject he was observing, the eyes moving back and forth. The discovery of rapid eye movement (REM), as it was called, was revolutionary, overturning all previous understanding of sleep. Prior to this, sleep had been assumed to be a passive state, a state of quiescence when both brain and body were "turned off," but here, suddenly, was this complex activity—and it seemed, most intriguingly, to be related to dreaming. More has been learned about sleep since 1953 than in all the centuries before, but scientists are still unable to say how we sleep, or even *why*. We eat to take in nutrients, we breathe to take in oxygen and expel carbon dioxide, but there is no comparable explanation for why we sleep. We spend a third of our lives in sleep (or most people do). Birds do it, insects, fish, and vertebrates do it, and they put themselves at considerable risk to do it, rendering themselves insensible and vulnerable to predators—and nobody knows why.

"The mystery of sleep function," says Allan Hobson of Harvard Medical School, "is still impenetrable." It's a mystery so deep that the most prosaic of scientists waxes poetic on it, comparing sleep to "an unplumbed ocean," "a subterranean terrain," "an undiscovered continent," "a last frontier," "a vast unknown," "an enchanted world," a (sigh) "virgin territory." Everywhere you turn in this field, there are questions. Why do we need two different kinds of sleep? REM and the rest of sleep (which is called nonREM sleep and includes deep sleep, as well as the shallower stages 1 and 2) are as unlike one another as sleep is to wakefulness. In nonREM, the muscles are relaxed, the breathing is regular, and the consumption of energy by the brain is minimal; in REM, where the most vivid dreams occur, the brain is as active as it is during consciousness, the breathing and heart rate are faster and irregular—yet for all this activity, we are paralyzed, except for the eye movements and the odd twitch. Why, after a certain time in REM, do we shift back into nonREM, then back into REM, then back and forth for four to six alternating cycles throughout the night, with longer periods of REM toward morning? How is each stage maintained for the time it is and then terminated? What are dreams for?

"It's a fabulous field to work in," says University of California sleep researcher Irwin Feinberg, "because so many of the important questions are still unanswered. It's especially interesting now, when new infusions from neuroscience and molecular and genetic biology are bringing fresh perspectives." As I head off each summer to another conference, I get caught up in the excitement, wondering what breakthrough discovery I'll be hearing about next. But when I get to the insomnia sessions, my heart sinks. In the hundreds of papers I sit through and read, I hear a great deal about insomnia as depression, anxiety, "dysfunctional beliefs and attitudes," but very little about the neurophysiology or neuroendocrinology or genetics of the problem. I find the same tendency to chalk it up to the *psycho* that I find in the doctor's office. The physiological is implied by the term *psychophysiological* insomnia, but it figures as *effect*, as the physiological reaction to the psychological or emotional upset that is thought to be the cause. Of course mind and body are not so easily differentiated; in fact, everything that's been learned in recent years suggests that they're so interdependent as to be inseparable—and this is especially so with sleep, which is, as James Horne calls it, "the meeting place for mind and body." But in practical terms, people have to begin somewhere in their thinking about origins or *etiologies,* and they begin from where they are: a psychologist comes at a problem from psychology, a neurologist from neurology. Nearly everyone who comes at insomnia comes from psychology, with backgrounds and training and degrees and publications in psychology—in *Freudian* psychology, in the early days of sleep research—which has given this field a certain slant.

"What the *physiological* side is, we haven't a clue," admits Clete Kushida, director of Stanford University Center for Human Sleep Research; "we feel it's there, but we haven't been able to put our finger on it." But how hard are researchers trying to "put a finger on it"? Of the $20 million spent on insomnia research in 2005, about $3.8 million went to investigations of the neurobiological mechanisms and pathophysiology of the problem, the kind of basic research that might lead to an understanding of the cause. The behavioral model *(change your attitude, change your ways)* "has had, perhaps, the unfortunate consequence of discouraging research into the neurobiology of the disorder," concludes a 2004 study that looked at where research has been directed.

And yet sleep is a physiological behavior. Its mechanisms are fundamentally biological, and as with any biological system, there's enormous variability. "Some people have better/stronger sleep systems, some weaker, just as there are short people and tall people," explains insomnia researcher Michael Bonnet. Babies are born with different sleep propensities, as parents well know, many of which are now known to be genetic. The sleep system is a physiological system and, like all such systems, deteriorates with age. Even elders who are free of psychological and medical problems lose the capacity for deep, sustained sleep—which suggests that some physiological mechanism wears out. And yet sleep also "lives in the world," as Brown University researcher Mary Carskadon says. It is shaped by psychological factors, by emotional, familial, social, cultural, and environmental influences, and by everything in our lives. It is infinitely complex.

Each year, scientists are learning more about the physiology of sleep, its neuronal and neuroendocrinal mechanisms, its genetic underpinnings. As sleep comes to be better understood, so will insomnia. "We used to think insomnia was something that happened only to crazy people," said a psychiatrist I talked to at a sleep conference, "but it's not possible to think of it that way anymore." "Where once we assumed it was depression that caused insomnia, we know now there's a *physiological* component," says sleep researcher Tom Roth. In the half decade I've been attending sleep conferences, I sense that change is in the air. But the tendency to psychologize insomnia, neuroticize it, pin it on the character, attitudes, practices of the sufferer, dies hard.

Against that mind-set, this book speaks out.

✸

In the pages that follow, I take you into this world of sleep research, a world most people do not know exists and one that I had no idea existed until I began this book, a world that's vitally important to millions of people. For the estimated 70 million people in the United States who have sleep disorders, the discoveries made here, the therapies developed or not developed here, the brilliance and blind spots of these researchers make the difference between whether we function in our lives, or not.

I start out, in chapter 2, by asking why a condition that affects so many people has been so long neglected. What is it about our culture that has made this long blackout, as it were, on an area so crucial to our well-being? For not only has insomnia been ignored, but sleep itself. "Sleep is for the weak," "sleep is for slackers," "the best don't rest"—such are the slogans heard from students in the college where I teach and from entrepreneurs in Silicon Valley, high-tech capital of the world. (Silicon Valley is home not only to the defiantly sleep-deprived but also, ironically, to Stanford, world center of sleep research; it is also where I grew up.) Sleep machismo is rooted in the Protestant-capitalist values by which we

Americans live, infecting even the doctors we turn to for help and some sleep researchers as well. No wonder insomnia isn't taken more seriously, when sleep itself is not.

"Sleep is for sissies," and people who complain they're not getting enough aren't cool. Insomniacs are people who complain they're not getting enough, and I find a strong strain of moralizing, even dislike, in the words researchers use for us. I find us described as "overly concerned about sleep," "chronic complainers," "neurotic," "self-absorbed," "obsessive," "histrionic," "hypochondriac," "chronic anxiety neurotics." "Though we want to be neutral in our feelings toward patients, we'll admit among ourselves," writes Dr. Atul Gawande, that some patients "are a source of frustration and annoyance: presenting a malady we can neither explain nor alleviate, they shake our claims to competence and authority." (Gawande is talking about people with chronic pain, but he might as well be talking about chronic insomniacs.) I look, in the third chapter, "Blame the Victim," at medical problems that were once pinned on the attitudes, habits, psychopathology of the sufferers but were later discovered to be organic—conditions like ulcers, migraines, multiple sclerosis—and argue that insomnia may someday be on this list, along with the several sleep disorders, narcolepsy, restless legs syndrome, REM behavior disorder, that already are. I bring myself into this chapter as a sort of case study, to show how a person's life and mind might get bent out of shape, might get bent *into* the shape of those negative stereotypes of insomnia, when she's unable to count on something so basic as sleep, so that when doctors and researchers see an insomniac who's stressed out, anxious, depressed, they may be looking at the *consequence* of a sleep disorder and mistaking it for the *cause*. Throughout the book, I bring you back to the lived experience of those who struggle with insomnia on a nightly and daily basis, juxtaposing the view from the inside with judgments made from without. The view looks different, depending on where you stand.

In "Sleepless in Seattle," chapter 4, I take you to the conferences, where I talk with anyone who will talk with me and eavesdrop on anyone who won't. I'm struck, right off, by the difference between what goes on at the insomnia sessions—where researchers are still telling us to change our attitudes, change our ways—and what goes on in sleep research, where hard questions are being asked about the physiological mechanisms of sleep and wakefulness, the neuroendocrinological and genetic basis of sleep disorders. I look, in "The Brain of an Insomniac," chapter 5, at what neuroscience and neuroimaging are turning up about these mechanisms and at recent discoveries that suggest there could well be a glitch in them that accounts for some kinds of insomnia—*some* kinds, that is, not all. Anything you can say about insomnia, you can only ever say about *some* insomnia, for this is a slippery beast that defies one-size-fits-all descriptions and prescriptions.

Stress is a catchall explanation that's often given for insomnia, an explanation that suggests we could get hold of this problem if we'd only relax (blame the victim, again). But it's not so simple, since insomnia itself is a powerful stressor. Studies are finding that exposure to stressors over long periods of time may ratchet the system up, that the stress systems of (some) people who have been exposed to early or prolonged stress may get stuck in the on position, leaving them more vulnerable to subsequent stressors, *physiologically* changed. I look, in chapter 6, at the *hyperarousal* researchers have been finding in insomniacs (*some* insomniacs, that is), the faster metabolism and heart rate and elevated blood pressure and levels of stress hormones that are evidence of a stress system on hyperalert. Research suggests a genetic component here, too, that the stress systems of some people, as of some animals, are more reactive than others'.

I turn, in the next chapters, to the treatments we're offered—drugs, behavioral modification, and sleep clinics—and the alternative treatments many of us seek out on our own. Are the drugs prescribed to us the drugs that are best for us, or are they what the pharmaceutical industry—one of the most powerful in the world—is pushing hardest? Or are they perhaps the drugs doctors feel most comfortable prescribing? *Hypnotics,* as sleep medications are called, after Hypnos, the Greek god of sleep, are *controlled substances,* governed by federal narcotics laws and monitored by the Drug Enforcement Administration: they can get doctors into trouble. How much easier to prescribe something that doesn't come under these controls—like antidepressants—which may be why these are so often given for sleep. I tell stories of people who've been messed up by drugs (myself included), and people who've been helped by drugs (myself included). I describe the new agents being developed that may someday give us a wider choice of medications that more precisely target our problem, and I look at a new and controversial drug that holds promise.

Behavioral modification, the subject of chapter 8, is the "nonpharmacological" treatment we are offered. It tells us to practice "sleep hygiene" and to regularize our schedules and restrict time in bed to the hours spent asleep, so that we'll consolidate our sleep into a solid block.

Insomnia researchers are keen on this approach and devote considerable research attention to it. It is effective with some insomniacs—*some,* again, though nobody really knows how many. It may actually be that the effort to get us to sleep in a single consolidated block is pushing against some deeply engrained natural tendencies. Studies that attempted to replicate preindustrial sleep conditions found that people tended to sleep in segments. Studies of sleep in earlier historical periods and the few investigations of sleep in other cultures that I find also suggest a biphasic or polyphasic sleep pattern. It may be that the shape sleep has today is a fairly recent development, an artifact of electric lighting and the industrial revolution. The sleep that is being studied in labs, the sleep of young, healthy, well-fed Western (male) subjects, may not be the "universal" it's cracked up to be.

Again and again, sleep turns out to be larger than our conceptions of it, more complex than our tools or technologies or the stories we tell about it. I take you, in chapter 9, through a night at a sleep clinic, a darkly comic experience, where I learn how difficult insomnia is even to diagnose, since the gold standard for measuring whether we're asleep or awake, the *electroencephalogram,* or EEG (which attaches electrodes to the skull to measure the electrical impulses of our brains), tells a very strange story about insomniacs, assuring us that we're asleep when we're sure we're awake. Insomnia is a subjective state. There's no blood test that it shows up on, no biopsy or x ray that picks it up, and it doesn't even show up on the EEG. You know that a person has it only *by what that person says,* which makes it, as James Horne says, "one of the few disorders where the diagnosis lies with the patient and not the physician." How much easier it is to tell us, as many clinics do, that we have "sleep disordered breathing," or apnea, a condition easier to treat.

Insomniacs turn to alternative medicine, the subject of chapter 10, in droves. Mainstream Western medicine is good at fixing things, but for chronic conditions (which are by definition conditions that can't be fixed), people seek out alternative therapies, where they find practitioners who take more time with them and who approach insomnia as though the body—the fluctuations of our hormones, the foods we eat—plays a part in the problem. Most of these methods, however, have had very little research. I turn, in chapter 11, to my own ways of dealing with the problem and the creative solutions others have found—tricks we've gleaned, techniques we've worked out, some from alternative medicine, some from knowing our bodies—many of which I've not seen written about elsewhere. (I'd originally titled this chapter "Outwitting Insomnia," but I came to feel as I wrote it that "Bedding Down with the Beast" was a more accurate description of what goes on at my house.)

I conclude, in chapter 12, with some speculations about what we might do to make change—and my "we" includes the professionals and the insomniacs together—so that there may come a time when more than a pittance is spent on this problem that affects so many millions, a time when the research is directed to a search for the causes, not the same old treatments.

✳

There's no end to books on insomnia. A look at some titles tells you the promises they make: *Conquering Insomnia, Overcoming Insomnia, Stopping Insomnia, Relief from Insomnia, Natural Relief from Insomnia, Learn to Sleep Well, Seventy-Five Proven Ways to Get a Good Night's Sleep, Sixty-Seven Ways to a Good Night's Sleep, Fifty Essential Things to Do to Get a Good Night's Sleep, Everything You Need for a Good Night's Sleep, Solve Your Sleep Problem, How to Cure Your Sleep Problem, Sound Ways to Better Sleep, How to Get a Good Night's Sleep, The Natural Way to Sleep, Don't Just Lie There, Sleep Better Tonight!, Get a Good Night's Sleep, Getting to Sleep, Learn to Sleep, Learn to Sleep Well, Nature's Answer to Good Sleep, Easy Sleep, Power Sleep, Say Good Night to Insomnia, Idiot's Guide to Getting a Good Night's Sleep.* (And there are many more.) I feel, as I make my way through this stack, like I'm reading the same book, hearing the same old advice: keep a regular schedule; avoid caffeine, alcohol, and sleeping pills.

More interesting are the books about the new sleep science. Some of these are written by the men who made sleep science: *Sleep: The Gentle Tyrant,* by Wilse Webb, research professor at the University of Florida; *The Secrets of Sleep,* by Alexander Borbely, director of the Sleep Laboratory, University of Zurich; *The Enchanted World of Sleep,* by Peretz Lavie, director of the Technion Sleep Laboratory, Israel Institute of Technology, Haifa; *Sleep and Dreaming,* by Jacob Empson at the Department of Clinical Psychology at the University of Hull; *Sleep,* by J. Allan Hobson, professor of psychiatry at Harvard Medical School and director of the laboratory of neurophysiology at Massachusetts Mental Health Center; and *The Promise of Sleep,* by William Dement, founder and longtime director of Stanford Sleep Research Center. There are also some fascinating popular science books: *Sleep and Its Secrets,* by Michael Aronoff, MD; *Sleep Thieves,* by Stanley Coren; *Counting Sheep: The Science and*

Pleasures of Sleep and Dreams, by Paul Martin. I love these books, and I devour them, but when I get to the chapters on insomnia, my heart sinks: "Keep a regular schedule," "Avoid caffeine and alcohol." But then, I remind myself, these books are not about insomnia—they're about *sleep.* When I look for the popular science books about insomnia, I find *Insomnia: The Guide for Troubled Sleepers,* by Gay Gaer Luce and Julius Segal, published in 1969. I find *Natural Sleep,* by Philip Goldberg and Daniel Kaufman, and *Creative Insomnia,* by Douglas Colligan, both published in 1978. A quarter of a century has passed since anybody wrote a popular science book on insomnia. What can that mean?

What is missing from everything I read about insomnia is—the insomniacs. We're there, of course, but only as numbers, figures, bars on charts or graphs, objects of scientific scrutiny. The electrical activity of our brains is monitored by the EEG, the results are recorded, tabulated, analyzed, but in all the books and articles I read, all the lectures and sessions I attend, I find us quoted three times (in 1976, 1978, and 2005). I find us referred to as *patients, insomnia complainers, complaining insomniacs, insomnoids*—and mostly, as *subjects.* But we're more like objects than subjects, really: we have no speaking part in this literature, no voice.

Where are the books on insomnia written from the point of view of the insomniac? I find powerful first-person accounts of depression— William Styron's *Darkness Visible,* Martha Manning's *Undercurrents,* Andrew Solomon's *The Noonday Demon*—that have done more to put a human face on this affliction than all the articles in the journals. But I find no such books on insomnia. Maybe the insomniacs are all too tired to write them, I think grimly, and decide, some years into writing this book, that it's probably true. Insomnia is not an easy subject to write about. It's an amorphous creature, *multifactorial,* as researchers say, meaning that there may be many factors working together to bring it on. It is difficult to get hold of, by researchers who research it, doctors who treat it, people who suffer from it—and writers who write about it. I can't weave a spellbinding tale around the race for the cure because there isn't one. Besides, as a friend once remarked, "who wants to read a book about a lot of sleepless nights? It's a real snooze." "Insomnia is a subject of keen interest to those who have it and great tedium to those who do not," writes Laura Miller in the *New York Times.* Insomniacs do not, as a rule, go through the dramatic breakdowns and breakthroughs that make page-turners. The real drama for us is getting through the day.

But by not telling our side of the story, by not owning up to our experience, we have left the describing to people who don't know what it's like to live with this condition, who do not, for the most part, know it from the inside. Nobody really knows what it's like to live inside another person's skin. I can't begin to guess what it would be like to lie down without earplugs and white noise machine and blackout curtains, to close my eyes and sleep till morning. "How do you do it?" I ask my partner, whose head hits the pillow and he's out. I want to pry open an eyelid, peer behind his eyeballs, find out what makes that curtain drop down on him but not on me. Insomniacs wouldn't presume to say what makes such restful slumber, but those who sleep well presume to know what's going on with us.

Everybody knows that worry, stress, depression can cause insomnia. That sleep is disrupted by "the throes of life" was written by Hippocrates in 4 B.C. People assume that since this is the sort of thing that keeps *them* awake, it must be the sort of thing that's keeping *us* awake: it's obvious, it's intuitive, it's universal. They don't get it that there are those of us whose sleep is never right, no matter what's going on in our lives, no matter what our lifestyle, habits, frame of mind. I sleep two, three, or four hours, sometimes five, and that's it. Too much happening in my life makes it worse, too little happening makes it worse; too much company, or too little; too much exercise, or too little; too much to eat, or too little. Any excuse my body can find not to sleep, it will find. Often, it needs no excuse at all. (Capricious, this sandman drops in from time to time, try as you may to entice him to stay the night: if this were a guy, you'd have ditched him long ago, but you need him too much, can't live without him, can't get through a day without him, and meanwhile, what's there by your side, lumpish, gray, and predictable as a scab, is—insomnia.) On those rare nights when I get seven unbroken, undrugged hours, I feel a rush of energy and optimism, like I could take on the world. You who sleep well and reliably have no idea what you take for granted. You cannot imagine.

In the 2005 study I referred to earlier, one of the three to quote insomniacs, University of Pittsburgh researchers brought together sixteen insomniacs in focus groups and actually *asked* them what they were thinking—unprecedented! The insomniacs expressed, above all, "the feeling that others (spouse, family, friends, co-workers, . . . professionals) could not really understand or minimized the impact of this experience" and that health professionals "either did not understand the full impact of insomnia on their lives or did not know what to do to effectively treat it." When I asked one of the researchers if anything had surprised him about these findings, he said, "The affect, the strength of feeling to what they said."

It doesn't surprise me. These are the sorts of things I hear:

Even when people are sympathetic, they're generally uncomprehending. . . . I've seldom appreciated anything as much as when an old friend told me he'd just gone through a few weeks of insomnia and had dimly begun to understand what I'd tried to tell him about for years.

I had two doctors who got it—when they had bad bouts of insomnia themselves.

I don't want sympathy but I want people to know this is terrible. I have friends who've survived horrendous things, like cancer, and they make me feel like such a wimp. Sometimes I wish they'd have a month of it, or even a week, then they'd know. I would wish on every doctor and every sleep doctor, that they should live with this and have to hang on to their jobs. Then we'd see some better treatments for insomnia, you bet.

I am really very tired of being told what it's like to live in my body by people who haven't a clue. I have come to feel that, when it comes to insomnia, there is truth to the old adage, *it takes one to know one.* As E. M. Cioran said, *I found everyone idiotic. Nobody understood what I understood. You see, there is a gang of insomniacs, there is a sort of solidarity, right, like people who have the same illness. We understand each other right away.*

✸

We know what it is to live in our bodies; we know where the ailing, failing parts are, we have ideas about what's gone wrong. We have inside information. Like the friend I had who drove a Jaguar that was always breaking down—he knew more about Jaguars than most mechanics. That's how it is with insomniacs and sleep. When there is something crucial to your existence that is constantly letting you down, you pick things up.

Anecdote is not highly regarded in scientific circles. Anecdote, say the scientists, is individual, particular, idiosyncratic, hit and miss. Science, they say, is systematic and general, a sure thing. Science produces, through methods of controlled experiments and statistical analysis, *evidence.* Anecdote is not evidence. Even a lot of anecdotes don't add up to evidence. But experience, say I (and others), has an authority, too, especially with a condition so subjective as insomnia. The inside story, the subjective account—what social scientists call an *ethnographic* perspective, a qualitative as opposed to a quantitative approach—is a useful counter to the "objectivity" of science, necessary for assuring that the thick, rich textures of individual lives don't get swept away by the broad brush of the statistical.

As a person coming to this subject from the alien field of literary studies, I find value in stories. Stories are how we get to know one another, how we glimpse the inner realties of one another's lives. I listen to what insomniacs have to say, their hunches and intuitions, what they think brought the problem on, what they know about dealing with it. I hear what they say, keeping an eye out for etiologies, trying to tease out patterns from the thicket of particulars, contrasting their accounts to the accounts of the researchers. I look for ways they corroborate the research, ways they contradict it, ways they qualify it. I find much in our experience that's explained by the research, but I find much that is not. I find more kinds of insomniacs, more richness and diversity in our characters and experiences than I find described in the scientific literature, which lumps us all together and tars us with the same brush. Researchers pay lip service to the idea that insomnia is multifactorial, yet they approach us as a homogeneous rather than a heterogeneous population and prescribe for us as though one size fits all. They have caricatured us, not characterized us. "Chronic anxiety neurotics," indeed.

Here's an anecdote.

One summer in the mid-1980s, when I was at my mother's, coming off the sleeping pills I'd get hooked on during the teaching year, she slipped me a clipping from a local paper: "Stanford seeking subjects for insomnia study." I called the number and asked what was involved.

"We take you for six days and monitor everything."

"Everything?"

"You know, temperature, heart rate, respiration . . ."

"Oh, good," I said. "Which six days?"

"What do you mean, which six days?"

"Which six days of the menstrual cycle?"

"Oh, we don't monitor for *that*."

"Well, you certainly *should!*" popped out of my mouth before I could do a tactful edit. We both beat a hasty retreat: they no more wanted to deal with somebody so uppity than I wanted to waste my time with these folks who were so in the dark ages that they didn't "monitor for that." If there was one thing I knew, it was that, just before my period, I got insomnia a pill wouldn't touch, and it happened invariably; if I ever happened to forget what time of month it was, the insomnia would remind me. *That* time of month wired me like strong coffee, not unpleasant, exactly—there was this amazing energy—except that I couldn't sleep. Then when my period came, I'd fall into a deep, blissful slumber—for about a night.

"It may not be news to many women that the menstrual cycle can independently affect sleep," writes William Dement, head of the Stanford sleep clinic at the time I had my brief conversation with somebody there, "but for sleep scientists it has been a relatively recent discovery." It was only in 1998, when a National Sleep Foundation poll found that 25 percent of women report disturbed sleep the week before their period, that researchers began to wake up to this association. If someone at Stanford had stayed on the phone and talked to me that day—or talked to any one of the thousands of women who've passed through their clinic—they might have got to this understanding much sooner. Women have always known this: *It's so obviously hormonal—a few days just before my period, I could jump out of my skin.* Says another: *One night a month it would be virtually impossible for me to sleep. No matter what I did—warm milk, reading* War and Peace, *occasionally reverting to Nytol—nothing seemed to work. Then, bingo! I'd get my period the very next day.*

"Couldn't be," said a doctor to my friend Roberta, when she told him she thought her insomnia had been triggered by birth control pills. Now there is evidence that she may have been right. Anecdote may not be evidence, but it may lead the way to evidence. How, but by listening, being open to the particularities of people's experiences, even when they go against the grain of received wisdom—or *especially* when they go against the grain—do scientists come up with new ideas to investigate? Where does science begin, but in observation?

One way that insomniacs are not all alike is that many of us are women. Scientists (most of whom still are not women) have been slow to recognize that many conditions and diseases look different, follow different courses, and respond to different treatments when the patient is female. A woman scientist whose biography I wrote, Dr. Alice Stewart, taught me how important it is to listen to the women. Stewart was a British physician who set out to discover, in the 1950s, why childhood leukemia was on the rise. (She was doing *epidemiology*, tracking the causes or origins of diseases, before it was even called epidemiology, as far back as the 1940s.) She had a feeling that the mothers might remember something their doctors had forgotten, so she devised a questionnaire that asked them about their exposures to a wide variety of things, automobiles, buses, hens, rabbits, dogs, colored sweets—and whether they'd had an obstetric x ray. (It was common practice in the

1950s to x ray women in the last trimester of their pregnancies.) "Ask the mothers? What can they possibly know?" objected her critics. But she persisted, distributing her questionnaires to the mothers of children who had died of cancer and the mothers of healthy children (these were the *case controls,* or comparison group). "Within 35 questionnaires," she told me, "the answer leapt out: those that had had an obstetric x ray were running two to one in terms of an early cancer death." Her study established that, when you x ray a pregnant woman, you double the risk of a childhood cancer, a discovery that revolutionized medical practice. This is why, before a woman gets an x ray today, she gets asked if she's pregnant.

Stewart advised her research team, "When you go to the mother, ask her questions about the child's illness, let her talk. You mustn't go and just ask the question you're interested in, you must get all the information you can. Take it down *verbatim.* Never cut your information off at the source. You must cast as wide a net as possible, remain open to what the data are telling you, let the data shape the question." I can still hear her saying this, in her stentorian British tones.

The researchers and clinicians who deal with insomnia have cut their information off at the source. They don't try to hear what their subjects have to say, to find out what we know. Most sleep studies still do not include women, and doctors' eyes still glaze when we say, "I think it might be hormones."

※

This is a somewhat cranky book. You can't live with this problem as long as I have, you can't be blown off and written off as many times as I have, and not get cross. It's a very personal book wrung out of my life's blood, but if I didn't think it was more than personal, I wouldn't have bothered to write it. My frustrations are shared not only by insomniacs but by people with other sleep disorders—narcolepsy, restless legs syndrome, *hypersomnia* (excessive sleepiness)—who tell me how hard it is for them to get their problems taken seriously. They are also shared by many sleep researchers who have been trying to get the world to pay attention to sleep, a thankless task, since the world goes its ways, beating sleep back into narrower corners of ever-more frenetic lives.

It's a cross book, but it's also a labor of love, for the many people I see suffering with this problem. People tell me their stories, and I'm in awe of what they go through, the spirit, valiance, grace under pressure.

If you want to see courage, try going without sleep, as an insomniac once said. I hear from many women who sleep worse than I do, who are raising children *and* holding down nine-to-five jobs (or worse, who are not). I hear from more women than men, which is not surprising, since "sleep complaints are twice as prevalent in women," as a 2003 NIH report states: in fact, "female sex is a risk factor for insomnia." Insomnia is a women's issue: it is not solely a women's issue, but it is certainly a women's issue. One reason insomnia has been so neglected is, I suspect, that it affects the neglected: the female, the elderly, and the poor.

I should say too that the book is a labor of heartfelt appreciation, if not love, for the researchers and physicians and psychotherapists who deal with insomnia, some of whom have made an enormous difference in the lives of insomniacs. I may be critical, but I'm also grateful to anyone who takes the problem seriously enough to try to help. I know that many researchers and clinicians will agree with me that, in the words of University of California at Berkeley researcher Allison Harvey, "we can't rest yet."

How we sleep, how much sleep we need, how we react to sleep loss, the rituals and practices we work out around sleep, the stories we tell ourselves are as individual and distinctive as our fingerprints. You and only you can know what works, because you're the only one who lives in your body. What works for me may be anathema to you, just as the drug that puts you to sleep may send me over the moon. I hope that this extended meditation on sleep and insomnia (for that's what the book has turned out to be) may encourage others to strike out in directions of their own, to come up with their own solutions—and to come *out* with these solutions, to share them with us all. I hope that it will encourage insomniacs to break the long silence about insomnia.

I've written the kind of book I wish I'd had, dealing with insomnia all these years. You might call it a field guide to insomnia, a user-friendly guide through a terrain most people don't know or admit exists, a guide to navigating the reefs and shoals of sleepless nights and sleepy days, a book of consolations for the large number of people suffering with this problem, thinking they are alone. You are not alone, and it may help to know this, because insomnia is the loneliest of conditions: you're awake when the rest of the world's asleep, no matter who's by your side, and then, when the world's awake, you're too wiped out to reach out and make contact.

If we find each other, we might help each other.

A How-To and a Who-For

This book is primarily for insomniacs and the people in their lives, but in the course of writing it, I began to hope that doctors and psychotherapists would read it, too. And the more scientific meetings I went to, the more I found myself wanting to enter into conversations with the researchers—conversations they were too busy to have with me. So I've ended up writing with several different audiences in mind, the insomniacs, the health care professionals who treat us, and the researchers.

This means that not everything in this book may be equally fascinating to everyone. So here are a few thoughts about reading it. If you're an insomniac looking for new ideas on how to deal with your problem and wanting to know how other people cope with theirs, the first three chapters will be of interest, along with chapter 7 (on drugs), chapter 8 (on behavioral modification), chapter 10 (on alternative approaches), and chapter 11, on "bedding down with the beast." If you're an insomniac who's curious about what the researchers are up to, you'll want to read the conference chapter, 4, and the science chapters as well (5, 6, and 12). I've been told that the conference chapter is very funny (if you bog down in chapters 2 or 3, skip to that). If you're a researcher wanting to know what your world looks like to an outsider (outsider to the field, that is, not to the condition), read that one, too, only don't take it personally. And, doctors and psychotherapists who deal with insomniacs (and that's every one of you), please read it all, know the experiential reality that lies behind a diagnosis of insomnia, know there are things you can do to help.

There's also a whole other discussion going on in the endnotes, material that I couldn't fit into the text because it took me in other directions. (A fuller version is on the Web.) I myself am fascinated by endnotes, since I know that writers sometimes bury their most interesting points there, where they think nobody is watching; but I realize that not everybody is. Dip into these as you please.

Dip into any part of the book as you please. "As needed," as it says on the pill bottle: the book is here to help. When I was a graduate student, my advisor tried to warn me away from writing a dissertation on Shakespeare, cautioning me that I'd have to "master all the scholarship on the subject"—which would have been impossible. That's when I learned the difference between *reading* a book and *raiding* it for what I needed. Feel free to raid this book. If you come across a passage or passages that bog down, just speed up and skim until you come to a part that's more engaging. If you're interested in insomnia, or in sleep, you'll find something in this book that's worth your while.

The book is, above all, for anyone who wants to understand what it feels like to live with insomnia, to move through the world and play by its rules with a serious and persistent sleep problem. Accordingly, I've sprinkled autobiographical accounts of my own experiences throughout, along with the words of many insomniacs I've talked to and corresponded with over the past five years, italicized, for an emphasis long overdue.

CHAPTER 2

Sleepstarved

How do people go to sleep? I'm afraid I've lost the knack.

Dorothy Parker, "The Little Hours"

I look at the clock and it is 6:05 A.M. The last time I looked it was 4:30, which, considering that I went to bed at 3:00, is not good. Must have been that cup of tea I had before class—no, one cup of tea doesn't do this. Maybe it was the wine I had with dinner—no, that was hours ago. It could be anything I did, it could be nothing I did, I have no idea—classes went fine, dinner with a friend, nothing on my mind. It's okay, really, it is okay, I can sleep in. No, it's not okay—it's torture. Actually, it *is* torture: sleep deprivation is a time-honored form of coercion. *Tormentum insomniae.*

Maybe I should take an Ambien. No, I've been taking too many lately. Maybe I should listen to a book on tape—sometimes, if I get my mind off my story onto somebody else's story, it lulls me back to sleep.

It does not. Two hours and two tapes later, I give up and get up, and it is bad, bad as the worst hangover, worse than jet lag. Head aches, eyes sting, I can't stop sneezing. Skin like parchment, but this is one of those don't-look-in-the-mirror days, and I can tell it's going to be one of those hungry days, an all-day hunger no food can feed. Back aches, hips ache, knees, muscles, joints, parts of me I don't know the names of. *Sleep, the balm of each day's hurt* (how do Macbeth's lines go?), *sleep that knits up the raveled sleeve of care—I heard a voice that cried, Sleep no more!* Macbeth, poor bastard. But he really did have something to keep him up nights. What I have done to deserve his fate, I do not know, but I'm sure I've spent as many sleepless nights as he.

And this was a day I was looking forward to, one of those rare, blissful days I'd set aside to write, no classes to teach, no errands to run, no traffic to hassle with, nowhere I need to be but to the pool fifty minutes before it closes. But now it hangs, useless, spent—no, *it* is not spent, I am.

No use trying to write—days like this, I can barely speak: *dog food* comes out *food dog,* sometimes entire sentences come out backward.

A chill day, the fog shows no sign of lifting. I find my slippers, wrap my bathrobe around me, fetch the *Times,* sit down at the kitchen table, move my eyes across the page. But the print lies inert, black, squiggly marks that make no connection with my brain. Okay, so this is one of those mind's-not-at-home days, there's a million mindless things I might do. I look around. Everywhere I look I see a mindless thing to do—sort through that pile of magazines, pay those bills. But these, too, seem beyond me. Motivation is one of the first things to go, say the researchers: the sleep-deprived may be capable of performing tasks, but they give up.

Well, at least this is a day I don't need to be anywhere, do anything. I have never, in more than forty years of teaching, missed a class on account of sleep loss—I say this with some pride—but there have been classes that never should have happened. Classes where I've felt like I was underwater, hearing what's being said but not taking it in, reaching for a word but not being able to retrieve it, groping for a fact to find that it's gone, and the drone of my voice tells me *I'm* gone, too—I'm on automatic. I stick close to the text, days like this, I hear the rote, formulaic things that come out of my mouth, but I don't dare begin a sentence unless I'm absolutely sure how it ends—I don't even dare write on the board for fear it will come out chicken scratch, badly spelled chicken scratch.

"Sleep-deprived people," summarizes Paul Martin, in his book *Counting Sheep,*

> perform badly on all aspects of creative thinking, including originality, flexibility, generating unusual ideas, being able to change strategy, word fluency. . . . Thinking becomes rigid. . . . They are more reliant on routine responses. . . . They also start using inappropriate, monotonous, or flattened intonation when reading out loud. Tired people are bad at finding the right words. Their language becomes less spontaneous and expressive, and they are less willing to volunteer information that others might need to know. All in all, they are worse at communicating their thoughts, feelings, decisions, and actions.

Bad news, if you're a professor.

I stare out the window at the blank, dead day. I tell myself, get a grip, this is a bad day, *it's not my life*—why, only a few hours ago, I was feeling fine, I will feel fine again. I tell myself, *it will look better in the morning*—*tomorrow* morning, that is, this day's a dead loss. For it's a cruel fact of life, you get only one crack at a day, and that crack is sleep:

what goes on or does not go on in sleep makes a day or breaks it. When you get out of bed, brain like a fried sponge, mood like something left out of the refrigerator too long, bad luck, write it off, just hope that the sleep fairy drops by the next night and sets the next day to rights. But meanwhile, there's this day to live through, this whole long day. How to kill the time? The newspaper? Tried that. E-mail? I don't think so. Run errands, shop for food? I'm not sure I want to drive. *Killing time,* what a travesty, when time is so short in a human life—might as well try to kill my life. When I think of the hours I've spent drifting around the house, flipping through magazines, doing my best to follow the plot of a dumb movie, nights spent half awake and days spent half asleep—they'd add up to years.

They call this a "sleep disorder," but it's actually an all-day disorder. Insomnia is not just something that happens to the night; it happens to the day, the whole of the day, and if it's chronic insomnia, it happens to many days. A half-life of ruined days.

Jacqueline

Jacqueline e-mailed me after hearing me on the radio. She came to my house to be interviewed. I don't know what I expected, but someone not quite so well put together. The woman who stood at my door could have been a model: tall, thin, pale, with long dark wavy hair, short black skirt and dark stockings, that understated elegance the French do so well. She is from Paris and now lives in San Francisco. She sat at my kitchen table and told her story.

I've had insomnia since I was a child, she began. *My parents talked about me as a baby not sleeping, but not crying. I was a happy little kid, you can see from the photos—I was laughing and smiling.* (I believe her: she emanates what we in California call "good energy," her voice and eyes are animated, her English is excellent.) *My mother said I hardly ever cried, though I was sick a lot. I still am—flu season, it doesn't matter whether I get a shot or not, I catch viruses back to back, just like my mother—she'd catch anything. She was insomniac too.*

I ask her about stresses in her family. *None that I can remember,* she says. *My parents were loving and supportive, they had a good marriage, no tension or yelling at each other, absolutely nothing to account for it, except the genetic.* I hear this often: *it runs in the family.* Yet I find, in all my research, maybe half a dozen familial studies of insomnia, and *one* study of its genetics. I also hear from many insomniacs that they've had the problem since childhood. Yet "childhood onset insomnia," as it's called, is claimed to be rare and is hardly studied. Researchers say insomniacs can't be trusted to remember their childhoods accurately. But I find Jacqueline's details convincing: *My mother would leave my play things around the bed because she knew how I was, plenty of books so I'd have something to read. She understood, she's lived with insomnia all her life.*

I ask her when she first perceived her sleep as a problem.

> *When I was eight and I went away to camp, I had to sleep in a room full of people—any bit of noise, and I'd be awake. It was awful. I remember being up and trying to do some knitting, and one of the counselors came and scolded, "What are you doing up?"*

But when it really began to undermine her was in school:

> *By the time I was in first grade, I had a hard time making it through the day. I'd be tired and sick—ear infections, high fevers, terrible headaches. I was an A student, but in France those days you went to school from 8 A.M. to 6 P.M. every day and Saturday, too, and there came a point it became harder and harder to learn. When I'm tired, I can't remember anything; with just a few hours' sleep, I can understand and memorize anything—I have a very good memory. The only way I could maintain being an A student was to study all the time, but as a normal rhythm I just couldn't keep it up, study at night and go to school all day. I knew this as soon as we started having a lot of homework, about third grade. At seventeen, the last year of high school, I was sick and missed a month.*

This, too, I hear again and again, how academic performance is impaired. Chronic sleep loss is, according to a 1990 study, "the most powerful predictor of school failure, more significant than parental education and profession." Researchers think it might also be linked to the attention deficiency disorders that are epidemic among kids today.

Jacqueline was able to graduate from high school because she was sent to a special school:

> *It was a school for people who had physical disabilities and were recovering from accidents. At the end of this year, I passed the exam and graduated. My first feeling of being normal was in that school, when my friends were in wheelchairs. I felt at home surrounded by disabilities. One of my best friends, in a wheelchair, said to me, "I don't think I'd want to switch with you." Because she'd see the way I would be.*

Feeling at home among people with physical disabilities, she began to think her own problem might be a disability. The Americans with Disabilities Act defines disability as "a physical or mental impairment that substantially limits one or more of the major life activities." "Walking, seeing, hearing, speaking, breathing, learning, and working" are counted as "major life activities"—but not sleeping. Insomnia is not a disability, according to the law, although it limits learning and working: we gauge our every move according to it, what projects we take on, what jobs we try for, or do not.

It has certainly been the strongest determinant in Jacqueline's life.

At that time, France didn't have any flex schedules, and I knew I'd be unable to work full-time. I decided to come to the U.S. and be an au pair girl, figured I'd be independent and become bilingual. The first family I took a job with, I had to be up every morning—it was horrible. Then I found a position with a divorced woman, a doctor. She was so happy to have me there, she'd drive her daughter to school herself, if I wasn't well enough to drive.

She stayed with this woman for several years. *I was great for her—I loved her daughter, and I organized her whole house. As insomniacs, we learn to be superorganized, we develop certain skills—well, you know how it is.* She describes this woman as *a doctor who didn't know what insomnia was and to this day she still thinks that sex will solve it.* Jacqueline has many doctor stories, some bad, some good, some about doctors who went out of their way to try to help her. She says the attitude of this doctor was *pretty typical: you know, just change your life, do something different, and you'll be fine. Like, get up at the same time every morning, all that. I did that, working at my first job, and I barely survived it.*

After this, she got what she calls "a real job":

I made sure I had a flexible schedule so I could come in late. It's not okay to tell people you can't sleep. But you know, even working only thirty-five hours a week, I had to be in bed at 8 P.M. every night and do nothing else. Nothing on weekends. And that was when I was twenty-five—now, at forty-one, I couldn't do it. I couldn't even do a part-time job. Thankfully, my husband . . .

I interrupted her and said, "I'm going to say to you what people are always saying to me—you don't look wiped out, you look fine." She shot back,

You don't see that I made sure not to do anything last night, that I made sure not to eat anything that might keep me awake, that I took a full-strength sleeping tablet so I could make sure I could drive across the

*bridge, and I took it early enough so I didn't get a hangover. You don't see
the way I live around this. I have six hours of livable time in a day.*

"Yes, I see . . ."

*No, you do not—you said you sleep three hours. If I get three hours, I cel-
ebrate, it means I have a good day, I can read a book or do something
intellectual, like learning PhotoShop or reading a difficult book. But if
I don't take a sleeping pill, I wake up every twenty minutes. And not
Ambien—it has to be long-acting. If I have two nights of no sleep in a row,
everything hurts, the brain burns, the head aches, I have burning inside the
joints, feet that become frozen. If I go for a week like this—well, you
know, you get suicidal. But that good feeling of wanting to go to sleep, it
rarely comes to me.*

I looked at this intelligent, attractive woman who has had such a
scraping-through life, and I felt blessed to be able to sleep three hours
straight, blessed to have a profession that allows me some control over
my schedule, blessed to have an empathic partner whose hours are also
flexible. I felt lucky to have an immune system that doesn't leave me prey
to every passing bug, though my immune system may be as dangerous.
Overactive rather than underactive, it plagues me with autoimmune
problems: Hashimoto's disease (a thyroid condition), gum disease, rashes,
allergies that just won't quit, and other indications of inflammatory responses gone awry. It seems to me that a lot of insomniacs have sluggish
immune systems like Jacqueline's or hair-trigger systems like my own,
that we are a population with a high incidence of chronic fatigue syndrome, fibromyalgia (a disorder of chronic musculoskeletal pain and fatigue), Graves' disease, and Hashimoto's. But this is only an impression.
I find no research on it.

Yet in many ways, Jacqueline's experiences mirror my own: the way
the problem's been there "just always," determining her every move, from
the minor to the momentous, shaping her sense of possibilities; the way
she lives around it, calibrating oh so carefully what drug she takes, how
much of it, and when. And the compensatory capabilities she's developed,
being "superorganized," knowing how to pull herself together and put on
a happy daytime face so the world won't see. And the way, once she begins talking about sleep, a floodgate opens and there's this pouring forth:
if you didn't know the experience from the inside, you might see her as
obsessed—and in fact doctors and researchers do call us obsessed. But
when there is something so basic to your existence that's not working—
well, as the proverb says, a starving dog thinks of nothing but meat.

I asked Jacqueline if there was anything she wanted to tell the world about insomnia.

When I heard you were going to be on the radio, I thought it was going to be the same old stuff, but when you started talking, I thought, Whoa, this is good, this is new. I told my husband, I'm going to go talk to that professor. I came here today, not to get sympathy or therapy, but because I hope you can be heard. I can't do it. I once had this idea of getting some people together to go on Oprah, but who'd listen to me? Maybe they will listen to you. . . .

I want you to tell the world what it's like to live with this curse, what it does.

What It Does, What It's Like

I don't think anyone can understand what it's like, the bone-aching awfulness, night after night, when all you want is sleep, when all you need *is sleep, so you can function the next day, but there you are "killing time" till you get sleepy or the night is over, whichever comes first.* So says my friend Roberta. Roberta and I bonded twenty-five years ago at a weekend faculty-trustee retreat when a meeting was announced for 7 A.M. and I heard a groan from the row behind; I looked back, caught her eye, we started talking—and we haven't stopped since. Roberta was my first insomniac, the first person I came out to, I mean, really talked to, about this problem. She was the only one who could truly understand what it was like to move through a life like mine, teaching classes, writing books, negotiating committee meetings on subsistence sleep, because this was her life, too. We aren't look-alikes—Roberta is tall, slender, and poised, with a blond pageboy, and her clothes never look rumpled—but we're sisters under the skin. (We share, too, a passion for horses—she still rides, in her midsixties. I do not. A fall from a horse when I was fourteen put an end to my riding—and a head injury may have dire consequences for sleep, as we'll see.) Roberta had a happy childhood, cookie-cutter normal, and she can actually remember a time when she could sleep. She traces her problem to birth control pills, which she feels threw her hormones out of whack, and to drinking in college, which she says "stripped the gears." She may be right, and for all I know, these things may have been factors in my insomnia, too.

What it's like is an acid test of sanity. When you spend night after night not sleeping, it undermines your hold on reality. "I can't tell you

how many lectures I give about this," says Ilene, another friend who figures prominently in these pages. A psychotherapist who's had bouts of
insomnia herself, Ilene has a both-sides view, as one who's suffered it and
who also treats it. Her eyes flash as she tells me about the sleep problems
she sees her patients put up with. "I tell them, 'When you don't sleep, it
erodes your ability to deal with things you can deal with otherwise.
Things you can deal with fine during the day get magnified when you
can't sleep—and it's not that you're crazy. It happens to everybody. The
demons come out at night.'"

What it does is make it difficult to function in the world. Studies show
that insomniacs have a hard time getting jobs, performing at jobs, holding on to jobs. Anecdotal evidence shouts this loud and clear:

> *I can't believe I'm fucking awake at this hour, and of course, I couldn't go
> to sleep once it hit 3:30 am for fear of not waking up at 7 am to get ready
> for my interview. somebody shoot me.*

> *Oh God, those days when I had a job I couldn't lose, and I'd just, finally
> drifted off to sleep. . . . If a gun had been handy, I think I'd have used it
> on myself. Sometimes my jobs required hard physical labor, all day, with
> the foreman watching every moment. You can imagine! In the evening, I'd
> feel desperately tired, but never sleepy.*

Sleep deprivation makes people indifferent and listless: subjects who
are sleep-deprived choose less difficult tasks and expend less energy. It
makes them stupid, too, bumbling and incompetent, as Stanley Coren,
author of *The Sleep Thieves,* found when he tried to restrict himself to
five and a half hours' sleep, night after night. Here are some of his journal entries: "It's not working. It's dangerous. It's making me stupid.
Today I showed sequencing and memory problems. For all purposes, I
became dyslexic at moments." He found himself writing down phone
numbers wrong, then dialing them wrong: "This scares me." When he
gave up the experiment and started sleeping again, "I recognized that I
had been ploughing my way through massive feelings of depression, anxiety, and helplessness. . . . The manuscript I had been working on . . .
was in really bad shape. There were hundreds of trivial errors, many of
them grammatical. Articles and other short words, like pronouns, were
randomly missing. . . . There were instances of repeated words (like 'the
the')."

(Welcome to my world. I can't type a line without making a half dozen
errors, my e-mails go out full of howlers, my typing's so inaccurate that

spellcheckers give up on guessing at what I mean, and word searches are useless because I almost never get all the right letters in the right order.)

Most workplaces are not insomniac-friendly, as Jacqueline discovered:

> I did sort of "come out" at that job. I told a few people about my problem, but it didn't really help—people can forgive you the first and second time, but not the third time, no. And I sort of understand. There was a woman at work who kept giving the excuse of a bad boyfriend—I was forgiving the first two times, but the third time I just felt, "Dump that guy"; so I understand how people feel, but it doesn't work that way. Insomnia is not something you can dump.

Job insecurity, the specter of job loss, looms large. *Who's going to pay the bills, who's going to pay the rent and feed my kids?* I hear this again and again.

"There's a built-in glass ceiling for people with severe sleep disorders," a psychiatrist friend told me. "Chronic insomniacs don't reach the top of their professions, assuming that they make it into a profession. You'll never get a constituency in Congress around this issue—they don't make it to Congress. Name one." It's true, how many members of Congress can you name who are insomniacs? How many CEOs? Short sleepers, yes, but insomniacs, no—or maybe there are a few and they just don't talk about it, but chances are, they get weeded out. Lord Roseberry, prime minister of England, resigned on account of insomnia. In 1903 he wrote: "I cannot forget 1895. To lie, night after night, staring wide awake, hopeless of sleep, tormented in nerves, to face the next day like a disembodied spirit, to watch one's own corpse, as it were, day after day, is an experience which no sane man with a conscience would repeat." The weeding out starts young. Here's Elaine, a student:

> I have a hard time staying awake in classes, and when I try to study after dinner, I just drop off, but then when I try to sleep, I'm wide awake. I've been this way since I was in high school, but college is a lot tougher. I'm not doing great in my any of my classes—yours isn't the only one. [She did not graduate.]

One woman told me she went back to school and got a degree to get a better job, but ended up staying at her old job: *I could barely meet the responsibilities of that job. I couldn't imagine a job that asked more of me.* Many insomniacs don't even trust themselves to drive to work: *I was afraid I might kill someone.*

No wonder so many of us find ways of living outside the nine-to-five world. *I never could keep the grades to graduate, but I did manage to start my own business. But now even that's going downhill—when I don't sleep I feel hopeless and put off contacting people and lose touch.* No wonder so many of us fall off the grid. *Drive a taxi, be a bartender—things you could do being an insomniac,* says a woman who became a freelance artist. Academia saved me, allowing me to structure my own hours. The first, and last, nine-to-five job I had, I got fired from—for coming in late.

Then, too, sleep loss hurts. *People don't understand that I'm in pain, sometimes severe pain,* as a woman wrote me. Sleep loss increases pain sensitivity, exacerbating existing aches and pains and creating new ones. If you deprive young, healthy adults of deep sleep for several nights, you can produce in them the pain, discomfort, and inflammatory skin responses of fibromyalgia; if you give arthritis sufferers sleep medication for a week, you improve their morning stiffness. Sleep loss produces headaches. *When I finally do get to sleep, I often wake up with this throbbing pain that lasts all day,* says a sufferer. With me, this kind of headache may last several days, like a dagger digging behind the eye. I can tell, from the way people scurry out of my way, that my face is scrunched up in an ugly squint. I'm not scowling, I want to say—I'm in pain.

"Nobody ever died of insomnia," we are told. We hear this from friends, family, physicians, psychotherapists, and researchers. We hear it so often that it has the ring of a proverbial truth. But recent findings suggest that it might not be true. People with fatal familial insomnia die of it; they stop sleeping in their fifties and they die within months, horrible deaths. This is a rare disorder that we don't need to spend sleepless nights worrying about, unless we've been born into one of the few families afflicted. But even shaving off a few hours of sleep a night has dire effects, as University of Chicago researchers Karine Spiegel, Eve Van Cauter, and Rachel Leproult discovered when they limited young, healthy males to four hours' sleep for six nights and produced in them the hormonal profiles of much older people. Subjects were less able to secrete *insulin* or respond to insulin, the hormone that allows glucose to enter and feed the cells, enabling us to utilize fuel. The University of Chicago team found that curtailing sleep for less than a week produced, in healthy young males, an *insulin resistance* like that found in the elderly and in people with diabetes. Researchers suspect that there may be a relation between the sleep deprivation that's a standard feature of life in industrialized nations and the epidemics of adult-onset diabetes and obesity that are sweeping these societies.

Spiegel and her colleagues also found that their sleep-deprived subjects had reduced levels of *growth hormone,* the hormone that's released in the deepest stages of sleep and that is essential to cell repair and restoration, and that they had elevated levels of *cortisol* and *norepinephrine* (adrenaline), stress hormones which, when elevated over a period of time, do damage. Stress hormones become elevated and growth hormone declines in the natural course of aging, which is why we lose muscle and bone density and put on fat. Anything that accelerates these processes makes us old before our time. Chronic sleep deprivation hastens the onset of age-related ailments, weight gain, diabetes, high blood pressure, hypertension, osteoporosis, memory loss—and it increases their severity. It compromises immune function and leaves us more vulnerable to disease, as we'll see. Then, having hastened our decrepitude, sleep deprivation makes us significantly less able, as elders, to live on our own. One study showed that difficulty sleeping was a "stronger predictor" of "nursing home placement and decreased survival time than any other factor considered."

"Sleep," says pioneer William Dement, "is the most important predictor of how long you will live, perhaps more important than smoking, exercise, or high blood pressure." A study that looked at healthy elders and followed them up four and nineteen years later found that those who reported sleep difficulties had mortality rates, within these years, almost double the rates of those who did not report such difficulties. Insomniacs have two to three times the rate of doctor consultations as people without sleep complaints, twice the number of hospitalizations, and more than twice the rate of auto accidents. So we may not drop dead of insomnia the next day, but chronic sleep loss may be cutting years off our lives.

The annual cost of insomnia, considering the drain on health care services, accidents on the highway, lost productivity due to absenteeism and workplace accidents, has been estimated to be as high as $100 billion. But nobody really knows how much insomnia costs, since nobody knows how many accidents it causes—exhaustion, unlike alcohol or drugs, leaves no trace. Besides, such estimates take into account lost productivity and accidents only among people who have jobs; of those who never make it into the workforce, there is no reckoning. Nor is there reckoning of the toll in suffering. "People with chronic insomnia are distressed," concludes a 2005 study. Their quality of life is worse than that of "patients with congestive heart failure, in terms of pain, emotional effect, and mental health."

Losing Sleep

It's a great mystery to me how something as crucial as sleep can inspire so little concern. Sleep is as essential to our survival as eating, drinking, or reproducing—and it's actually the strongest of these instincts, since you can voluntarily refrain from the others but you can't from sleep. Yet it was not until 1953, the year James Watson and Francis Crick described the DNA double helix, that sleep even became the subject of serious scientific inquiry. It's an "astonishing anachronism" in the history of science, says science writer Chip Brown, that the structure of DNA was unraveled "before virtually anything was known about the physiological condition in which people spend one-third of their lives." "It's as though we'd flown to Mars with a third of the earth's surface still unexplored," as a sleep researcher once commented.

"Nothing wrong with you except you can't sleep," said a doctor, reading me the results of my physical. I didn't know whether to laugh or cry. I tried to imagine this doctor saying, "Nothing wrong with you except you can't breathe."

The indifference is everywhere, from research-funding priorities to dinner party chat. The National Institutes of Health (NIH), which funds most biomedical research in this country, spends more today than it ever has on sleep research ($188.7 million in 2005, up from $76.1 million in 1996). But it was only in 1993 that the National Center for Sleep Disorders was established at NIH—and to this day, it has no funding. The Center for Sleep Disorders is housed in the National Heart, Lung, and Blood Institute, one of several institutes that supports sleep in the vast, sprawling parklike complex outside Washington, D.C. "Heart, Lung, and Blood" is not the first place I'd think to look for sleep, but it's there because of the link between sleep problems and breathing disorders.

When I bring up sleep at a dinner party (as I often do these days, in search of stories), what I mostly get is the kind of well-intentioned, useless advice I've just described: "Oh, I had insomnia once, I just . . ."—whatever. Sometimes there's a nervous laugh and a change of subject, as though sleep is too private, or too trivial, to be a topic of conversation. Sometimes I get the sense that insomnia makes people uneasy, as though they think it might be contagious. Actually, I bring it up not to vent but to find out how others sleep, but I still feel like the ancient mariner dragging a rotten albatross to the table.

It's not only in the reactions of friends, family, and doctors, this dismissal, but in the books we read. How many novelists let you see how their characters sleep? How many biographers let you in on the sleep life of their subjects? In a recent four-hour PBS special on Mark Twain, who was famously insomniac, there was one passing reference to his difficulty sleeping in old age. Anthropology, the study of the human condition, has barely looked at sleep behavior. Nor have historians dealt with it. Doctor Samuel Johnson asked, in 1753, why "so liberal and impartial a benefactor" as sleep should "meet with so few historians," a question he might ask today. There have been histories of hygiene, dress, illness, child care, and eating; I find maybe a half dozen articles (and no book) on the history of sleep. As for the social sciences, "Sociology is concerned with only two-thirds of the lives of its human subjects and has systematically ignored one-third of them," as Brian Taylor says. Standard textbooks in physiology and psychology, even many medical textbooks, leave sleep out.

It may be that sleep is so much a part of the fabric of our everyday lives that it gets taken for granted, fades into the woodwork. Familiarity breeds contempt, as with housework, though even housework has had its historians. But I think there's something deeper going on that accounts for this indifference to a realm of experience so vital to our being. It's as though we'd like to deny that we need sleep, as though our dependence on it is a weakness of the will, a failure of character, a threat to those prized values of control and rationality that are the bases of selfhood in the West. "Sleep is the most moronic fraternity in the world," writes Vladimir Nabokov. "It is a mental torture I find debasing. . . . I simply cannot get used to the nightly betrayal of reason, humanity, genius. No matter how great my weariness, the wrench of parting with consciousness is unspeakably repulsive to me." Sleep, says Edward Said, the celebrated literary scholar, is "something to be gotten over as quickly as possible. . . . For me, sleep is death, as is any diminishment in awareness. . . . Nothing invigorates me so much as immediately shedding the shadowy half-consciousness of a night's loss." Our culture is in awe of people who don't need sleep—Thomas Edison, Winston Churchill, John F. Kennedy, Margaret Thatcher—as though they've mastered a weakness we despise in ourselves. "Sleep puts even the strongest people at the mercy of the weakest and most feeble. Can you imagine what it must be like for a woman of Mrs. Thatcher's fibre, her moral character, to be obliged to prostrate herself every day in that posture of abject submission? The brain disabled, the muscles inert and flaccid? It must be insupportable," says a character in Jonathan Coe's wickedly funny *House of Sleep*.

To those who base their identity on a sense of control, it is terrifying, this nightly annihilation of consciousness, this disappearance of the self. To those wedded to the idea of their own specialness, it is humbling to find ourselves all alike and all subordinate to the need for sleep. Sleep is the great equalizer, putting kings on a par with beggars, men with women, men with beasts. It is "the indifferent judge between the high and low," writes Sir Philip Sidney. "Sleep is something we share with the unreasoning brute," says Marcus Aurelius, who encourages, therefore, wakefulness.

Sleep is a nightly reminder that we are beholden to our bodies, that we *are* our bodies, and that one day we will die. It puts us at the wrong end of the mind-body dualism that has, from Plato through Descartes, raised mind over body. It's a blow to our dignity, a reminder, like sex, that we are (to borrow a phrase from Shakespeare) "stinkingly dependent." Sleep, like sex, is done in the dark; it is, as sex was once thought to be, a "little death." You yield to sleep, "cross over," as it is said of death, though sleep, unlike death, is a realm from which you *do* return. Yet it's as incomprehensible, as baffling, in its way—you sleep, you die, except that *you* are not there to experience it, which calls into question the very notion of *you*, the very notion of the *self*. "The individual who lives out his allotted seventy years only remembers forty-seven of them," writes Phyllis Rosenteur, chillingly, in *Morpheus and Me*. Where were we the rest of the time?

"Don't go there," said Mark Twain, "people die there." People dream there, too. Sleep is the gateway to those nightly visitations of the irrational, the incomprehensible; sleep is where nightmares come from. In Greek mythology, Night gave birth to twins, Thanatos, the god of death, and Hypnos, the god of sleep. Hypnos was the gentlest of the deities, a giver of health and friend to man, but no cults grew up to worship or sacrifice to him, no temples were built to him. Even in classical Greek and Roman times, sleep was accepted as a need, but it was never honored, as Stanley Coren says. Nor does the Judeo-Christian tradition hold it in high esteem. The Bible cautions against it: "Love not sleep, lest you come to poverty; open your eyes, and you will have plenty of bread" (Proverbs 20:13). "Awake, O sleeper, and arise from the dead, and Christ shall give you light" (Ephesians 5:14). To awake is to be enlightened; to sleep is to be benighted, slothful, damned.

The Protestant-Puritan-capitalist ethic puts its own spin on this, defining time as money and sleep as a waste of time. More than 80 percent of Americans believe you can't be a success at work and get enough sleep. "Guys like General Electric's Jeffrey Immelt boast they can survive on five hours a night and still run a dozen multibillion-dollar divisions," reports *Forbes*. "In the corporate world . . . to get by on five hours of sleep or less is a badge of honor, a mark of the Olympian executive who can straddle time zones, bridging the NASDAQ and the Nikkei," writes Jerome Groopman in a *New Yorker* article on the new wake-up drug Provigil (Modafinal).

Americans work harder than anyone, even the Japanese. Since 1969, we've added 150 hours to the work year. Cell phones, laptops, Palm Pilots mean we never have to leave work behind, we can take it anywhere, any time—and we do. One-fifth of the workforce does shift work. We live in cities that never sleep, with Home Depots, Wal-Marts, and health clubs that stay open round the clock. Our 24/7 society needs 24/7 workers, factory workers, airline workers, telephone exchange workers, police, emergency services, military, doctors, nurses, sleep lab technicians. A new principle of "incessance" informs our activities, and a new principle of speed: time is now the scarcest commodity in the world. Everybody complains that there's not enough of it, nobody knows what to do about it—except to cut back on sleep. In 1910, people slept an average of nine hours a night; it's now estimated that we sleep less than seven.

"I'll sleep when I'm dead"—so say my students.

Sleep Is the Enemy, the name of a 2006 album by a Canadian rock band, says it all: sleep is to be outwitted, conquered, overcome. Coffee is the second-most traded commodity in the world, second only to oil, and the United States is, not surprisingly, its largest consumer. Starbucks, morphed from an eleven-store chain in 1987 to an international phenomenon and a household word, is everywhere, at the supermarket, at the shopping mall, at the airport. "Energy drinks are a $3.7 billion industry whose revenues have increased by 51 percent in the past year [2006] alone," reports the *New York Times;* a new drink, called "Cocaine," contains 280 milligrams of caffeine. The wake-up drug Provigil, approved in 1998 by the FDA for daytime sleepiness associated with narcolepsy, had worldwide sales around $575 million by 2005, with 90 percent of prescriptions *off-label*, that is, for purposes other than that for which it was approved. It is now regularly taken by students, long-haul truck drivers, computer programmers, and insomniacs.

The physicians we turn to are themselves caught up in this madness.

"You would think that the tangible close-to-home experience that physicians have had with sleep deprivation during their training should make them more sympathetic with their patients who complain about sleep problems, but it doesn't seem to," said Vaughn McCall, medical director of the Sleep Center at Wake Forest University. A national survey found that it's common for residents to work 100 to 120 hours per week. "I have heard doctors say, 'I went through it. I don't see why [residents] shouldn't have to go through it, too,'" confided the dean of a major medical school to Stanley Coren, author of *Sleep Thieves*. "Publicly, doctors tell you that the residents have to put in this time so that they can see as many diseases and injury states as possible during their training," but privately, they view it as "a sort of trial by fire," said the dean, who admitted to sharing this view: "I think that patients really benefit from doctors that have been toughened and tested this way." Do patients "really benefit" from the medical errors caused by physician fatigue, I wonder. A 1999 report from the Institute of Medicine, a branch of the prestigious National Academy of Sciences, attributes approximately forty-four thousand deaths per year directly or indirectly to medical errors, citing "reduced vigilance and fatigue" as major problems.

As recently as 1977, British sleep researcher Ray Meddis argued that "sleep serves no important function in modern man. In principle at least, man is capable of living happily without it." That myth was exploded in the late 1980s, when Allan Rechtschaffen, one of the most distinguished figures in the field, subjected rats to total sleep deprivation, and they died within three weeks. Their heart rates and stress hormones soared, their body heat plummeted, their weight dropped, though they were increasing their food intake as much as 80 to 100 percent; they became uncoordinated, their skin and paws ulcerated, and they died of causes unknown. Later work suggested that they might have been overwhelmed by bacterial strains in their blood that the immune system normally keeps at bay.

At about this same time, scientists in Bologna were analyzing the first cases of fatal familial insomnia. Thirty or so descendents of a man named Giacomo, born in a small town near Venice in 1791, have been afflicted by this curse: they stop sleeping in their early fifties, and they die within months, hallucinating, losing control of their faculties, jerking and flailing about. One of the sufferers found his way, in 1984, to the clinic of Professor Elio Lugaresi in Bologna. Lugaresi could do nothing for him but watch him die, but he succeeded in getting his brain immediately to a neuropathology lab, where a postmortem examination revealed the

lesions that destroyed his sleep. Later work was able to pinpoint the genetic mutation that is the source of the problem.

The discovery of fatal familial insomnia and the death of Rechtschaffen's rats put an end to the idea that we can live without sleep. Like it or
not, sleep is a biological imperative. All the will in the world will not make
it go away.

Finding Sleep

Sleep researchers have been campaigning valiantly "to wake America to
the importance of sleep," in the words of the slogan of the National Sleep
Foundation (NSF), which was established for that purpose in 1991. The
NSF does yearly surveys that reveal shockingly high numbers of people
who go around sleepstarved, either by choice or on account of the demands of their lives or because they just can't sleep. In 2006, the Institute of Medicine issued a report describing sleep deprivation and sleep
disorders as a public health crisis of enormous proportions. It warned
that chronic sleep loss puts people at risk of diabetes, obesity, heart attack, stroke, and accidents, and that it will, with our aging population,
heap untold burdens on our crumbling health care system.

But researchers are swimming against a strong tide with this campaign, as they well know. Sleep, insofar as it figures at all in our 24/7
society, figures as a power tool, as the *Power Sleep* promised by a 1998
mass-market book of that name. So as I make my plea that insomnia be
recognized as a debilitating, disabling, and perhaps even life-threatening
condition, that there be more research on it and greater understanding
of its sufferers, I join the researchers, shouting into the wind. But maybe
it takes a person who's chronically sleepstarved—and *not* by choice—to
fully appreciate what the sleep-sated take for granted, to tell the world
what it so carelessly tosses away.

I love sleep, with the passion of a lifelong unrequited longing. I am
fascinated by it. All those hours I've had to contemplate sleep, drifting
in and out, all those days I've made do without it, stumbling through on
the barest bones of it, give me a keen appreciation of what it can do. And
I hate sleep, resent that it takes so much time and life, understand why
you'd want to do away with it. Why do I have to stop whatever I'm doing
and thinking and lie down for it? Why can't I just go on, if I want to or
need to, through the night and the next night and the night after that—
why does it demand that I put aside everything, go through the whole
complicated rigmarole of preparing a dark, quiet place (which, if you're

built like me, had better be like a tomb), of setting aside eight hours in every twenty-four to withdraw from the world, make myself quiet, make my mind go blank, just so I can refuel? Why can't it be optional? Why can't it be as quick and uncomplicated as a meal? It asks too much.

"The gentle tyrant," sleep has been called, only it's not so gentle. Just try doing without it, and it takes you apart, piece by piece. On days when I've slighted sleep (or more often, when it's slighted me), it eviscerates me, hollows me out—we're back to those terms insomniacs use, *sucked dry, eaten away, unglued, not myself. Zombie, zomboid, zombied out* are words we reach for to describe this feeling that our souls and spirits have taken leave, only our physical shapes are left stumbling around, as in that old movie *The Night of the Living Dead.* Other terms we use, *comatose, spaced out, running on empty,* also suggest this sense that we're *not all there.*

What goes on in the brain of the sleep-deprived to produce these effects can actually be *seen.* Neuroimaging shows that the *frontal cortex,* the region behind the forehead (sometimes called the *frontal lobes*), is what's most affected: it doesn't light up, as it does in the scans of people who've slept well. This is the seat of "higher order" mental abilities, the most recent addition to the human brain, in evolutionary terms; on this, the so-called *executive functions*—selective attention, problem solving, decision making, organization, judgment, reason, abstraction, language— all depend. This is where humans are thought to "form their sense of who they are—their self-awareness and their self-consciousness"; this is where the self resides. And this is what's most clobbered by sleep deprivation. Creative thinking, what researchers call *divergent thinking,* takes a beating, too: if you give sleep-deprived subjects tests that require flexibility, the ability to change strategy and generate unusual ideas, you'll see that these are impaired.

But if lack of sleep takes us apart, sleep puts us back together again, knits the raveled sleeve. On days when I wake up after seven to eight hours of sleep, my mind and body and mood feel mended, stitched back together. My head doesn't ache and my heart doesn't pound and my skin's not parched and my eyes don't sting and tear, and the world comes into focus. I can face the stacks of papers strewn all over my desk and floor, I can tackle the thorniest parts of this book, I know what goes where and how it fits together; and I have energy to take it on. I step on the pedal and there's fuel.

When we restrict sleep to five or six hours, what we mainly lose is dream sleep, the REM sleep that occurs in the later hours of sleep. We dream in every stage of sleep, contrary to what was once believed, but

REM is where the most vivid dreams occur, and certainly the most memorable, since this is when we're closest to consciousness. Nobody knows what dreams are for, but something in nature wants us to dream, since between a quarter and a fifth of our sleep is spent in REM; if we live ninety years, six or seven of them will be spent in REM. And when we're deprived of REM, the brain makes up for it: there is *rebound,* an increase in the amount and intensity of REM equivalent to the duration of the deprivation. I'm probably in perpetual REM rebound, since the second part of the night, when most REM occurs, is when it's hardest for me to sleep: I can feel my poor brain snatching at each patch of sleep to spin a dream.

I may have fewer dreams than most people have because my sleep is so broken, but I probably remember more of them; insomniacs tend to remember lots of dreams because they're always waking out of them. This is one of the few things I like about being an insomniac—I'm in close touch with my dream life. Within recent memory, I have traveled to a distant galaxy to be greeted by friendly creatures who looked human but were really lizards in plastic people suits; I have been captain of the *Nautilus;* I have been Elizabeth Taylor, being wheeled in for brain surgery. And there's something about all this wackiness—not the insight that comes from analyzing the dream, because often I haven't a clue "what it means," but something about the *process* of dreaming—that seems to clear my head, give me dream energy, fuel for thought. There are also, of course, those troubled and muddy dreams that cast a cloud from which the day doesn't recover. . . . There are all kinds.

What are they for, these phantasmagoric images and stories that play through our heads each night—whether we remember them or not? Sometimes I think I dream to amuse myself, sometimes I think I dream to confuse myself. Sometimes I think I dream to escape from myself, sometimes I think I dream to confront myself, to take on issues too charged to face while I'm awake, for dreams can be as brutally honest as they can be cunningly disguised. There are deep dreams and trivial dreams, dreams as piddling as, did I pack the dog's dish, and dreams that plunge me into seething cauldrons of memory and desire. There are dreams from yesterday and dreams that reach way back. There are dreams so transparent that I know their meaning instantly (an old rival turns up, fat and with bad hair) and dreams so opaque that I can find no way in.

Some dreams feel like a sloughing off of the impressions of the day, like the day's detritus shuffling itself off, the needling little annoyances I didn't have time to attend to come back to claim their due, and sometimes they're back with a message: but you never *liked* that man you just

agreed to team-teach with. But there are also those dreams in which I
return to the house where I grew up, and my mother and aunt are sitting
at the kitchen table, the dog plotzed on the kitchen floor, and their presence is so vivid that it stays with me the whole day—visitations, these feel
like, conjurings of the dead. When I dream like this, I could almost believe that dreams are a response to separation, that their function is to
reunite us with the dead or the distant, to assuage loss and loneliness.
And who knows but what they began, evolutionarily, when our lives
took us away from the packs and tribes we once lived in, and that's when
we became dreamers? But that can't be, because animals dream and babies dream and even late-term fetuses seem to dream—about 60 to 80
percent of their sleep time is spent in REM. Whatever about?

H. P. Roffwarg, J. Muzio, and Dement proposed in 1966 that in utero
dreaming may develop the nervous system and brain, taking the place of
external forms of stimulation to develop neuronal connections, so we're
born with certain instinctual behaviors in place. The species whose young
are born the most helpless and immature, with the most to learn, are the
species that have the most REM, not only early in life but throughout,
which argues for the role of REM in learning. And yet people who take
antidepressants that wipe out REM seem to go about their lives
unimpaired—so it's not only REM but nonREM sleep too that's involved
in learning.

But when researchers wake people out of REM and give them a
word to associate to, they find that their associations are more novel,
original; they "ignore the obvious and put together things that make a
kind of crazy unexpected kind of sense," says Robert Stickgold, a foremost authority on sleep and learning; they "search out and find potentially valuable new associations" in a way that may "foster creative
processes." Dreams are where we pull things together, make startling
connections, culling from the disparate parts of our lives and imagina-
tions to forge new combinations. Dreams are where we see patterns,
parallels, relationships unseen before. This is what metaphor is, bringing things together, making new combinations. Aristotle said the genius for metaphor was the one thing that could not be taught, that a
writer either has it or does not; but it seems we all have this gift tucked
away in our skulls. I have had dreams so cunning in their wordplay, so
stunning in their associations, so far beyond anything my conscious
self could conceive that I've sometimes felt, if I could access what's
going on in there, I could make art. In our dreams we are artists, and
our creations delight and instruct, as art was once said to do, though

they may horrify, too. And like art, they shift us around, jolt us into new ways of seeing.

I can't tell you what dreams are for, but I do know that when I dream deeply and sleep deeply I come to with my mind firing on all cylinders, culling from here, there, everywhere, drawing on its own stores of knowledge, the past, the present, the possible, seeing connections, weaving things together, making new combinations. Those are the days that the words and images come, only this doesn't begin to describe it—they tumble out so fast that they trip over each other, my fingers on the keys have a life of their own. This is what creativity is, as Stickgold says, "putting things together in fresh ways."

Stickgold guesses that REM may be more involved in creative problem-solving, and nonREM more involved in consolidating or fixing memory. Also, *procedural memory,* learning a skill such as playing the piano or riding a bike, seems to be affected by REM, whereas *declarative memory,* remembering a fact or a word, seems to be less affected by it. Studies suggest that different kinds of memory are dependent on different kinds of sleep. But it does seem to be that when animals or humans are taught a new task, whether it's memorizing facts or mastering motor skills, they learn it better when they're allowed to sleep than when deprived of sleep—and the more sleep they get, the better they learn it. The sleep best for learning, then, is a full night's sleep, a night that encompasses all stages of sleep—the kind insomniacs almost never get. Maybe this is why so many of us have, by our own accounts, bad memories. Maybe it's also why memory problems come on with age, as people lose the capacity for long, deep sleep.

All this is highly speculative and the subject of heated debate. There is "precious little on which dream researchers agree," as Stickgold says. But the connection between sleep and learning, between sleep loss and forgetting, feels, experientially, right to me and to many insomniacs: *when I'm tired, I can't remember anything,* as Jacqueline says.

Memory is related to *plasticity,* the amazing ability of the brain to reconfigure itself in response to new stimuli. When we're born, our exposure to the light, shapes, smells, tastes we come in contact with, our mother's voice and touch, the nutrients we take in, determine which neurons get pruned and which *synapses* (circuits connecting neurons) get strengthened. The brain is continually revising itself in response to new experiences, laying down new neural pathways, and the process goes on throughout adulthood as we evolve and adapt to new environments—such that the brainscan of a London cabbie will show disproportionately large areas devoted to spatial relations.

Researchers now believe that plasticity is dependent on sleep. When we're awake, there are too many signals competing, getting in the way, to allow the consolidation of memory. "We are taking in so much information through our senses," says Stickgold, "that we don't have time to process it all while we're awake. . . . We need to shut down that external input so that we can replay the tapes and mull over the day's activity. It's sort of offline memory reprocessing." Sleep allows us to organize and reorganize the impressions of the day—to lay down new tracks.

But we need not only to be able to adapt to changing circumstances, to move with the new; we need also to maintain continuity with past selves and experiences, to remain who and what we are. In the face of the new stimuli we encounter each day and the constant remolding of our brains, the enormous changes we go through in time, we need also to retain memories from years ago, memories that may lie dormant and unreinforced by experience, year after year, such as riding a bike and speaking a foreign language. How are those memories preserved when they are not being used? How but through dreams and sleep. Stickgold has found that when subjects learn something new it will trigger a dream about a related experience in the past. Subjects who've been taught the arcade game Alpine Racer II, for example, a game that simulates skiing, may start dreaming about actual skiing from the past. Dreams, says Stickgold, "review and recombine memories from both the recent and the distant past." Dreams are the way our brains identify patterns and fit those patterns into patterns from the past, processes he describes as "arguably among the most sophisticated human cognitive functions."

Sleep and dreaming, then, not only enable us to lay down new tracks, they reinforce old tracks. They allow us to incorporate past and present selves and experiences as we move through time, to remain who and what we are in the midst of change. And the learning at stake here—the sorting through and fitting in—involves more than the French phrases we try to cram into our memories on the flight to France. It's about extracting meaning from the world around us, making sense of our experiences, making judgment calls, negotiating a delicate situation with a colleague, say, or heading off a divorce. Anything that undermines this process undermines us thoroughly, compromises our ability to deal with our lives.

Researchers say there are people who don't even know they have a sleep disorder. Meir Kryger, director of a sleep disorder center in Winnipeg and lead editor of *Principles and Practice of Sleep Medicine,* the major sleep text, describes a nurse who lived for more than twenty years on a schedule that left her so tired she could barely stay awake, but who "didn't make the connection that when you sleep five hours or less you'll feel sleepy the next day and unable to function." I find it amazing that anyone could miss that connection. To me, this would be like not noticing that the reason I'm having trouble typing today is that, uh, one of my fingers has gone missing. But when you're running on caffeine and cortisol, bludgeoning yourself into insensibility with a killer schedule, deluding yourself that you can get by on subsistence sleep, you may be forgetting what it's like to be *all there*.

Sleep, like insomnia, is not just about what happens at night: it's about what happens to the day. When you lose sleep, you lose the better part of yourself. You're *not all there*—as insomniacs know, as we say with the terms we use for ourselves: *zombies, the living dead, nobody home*. It seems ironic that sleep is feared as the loss or disappearance of the self, when it may actually be the way we become most fully ourselves, maintain the continuity of past and present selves, retain our identities through time and change, become our most creative, intelligent, and alive. Sleep is how we manage to be *all there*. You might even say, *I sleep, therefore I am*.

Insomniacs know these things. We seem to be more finely tuned to the ravages of sleep loss than others are—*too* finely tuned, we are told. One of the criticisms researchers and clinicians level at us—one of many, as we'll see in the next chapter—is that we are overly concerned about our sleep, all worked up about losing a little sleep. But we get it, what sleep loss does to us, what sleep does for us. The researchers could use us to make their case.

CHAPTER 3

Blame the Victim

They told me I was doing it to myself, and that it was in my head and I could stop it if I really wanted to. They told my husband that I was doing it for attention.

No one does this to themselves. There are more fun ways to self-destruct, like drinking or doing drugs. It doesn't make sense.

When Macbeth can't sleep, we know it's because he's done something really bad—he's murdered his king, kinsman, countrymen, and, along with them, sleep. When King Henry IV cries, "O sleep, O gentle sleep . . . how have I frighted thee?" we know that he, too, has blood on his hands. Storytellers from Shakespeare to Dostoevsky have moralized insomnia, associating it with the guilty conscience, the tormented soul. But physicians, psychotherapists, and researchers moralize it, too, when they tell us it's something we bring on ourselves that we could change if we would, and if we can't we probably don't need all that much sleep anyhow.

When a problem doesn't show up in a blood test, a tissue sample, or an x ray, when you can't see it, palpate it, measure it, there's a tendency to refer it to the neurosis or psychopathology of the sufferer. "When all else fails, invoke a psychoneurosis," says Michael Gershon, who has done groundbreaking research on the enteric nervous system, the nervous system in the gut ("the second brain," as he calls it): "Where primitive peoples use a variety of gods to explain the inexplicable, modern humans use psychiatric illness." People with *irritable bowel syndrome,* a condition that, like insomnia, provides no telltale signs, are often told that their problem is psychoneuroses. Their GI tract looks normal, no lesions show on an x ray or an endoscopy, yet they're doubled over in pain—so the problem is said to be *psychosomatic,* originating in the psyche and manifesting in the body. Such people are often, in fact, anxious and de-pressed. "If you were chained by bloody diarrhea to a toilet seat, you, too, might be depressed," says Gershon.

"When I was a medical student," Gershon told me, "we used to be taught that there was an ulcerative colitis personality. We now know that ulcerative colitis is an autoimmune disease, like rheumatoid arthritis." People with ulcers used to be told that their problem was neurosis or stress and were advised to take a tranquilizer or a vacation. Then in the mid-1980s, the bacteria found in ulcer lesions, *Helicobacter pylori,* were discovered to be not just coincidental with the condition, but causal. "We now know this is not a psychosomatic disease," says Gershon, whose re-search is yielding evidence that irritable bowel syndrome may also orig-inate in the gut rather than the attitude of the sufferer. "The more you learn about syndromes, the less they become psychosomatic."

"When All Else Fails, Invoke a Psychoneurosis"

In the past few decades, many conditions once thought to be *psy-chogenic,* originating in the psyche or mind, have come to be understood as *neurogenic,* having neurobiological origins or bases. "Migraine, we used to believe, was a disorder of anxious, neurotic women whose blood vessels overreacted," said Stephen Silberstein, neurologist and cochair-man of the U.S. Headache Consortium, in 2002. "Migraine is not that. Migraine is a neurological disorder of the brain." Obsessive-compulsive disorder was described by a Freudian, Otto Fenichel, in 1934, as "the ego having already begun to adopt protective measures at the time of the original anal sadistic level of libido organization, so that the patient never reached the phallic Oedipus complex." In 1996, the acting direc-tor at the National Institute of Mental Health announced that obsessive-compulsive disorder is a "neurobiological illness": "What was previ-ously thought to be due to punitive toilet training is now known to be associated with changes in brain chemicals and patterns of responsive-ness of glucose metabolism."

Schizophrenia was once blamed on the cold, rejecting mother. The schizophrenic is "painfully distrustful" and resentful of others "due to the severe early warp and rejection he encountered in important people in his infancy and childhood, as a rule, mainly in the schizophrenogenic mother." The cure was a long therapy directed at excavating repressed fears, guilts, and desires thought to be buried in the unconscious. The analyst was silent while the schizophrenic lay on a couch and "free associated," analyzing dreams and desires, primarily of a sexual nature, and "transferring" his or her neuroses onto the analyst. "We would have all these erudite conversations, talking about interpretations," says Dr. Thomas McGlashan, the first psychiatrist who dared stand up against his profession and say the treatment wasn't working, "and meanwhile the patient is crumpled in the corner of his or her room." Then new techniques for imaging the brain turned up organic abnormalities in the brains of schizophrenics, and studies of identical and fraternal twins who were raised together and apart indicated that the heritability of schizophrenia is "roughly 80%, or about the same heritability as body weight." By the late 1990s, schizophrenia was recognized as a problem of genetically based developmental changes in the brain.

"We used to believe," "It was once thought," "We were taught in medical school": I keep hearing these phrases in these discussions. I hear them a lot these days in relation to sleep disorders.

Narcolepsy is a disabling and often a dangerous condition that affects about one in one thousand or two thousand people in the United States. Sufferers experience extreme daytime sleepiness and, in some cases, episodes of muscle paralysis called *cataplexy:* the jaw sags, the head and eyelids droop, the knees buckle, and the person collapses, sometimes while hallucinating. In the nineteenth century, the condition was attributed to "an excess of masturbation and deviant sexual behavior"; in the more enlightened twentieth century, the afflicted were told they were lazy or crazy. "I was sent for psychotherapy to try to determine what deep, dark secret I was trying to escape through the defense mechanism of sleep," writes Marguerite Jones Utley in *Narcolepsy: A Funny Disorder That's No Laughing Matter.* Since cataplexy is triggered by anger, fear, embarrassment, sexual excitement, laughter, narcoleptics were said to have a problem with emotion. Then, in the late 1990s, a series of groundbreaking studies discovered that the brains of narcoleptics have too little of the "wake-up" neurotransmitter *hypocretin,* also called *orexin.*

Work leading to this discovery began in the early 1960s, when William Dement, newly arrived at Stanford from the University of Chicago, founded a center for treating and studying narcolepsy. Hearing that dogs, too, had these symptoms, he bred a colony of narcoleptic dogs and began to look for a physiological basis of the disorder. (These dogs are famous: I've seen films of them, bounding, leaping, then collapsing to the ground paralyzed; they look sort of bewildered, but, being dogs, pick themselves up when the attack has passed and go on playing.) Emmanuel Mignot, who came to Stanford from Paris in the early 1980s to work on the dogs, identified, through a series of elegant investigations, the neurochemical elements in the dogs' brains that were responsible for the narcolepsy. Mignot's search for genetic abnormalities in the dogs led to the discovery, in 1999, of a mutated gene that affects receptors related to the neurotransmitter hypocretin, or orexin. (*Receptors* sit on the surfaces of neurons; when a neurotransmitter binds to them, it acts like a key opening a lock, stimulating the cell to activity.) He and his research team found receptors altered in a way that kept them from receiving the wake-up messages of hypocretin, or orexin.

Within weeks of Mignot's study, in one of those coincidences that sometimes happens in science, a group headed by Masashi Yanagisawa at University of Texas Southwestern Medical Center turned up further evidence of the link between the hypocretin/orexin gene and narcolepsy. They called it orexin because it was known to affect appetite *(orexin* comes from the Greek *orexis,* appetite, as in *anorexic).* Yanagisawa and his team, investigating the gene's role in feeding behavior, developed a strain of mice whose orexin genes didn't function, and much to their surprise, the mice began collapsing into sleep attacks. "We didn't aim at, or expect, sleep to be involved," says Yanagisawa, but "if you think about it . . . it makes sense—sleeping and eating are linked behaviorally and evolutionarily. . . . Now it appears [they] are linked genetically as well."

("Chief nourisher in life's feast," Macbeth calls sleep, lamenting that he has murdered his, his metaphor pointing to this connection between sleep and nourishment.)

The next year, in 2000, Mignot's group made the leap to humans when they looked at the cerebrospinal fluid of narcoleptic patients and found that it contained no orexin. Then he and his team did something unprecedented: they did postmortem examinations of narcoleptics' brains, of slices of brain tissue. ("You don't want to hear this part," he warned. Mignot, a short, blond, curly-haired man with a boyish exuberance and Gaelic charm, was more than generous with his time and indefatigable in our conversations, still going strong after hours—I had to steer him off the subject of Shakespeare when he learned that was my area.)

Sure enough, the cells that make hypocretin, located in a part of the brain called the hypothalamus, were either completely missing or the few cells that remained were not producing the neurotransmitter. Mignot compares this deficiency to the loss of insulin-producing cells in diabetes and the loss of dopamine-producing neurons in Parkinson's. "We think that there's something that specifically kills the cells that make hypocre-tin, possibly an autoimmune disorder," he says. Hypocretin (I'll refer to it now by the word the Stanford researchers use) is turning out to be, as Mignot suspected, a mastermind that has links to other cell groups and systems involved in wakefulness, such as *histamine,* another wake-up neurotransmitter. Within a few years of its discovery, hypocretin has remapped scientists' understanding of the sleep-wake system.

Another major breakthrough has taken place in relation to *REM behavior disorder* (RBD), where men try to act out their dreams, leaping from bed in their efforts to slay dragons and wild beasts, kicking, punch-ing, and throttling their wives (it generally affects men over fifty). Until the late 1980s, people who had this problem were thought to have a screw loose. "We were taught in medical school in the 60's that sleep-walking and sleep terrors in adults were associated with significant un-derlying psychiatric disease," said Mark Mahowald, neurology profes-sor at the University of Minnesota and director of the Minnesota Regional Sleep Disorders Center. But in 1986, Mahowald's findings re-defined RBD as a physiological disorder affecting the brainstem, the part of the brain that connects the spinal cord to the cerebral hemispheres. With normal REM, the brainstem blocks the messages that move mus-cles, and the body is paralyzed, which is why we don't act out our dreams, but with this disorder the messages get through and the muscles react. The fact that most cases occur in men of a certain age suggests that there may be a hormonal component. (No, they are not unhappily mar-ried: in the dreams they're acting, they're usually trying to *defend* their wives from harm.)

As I write, discoveries of this sort are being made. *Restless legs syn-drome* (RLS), an irresistible urge to move the legs, afflicts 6 to 15 per-cent of the population. It is a torment that drives people to spend night after night pacing the floor; it has ruined the lives of two people I know, and their spouses' as well. This is another of those syndromes that has had no organic markers, whose sufferers are, as Virginia Wilson says in *Sleep Thief,* "judged as psychotic, hypochondriacs, malingerers, and just plain crazy"; they're told that they're making up "imaginary ills . . . to get attention" or concealing some deep, dark deed. But in 2003, in the first study that looked at postmortem brain tissue of people with RLS, researchers discovered a deficiency in a specific receptor for iron trans-port: "The missing iron may cause certain neural signals to misfire, lead-ing to the classic RLS sensations of an irresistible urge to move the legs."

But there have been no such breakthroughs with insomnia.

Insomnia as Psychoneurosis

It was Freud and his followers who gave intellectual respectability to the neuroticization of practically everything. Though earlier in the century there had been an interest in the *brain* as the basis of mental illness, the Freudianism that took hold in the early 1940s—as Freudians moved into the most prestigious chairs in psychiatry in university departments— shifted the terms of discussion to the *mind*. Mental illness, and much physical illness as well, came to be seen as psychogenic. Freud saw mental disorders as arising from the unconscious, from repressed childhood experiences and conflicts primarily of a sexual nature.

"Freudian psychology and its offshoots held an intellectual monopoly on the study of the mind," says Dement, recalling how, when he arrived as a graduate student at the University of Chicago in 1951, he aspired to be a Freudian psychoanalyst. Papers in respected journals "would start out with something like 'In 1917 Freud said . . .' as if they were quoting from holy scripture": "Today this would never pass for hard science." "There was a belief," says Dement, that Freudianism "could explain every aspect of our problems: fears, anxieties, mental illnesses, and perhaps even physical illness," and that it could "cure all manner of psychological problems, neuroses, and even psychoses."

Freud and his followers explained insomnia as neurosis or symptom of neurosis. "The disturbance of sleep is a neurotic symptom," wrote a Freudian analyst in 1942. "Like alcoholism or homosexuality, insomnia is not a disease entity but merely symptomatic of some underlying neurosis," said F. S. Caprio in a 1949 article, "Bisexual Conflicts and Insomnia." Causes included repressed fears of death, fears of homicidal wishes, of suicidal wishes, of sexual impulses, guilt over sexual impulses, guilt over Oedipal jealousy, masochistic impulses, inferiority complex, and paraphilia (sexual perversions). Diagnoses included "schizoneurosis, with anxiety-hysteric, dissociated trends, passive dependency reaction, . . . anxiety state with passive dependency reaction" (these from Valentine Ujhely's "Oedipal Jealousy and Passive Dependency States in Insomniacs"). Ujhely said of a patient, "She dared not sleep for fear of killing her mother." Caprio analyzed one of his cases as "the struggle between her id or homosexual cravings and her superego or moral censorship, that awakened her." Otto Fenichel explained that "the autonomy of the cathexis of the repressed, acting in opposition to the wish to sleep, either makes sleeping impossible or impairs its refreshing effect." "Here we have a veritable catalogue of psychopathology," wrote Dr. Jacob H. Conn in "Psychogenesis and Psychotherapy of Insomnia."

Here we also have a salutary reminder of how rapidly the certainties of one age become the absurdities of the next.

Strip away the verbiage, and you find essentially two explanations. There's anxiety, on the one hand—the insomniac is afraid to relax his guard and go to sleep, for fear of yielding to repressed impulses and "do[ing] something crazy," says Dr. Conn (no, I did not make that name up). And there's depression, on the other hand: "The almost universal tendency of insomniacs is to show depressive symptoms or mood (affect) disorders; rarely does one find an exception to this." Even when the insomniac insists he is not depressed, he's depressed, pronounces Leonard Gilman in "Insomnia in Relation to Guilt, Fear, and Masochistic Intent": "There is always a reason . . . for insomnia. Yet the patient often denies any disturbing or unpleasant thoughts . . . [insisting] that there's nothing in his mind but an extreme desire for sleep."

The cure for insomnia, as for any neurosis, was a long therapy, and since people see what they believe, Freudians saw that this method was successful. "Psychotherapists have ample case material to prove that when the psychodynamic factors motivating the insomnia are made known to the patient and are properly treated, sleeplessness as a symptom disappears," claims Caprio. "By exposing the root conflict and working it out with the patient in psychotherapeutic sessions, the insomnia gradually dissipates itself" (that sentence is why people who want writing to make sense rail against dangling participles: it has "the insomnia" "exposing" the conflict and "working it out" with the patient). Of another patient, Caprio writes, "The guilt was dissipated during [the patient's] free association sessions. . . . The insomnia disappeared and I later learned she was making a normal adjustment to the opposite sex, having been able to experience a coital orgasm for the first time . . . [and was] planning to remarry." In the 1950s, "adjustment" was the highest ideal, and marriage was the highest goal for a woman, as I can tell you, having come of age in that decade. In the case of a woman of thirty, single and "highly successful in the business world," who "derived much satisfaction and pleasure from her work" but was not interested in marriage, "the psychopathological basis [of insomnia] was obvious," writes Freudian F.R. Riesenman: "When insight into her illness had been established . . . eventually her emotional needs for love, home and family received expression through marriage."

The analysts were confident about their diagnoses, sure that their methods worked. Meanwhile (like the schizophrenic who remained huddled in the corner) the insomniac went home to her crumpled sheets.

In the 1960s, the hold of Freudianism began to weaken. As the biochemistry of the brain began to be better understood, as antipsychotic drugs were discovered that were effective with schizophrenia and depression, explanations for mental disorders began to shift from the psychogenic to the neurogenic. As more refined techniques of neuroimaging yielded more detailed information about the brain and as neurotransmittal systems came to be better understood, the biomedical model of explaining mental illness gained ground. Depression, which had once been explained as anger turned inward, "a despairing cry for love," came to be understood as having a biochemical basis. Prozac, which arrived on the scene in the late 1980s and was followed by other SSRIs (selective serotonin reuptake inhibitors), such as Zoloft and Paxil, tipped the scales further toward the biomedical model and shifted treatment toward medication. It became difficult to believe in the value of a long Freudian analysis when Prozac could do the trick. In the past few decades, as Harvard sleep researcher Allan Hobson says, "nearly all of Freud's central concepts—his theory of dreams, the Oedipal complex, infantile sexuality, penis envy, childhood repression," have been "placed in the same sort of scientific limbo as astrology."

And yet with insomnia, psychogenic explanations are set in stone.

"Physiological factors are seldom the primary cause of insomnia," write Anthony and Joyce Kales. Anthony Kales, founder of the first sleep lab in the country and author, with his wife, of the influential *Evaluation and Treatment of Insomnia,* 1984 (revised 1990), is one of the foremost insomnia researchers of the twentieth century. "The majority of chronic insomniacs . . . are anxious, ruminative, apprehensive, neurotically depressed, or somatically preoccupied," write the Kaleses. Insomniacs feel "inadequate, insecure, and dependent" because they've been "emotionally deprived in childhood. . . . Having experienced depression, self-doubt, and inferiority, . . . they need and demand sympathy and support, but are often too self-preoccupied to be attentive to the feelings of others"; they have "feelings of entitlement and expect to be nurtured and cared for by others." Insomniacs "tend to be obsessional. . . . Not only do these patients manage stress ineffectively, they have high levels of psychopathology" and are "possibly schizoid." "The well-established importance of psychiatric factors in the etiology of insomnia," says Alexandros Vgontzas, "suggests that, with our current level of knowledge, the clinical skills of the psychiatrist are the most important tools in the effective diagnosis of chronic insomnia."

Throughout the twentieth century, these are the terms and explanations that prevailed—which is why, at the beginning of the twenty-first century, an insomniac seeking help from a doctor still gets shunted to psychiatry. Insomniacs are "tense, complaining, histrionic individuals, who are oversensitive to minor discomforts," says Quentin Regenstein, former director of the Sleep Clinic at Brigham Hospital, Boston. Insomniacs have an "internalizing or obsessive personality style," say Cynthia Dorsey and Richard Bootzin. "Good sleepers appear busier, more active, and more involved in their work and with other people," writes another researcher. "Insomniacs seem more preoccupied with self."

Insomniacs score high on the *neurotic triad* of the Minnesota Multiphasic Personality Inventory (MMPI), "hysteria, depression, and hypochondriasis," according to some studies (though not all). The MMPI is one of the most frequently used personality tests, though a psychiatrist I respect described it as "the most overrated tool in the business—it has no predictive value whatsoever." Critics point out that it was devised in the 1940s, on the basis of 724 Minnesotans, all white, mostly Protestant, rural, and of Scandinavian descent; the answers given by the majority of these "Minnesota normals," as they are sometimes called, became the basis for discriminating normal people from those with psychiatric problems. Critics question whether the Minnesota normals are all that representative.

Insomniacs are said to be "emotionally seclusive and socially withdrawn, . . . mentally and physically inactive, uncomfortable, sleepy, indifferent, not enjoying themselves, and depressed." They appear to be a "distressed, pessimistic, worried group who face the world with apprehension, anxiety, and self-deprecation." They have "greater difficulty in interpersonal relationships, . . . impaired social skills or negative social attitudes." Since insomniacs have a tendency to deny psychological problems, "essentially considering sleeplessness to be the entire problem," they have a "strong resistance to the physician's exploration of problem areas; a need for control, as expressed in manipulation of medications and lack of compliance with general measures." Even when they deny that they're depressed and insist that sleeplessness is "the entire problem," say Kales and Kales, they are depressed, and a thorough history will ferret this out.

Few psychotherapists today talk about Oedipal complexes or egos at war with ids, but to say that we can't sleep because we're depressed or distressed comes to much the same thing: the emotional upset is differently described, but it's still the emotional upset, the internalization and repression of emotion, "stress-related psychophysiological problems," as Kales says, that's the source of the problem. The behaviorists deneuroticize the problem, somewhat, attributing it to bad conditioning and inadequate coping mechanisms, but they still explain it in terms of the emotional upset of the sufferer.

The *physiological* side of psychophysiological insomnia is always, when you look at what's being said, an effect of the *psycho*.

Language with an Attitude: The DSM

Psychological explanations are inscribed in no less an authority than the *Diagnostic and Statistical Manual of Mental Disorders* (DSM-IV, i.e., fourth edition), the American Psychiatric Association's compendium of definitions of behaviors deemed abnormal enough to be described as disorders. These are the terms and categories that are recognized by insurance companies, funding agencies, and government entities such as Medicare. This is where medical professionals turn for a diagnosis if they want reimbursement for themselves or their patients.

Primary insomnia is the DSM-IV category for insomnia that is not secondary to a mental disorder or a medical problem such as apnea, restless legs, or pain. (Not until this fourth revision, in 1994, was insomnia granted a "primary" status and acknowledged as a possible disorder in its own right rather than a problem secondary to some other thing. "It was a major victory getting that through," Peter Hauri told me.) The DSM-IV defines primary insomnia as difficulty initiating or maintaining sleep, or nonrestorative sleep that goes on more than a month. Here's the language:

> Primary insomnia is often associated with increased physiological, cognitive, or emotional arousal in combination with negative conditioning for sleep. A marked preoccupation with and distress due to the inability to sleep may contribute to the development of a vicious cycle: the more the individual strives to sleep, the more frustrated and distressed he or she becomes and the less he or she is able to sleep. . . . Individuals . . . may thereby acquire maladaptive sleep habits (e.g., daytime napping, spending excessive time in bed, following an erratic sleep schedule, performing sleep-incompatible behaviors in bed).

"Emotional arousal," "distress," "frustrated"—these words give the problem a psychological cast. "Negative conditioning, "maladaptive sleep habits," "behaviors"—these words tell us that it's *conditioned*. The DSM-IV has no separate category for psychophysiological insomnia: psychophysiological is "subsumed" under primary insomnia, and not only subsumed, it is *equated* with it. The terms are used—here and by most researchers—to mean the same thing; in fact, many researchers fuse them into a single term, *psychophysiological primary insomnia*. This means that—bear with me here, this is not just quibbling—primary insomnia is defined as psychophysiological insomnia which is defined as conditioned insomnia. This conflation of *primary* and *psychophysiological* implies that *all* insomnia that is not secondary to some other cause has behavioral and ultimately *psychological* origins. It crowds out any possibility that insomnia might be other than psychological, leaves *no room in the language itself* for the physiological, except as an effect of certain medical problems that are known to disrupt sleep, such as apnea, restless legs syndrome, Parkinson's, and so on, or of the negative conditioning that's assumed to keep us riled up. It would be more appropriate to call it *psychobehavioral* insomnia (as Kales calls it) than psychophysiological, because the *physiological* plays no part.

This is language that's loaded, language that's laden with a view of insomnia and its causes. A physician who looks in the DSM-IV for a term to diagnose a patient (and all physicians must look here, since these are the accepted categories) is told, in effect, that primary insomnia is conditioned behavior, and is given no hint that there might be any other way of looking at it. A patient who's diagnosed with *primary psychophysiological insomnia* is told in effect that her problem is a conditioned behavior, a learned association of the bedplace with wakefulness. No wonder doctors tune us out when we try to tell them about our hormones.

One of the weirdest moments I had writing this book was while I was trying to make this point to Peter Hauri, founder of one of the first sleep clinics in the country and lead author of the best-selling *No More Sleepless Nights,* and he informed me that it was *he* who had written the DSM-IV description. Hauri has done some of the most interesting research in the field, as we'll see; he gave me a long, cordial interview in his office at the Mayo Clinic, in Rochester, Minnesota, and won my heart by admitting that his interest in insomnia was to some extent motivated by his mother's insomnia and his own. I was trying to make the point I've argued here, that to equate *primary* with *psychophysiological* leaves no room for the *physiological,* but we had run out of time and I had run out of nerve, having just learned that it was *he* who had written the description I've just critiqued. But I made myself speak up, as he was ushering me out the door, and asked, "Don't you think there might be a problem, equating *primary insomnia* with *psychophysiological insomnia,* defining all primary insomnia as behavioral?" After what seemed a long pause, he said, "I see. You are saying, this might be a case of—premature closure?"

Premature closure is exactly what I think it is: Hauri gave me the term I was groping for, to describe my sense of "case closed" on insomnia.

The other terms used for insomnia, *symptom* or *complaint,* are also problematic. In medicalese, a *symptom* is a subjective feeling reported by the patient. Insomnia is, as we've seen, a subjective condition that depends on the sufferer's report or complaint. (It's like pain, in this respect, which also depends on the patient's account: "my chest hurts" is a symptom; coughing up blood is a *sign* or objective indication.) But in everyday English, the term *symptom* suggests something that is *merely* symptomatic of or *secondary* to something else, which demotes the problem to *secondary* status and doesn't make a lot of sense when you're talking about *primary* insomnia. *Complaint,* in the language of medical professionals, is used interchangeably with *symptom* (though these words don't mean the same in any English I know); it refers to the *subjective* sense of having not slept well or enough. But in everyday English, a complaint is a lament, a protest, a reproach, a remonstration, an accusation; to complain is to grumble, gripe, whimper, whine, moan, snarl. Insomniacs are thus, by definition, complainers: the negative baggage carried by this word lands on us. This is language with an attitude.

In 2004, insomnia was promoted from symptom to syndrome. A *syndrome,* as in restless legs syndrome, irritable bowel syndrome, chronic fatigue syndrome, is a pattern of symptoms and signs, "used especially when the cause of the condition is unknown." Insomnia can't be termed a disease, because a disease is defined as having a known etiology. Syndrome has greater legitimacy than symptom—insomnia is moving up in the world—except that the change occurred only in the *International Classification of Sleep Disorders* (ICSD), the system of categorization used by sleep specialists, but not in the DSM.

Why does it matter whether we call insomnia primary or secondary, symptom or syndrome or disease? "The naming of diseases is a powerful social act that in turn can dictate social behavior," writes David Shenk in *The Forgetting, Alzheimer's: Portrait of an Epidemic.* "It therefore behooves the public to keep a close watch over the definition of diseases." The name, says Shenk, is a "public recognition of a shared affliction. The name says, *THIS is what you're suffering from. You are not alone. Others are suffering from the same thing. . . . We're going to fight this thing. . . .* Naming a disease is tantamount to launching an assault against that disease. . . . As a matter of social reality, no disease exists until it has [a name]." Shenk notes that Alzheimer's was long thought to be "just senility," something that came with the territory of old age, which might occasionally affect a younger person; there was reluctance to challenge centuries of thinking and call it a disease, which it is now known to be. So for decades after Dr. Alzheimer discovered the plaques and tangles that ravage the brains of the afflicted, "the question of what Alzheimer's disease was" remained "a great sad muddle."

The terminology for insomnia is also a great, sad muddle. Insomniacs know it: *They don't even call it a disease. They call alcoholism and obesity and drug addiction diseases, but they call insomnia a symptom. It's like they think if they don't recognize it, it will go away. It's like they'd like us to go away.* And researchers know it. "The inability to accurately define insomnia within established disease classification," said James Kiley, former director of the National Center for Sleep Disorders, "has been one of the impediments to progress in insomnia research." Lacking a name, or having too many names, or having names that are loaded, insomnia fails to rally support. There is no public recognition of a shared affliction and no assault being launched against it. There is nobody saying, "we're going to fight this thing."

Let me state, for the record, what my definition of insomnia is, the meaning I'm assuming in these pages. It's simple: insomnia is when you can't get the sleep you need to feel good, for no reason other than you can't. Some researchers define insomnia as taking thirty minutes to fall asleep and/or waking up and taking thirty minutes or more to fall back to sleep. I'd say that the minutes matter less than the way you feel. Chronic insomnia (and I'm talking about chronic insomnia in this book, not the occasional bad night or bad patch) is feeling starved for sleep, continuously, over a period of time. My definition does not shed light on what name to call this beast, but it does address questions people ask. No, you're not an insomniac if you wake up several times during the night but fall readily back to sleep and get enough sleep to feel okay. And no, you're not an insomniac if you sleep five hours and feel fine. Insomnia is when your sleep leaves you feeling not okay—with a complaint, if you will. I don't like that word as a definition of insomnia, but I'm not sure I have a better one.

Blame the Insomniac

Referring a problem to the neurosis or psychopathology or the attitude of the sufferer is a way of shifting responsibility to the sufferer—a way, in effect, of blaming the victim. If you're obese on account of a metabolic condition, you don't get blamed, but if there's no physiological problem anyone can find, you do: you could get hold of this problem if you were a better or a stronger person. I'm not sure it makes sense to blame people more for problems that are thought to be "psychological" than for those that are demonstrably physiological, but people do think this way, and such thinking drives policies. Health plans give less compensation for mental than for physical problems, and many disability policies refuse reimbursement for cases involving the psychological. It is deeply engrained in the American psyche, as Andrew Solomon says, that we need not treat an illness that a person has brought on himself or developed through weakness of character. A disease that is clearly organic "must be treated and insurance companies must provide coverage"—even if it's lung cancer brought on by a lifetime of heavy smoking—whereas a problem that's rooted in character receives "no more protection than does stupidity."

"Patients who present themselves to doctors with problems that are insoluble are perceived as threatening and often dismissed as mentally unbalanced, with the epithet 'crocks' whispered behind their backs," says Gershon, on the basis of the way he's seen irritable bowel syndrome sufferers treated. "There is little sympathy for people who have problems for which no anatomical or biochemical abnormalities have been identified." People I know who have chronic conditions for which there is no cure, such as IBS, headaches, backaches, arthritis, tell me their doctors just want them to go away. "We're a walking reproach, and a time sink to boot," says a friend who has chronic fatigue syndrome. Insomniacs feel this, too. *I feel like we actually sort of embarrass doctors, and so they turn it around and blame us. They know nothing about insomnia, and they don't like looking foolish in front of their patients. I think this is why they're so rude sometimes.*

Here are some attitudes I come across at the sleep conferences. "An insomniac comes in and we dread it, it opens a huge can of worms," says Dr. Jed Black, director of the Stanford Sleep Disorders Center, urging his audience *not* to take this attitude. Another speaker comments, "Physicians don't want to get into it, because it seems to open a can of worms that might bring up psychological issues they don't want to go into." (*Worms,* again.) A comment overheard: "The only thing I like to see come through my door less than a kid with ADD is an insomniac." "I used to think they were all crazy," said a sleep doctor I talked to, "so when I set up my clinic, I hired a psychologist to deal with them. Well, *that* didn't work."

The *psycho* in *psychophysiological* insomnia does not actually mean *wacko,* but I think sometimes it might as well. I can guess why: by the time we get ourselves around to seeing a doctor, after a bad spell of insomnia, or a lifetime, we're not in the best of shape. We may well be strung out, unhinged, querulous, whining, petulant, panicked at what's happening to us. We've tried lots of things that haven't worked, and we aren't thrilled to hear these things suggested as though they're new and wonderful; nor does it help that we come in asking for drugs doctors hate to prescribe. We're "difficult" patients: "Insomniacs have a tendency to . . . appear insistent and tiresome to their physicians, to feel neglected," I read in a 2002 study. "Poor sleepers tend to have weak and negative personalities," writes Ray Meddis in *The Sleep Instinct.* "Doctors and researchers often claim that insomniacs are complainers and hypochondriacs."

Since insomnia affects nearly twice as many women as men, it gets pegged as "a woman's thing." Women's problems are more likely than men's to be attributed to emotional and "mental" causes, to hypochondria or hysteria (*hysteria* comes from *hyster,* or womb, which was thought to wander around the female body and interfere with thought). Hot flashes and premenstrual syndrome were once said to be "hysterical." Multiple sclerosis was once called "hysterical paralysis." And when a condition gets thought of in these terms, it loses credibility and funding.

Hauri recounts approaching a psychiatrist to ask him if he'd ever used his relaxation technique on insomniacs and being told, "in essence, that insomniacs were a bunch of chronic complainers that one best kept away from one's practice." An appreciative chuckle ripples through the audience when a speaker refers to "the, shall we say, personality problems of insomniacs." A friendly laugh goes to a speaker who describes a questionnaire designed "to find out what's bugging them." These responses tell me that health care professionals have certain shared assumptions about insomniacs—that we're a pain in the ass.

"No, I don't like insomniacs," said a young man standing by his poster of a study of the new wake-up drug modafinil. I'd asked if he'd thought about studying whether this drug would help insomniacs survive sleepstarved days.

"You don't *like* insomniacs?" I echoed.

"Insomnia," he said, sensing my bristling. Then he added, "Well, you know, it's a swamp—I have other things to do."

Bringing It on Ourselves

"It is clear," says Dr. Julius Segal, formerly at the National Institute of Mental Health, "that much of the insomnia we suffer is voluntary—that many of the sleep problems that beset us are of our own making." (What *we* are we talking about, I wonder.) Insomniacs often bring their insomnia upon themselves, are their "own worst enemies," says Douglas Colligan in *Creative Insomnia*. "Some people really produce the whole problem by worrying," says Dr. Ernest Hartmann, former director of the Sleep Clinic at Boston State Hospital.

Not only do insomniacs bring the problem on themselves, they use it to their advantage. "There are people who exploit their insomnia. They feel injured by life and carry the martyrdom of insomnia for all to see, as a kind of plea for sympathy. . . . [They] pay undue attention to it rather than to their work, hobbies, or outside interests." "Those are persons for whom sleeplessness has become something of a status symbol . . . a badge of success," says Segal. "Insomniacs are usually highly invested in and preoccupied with their symptoms, and they derive a great deal of secondary gain from them," using them to gain "sympathy and attention" and withdraw from "normal daily functioning," to "detach themselves from parental responsibilities and marital and sexual interactions," say the Kaleses. "At work they typically function at a level much lower than normal." Insomniacs "avoid family and social interactions routinely by insisting they are too tired or by protesting that a certain activity will disturb their sleep"; they "may even demand that the spouse sleep in a separate bed or separate room."

The Kaleses' idea of *secondary gains* (it is Freud's, actually) is widely accepted. "Some people find it difficult to give up their sleep disorder, for it serves them in their relationships with other people," writes Peretz Lavie in *The Enchanted World of Sleep*. To illustrate "the use to which sleep disorders can be put," Lavie quotes Proust's aunt, who is heard muttering to herself mornings, " 'I must not forget to mention that I never slept a wink. . . .' Never sleeping a wink was her great claim to distinction, and one admitted and respected in our household vocabulary." "Using their insomnia as a lever," says Lavie, "insomniacs bend everyone around them to their will. The whole family is in a state of permanent anxiety. . . . People suffering from a sleep disorder are always the centre of attention. . . . Their status would change if the insomnia disappeared, and so it is difficult for them to give it up."

Does Lavie really know a lot of people like Proust's aunt, I wonder, this malingering aristocrat on her great estate, surrounded by extended family and servants that hop to her every whim? I don't know such people. The insomniacs I know are pedaling as fast as they can to keep up with the demands of modern lives, bearing their insomnia not like a badge of honor but like a dead limb.

It is difficult to read such descriptions and not take them to heart. Such terms are powerful, and they are predisposing: they determine the way we are seen and the way we see ourselves. If I come to you with a label that says *psychopathological,* chances are, you will *see* psychopathology, since we see what we believe. And even if I insist I am not depressed or anxious, except about sleep, a thoroughgoing psychological history will, as the Kaleses say, ferret the psychoneurosis out. But you can find psychopathology in anyone if you dig deep enough, or not find it, if you do not. A Harvard study gave doctors the case histories of patients who had committed suicide; some of the histories included the fact of the suicide, others did not. Of the doctors who were told of the suicide, 90 percent found evidence of instability; of those who were not, only 22 percent detected instability. In our readings of others, we read back from the ending—and a label is a kind of "ending," a sum total of what a person has been judged to be. Since people see what they expect to see, and "insomniac" is a label that says *psychopathology, psycho* is what they see.

But some of the nuttiest people I know sleep like babies. I had a roommate who spent years obsessing with her second shrink about whether she should tell her first shrink she was seeing a second shrink. I had a roommate who conversed with aliens. These women slept well. I have a friend whose love life and work life tie her in knots of rage, and another who drinks himself into nightly oblivion and seems intent on ruining all the good things in his life. I know a woman who obsesses about things that happened fifteen years ago, grinds her teeth in her sleep, has anxiety attacks if her husband's away from home for more than two nights. They sleep well. And, conversely, some of the sanest and stablest and most laid-back people I know have sleep patterns like mine: a neighbor who wins prizes for his horses, a friend who teaches yoga and takes long, interesting, restful vacations, both of whom are in long, happy marriages and nonstressful jobs and eat and drink healthfully. I also

know insomniacs who are type A and stressed out, and I know insomniacs who are as neurotic as hell. But we are not so easily characterized—
or caricatured—as the literature suggests.

Inside, Looking Out

I hold up each term, each description, and look at it in relation to myself. Tense, complaining, histrionic, hypochondriac, self-absorbed, passive, socially withdrawn, depressed, miserable, self-pitying, neurotic,
attention-seeking, inhibited, anxious, worrisome? Is this what I am? And
the insomniacs I talk to and interview and whose postings I read on the
web—is this what they are? This assault, for it feels like one, makes me
want to cry out that *these qualities, insofar as they exist, might be the
consequence and not the cause of insomnia.* I can't "prove" that it's as
likely to be the sleep problem that warps the personality as the personality that warps the sleep—I can't refer you to studies, since they have not
been done. But I can show you how these things work in my life, how
much of who I am and how I live has been shaped by my problems with
sleep. This is anecdote, but it's a story with a point.

"Socially withdrawn"? "Impaired social skills"?

"Social butterfly," my mother used to call me. Such a social animal I
was, she could never get me to come home from school. "Did I have a
sleep problem when I was a baby?" I asked her, more than once. "No-
o-o," she'd say, hesitating a moment too long, "but I could never get you
to sleep." She told me she'd put me down for the night and I'd get up on
all fours and shake the crib so it walked around the room. Born at 10:30
P.M., I began my day just as everyone else was ending theirs, a pattern
that's persisted. She was at the beach that day, a June day, just past the
solstice. I think I imprinted on the summer light, since summer and the
beach are where I'm happiest. In high school, I'd put down the top of the
little convertible my father gave me, load my friends in the car, and head
for the coast. If I was depressed in high school, I was too busy to notice,
though when I was sixteen I won a prize for a story told from the point
of view of a woman locked in a loony bin for killing her husband (though
I also wrote happy stories about horses and dogs). What I remember most
about high school was the agony of getting up mornings, slogging
through classes in an exhausted haze, bingeing on candy bars at recess.

"*Am* I depressed?" I've asked myself, more than once. It's a sloppy,
catchall term, a term I distrust, but I think I've been there. (I'm not talking

about major depression—that's in another league; I'm talking about feeling down.)

I was depressed in graduate school. I'd set out for New York City when I was twenty-three, armed with a master's degree from Berkeley, in search of "the real world." I got a job in publishing, then I got promoted, then I got fired—for coming in late—and I jumped back into school. I found a part-time job at Queens College and discovered that I loved teaching, but the job market crashed just as I got to graduate school, so there I was working for a degree for a job I was sure didn't exist. I knew I was depressed because I was attending daytime movies, which I've never done before or since: I'd take in a double feature Saturday afternoon and sometimes another Saturday night, and on really bad weekends, I'd do one Sunday, too; and I was eating vast amounts of chocolate. I was sleeping badly, though no worse than I had in high school. I'd wad cotton in my ears to shut out the sound of the wind that whipped off the river and whistled through my drafty old Upper West Side bedroom, rattling the panes like kettle drums. It was a room with a view, terrific for writing but not so good for sleeping. I learned to sleep with a long black sock draped over my eyes and hooked around my ears, which I do to this day. I popped over-the-counter pills like Sominex and Sleep-Eze, which didn't do a thing. I went to a psychiatrist, who didn't do a thing but write me a prescription for Elavil, one of the oldest of the antidepressants, which gave me dry mouth and constipation and fogged my brain and made it difficult to work. That's when I started seriously swimming. I was, at my worst, swimming up to two to four miles, twice a week.

I could have spared myself the worry about the future—I got a good teaching job back in California and had a happier professional life than I could have predicted in those graduate school days. But I do know about depression. It moved in again after my brother died, after my father died, and after the deaths of my mother, my aunt, and my dog Nellie. Death is depressing, nothing worse, draining, debilitating, distracting— you go around bumping into things, not all there, not even knowing you're not all there, until finally one day the cloud begins to lift and parts of you come back to life. Depression moves in on me at points like this, and at points when I'm physically run-down or starved for sleep—but it moves on when the circumstances change, and it's never made all that much difference to the way I sleep.

I know what it is to feel depressed, and it's not what I feel most of the time.

At sixty-four, I'm not the party animal I once was, though I don't think I've ever left a party in full swing. But it's a pared-down, stripped-back kind of life I lead, more socially withdrawn than I'd like. I start the day late and I run late. I don't do lunch, and often I don't do dinner—I graze while I work—and though I have hours after midnight, they are not my best, and they are solitary. I'm sure it looks strange, the way I live, hyperorganized, as Jacqueline describes herself, but it's a time-devourer, insomnia. I have half a day to other people's days, and I never know when I'll have no day at all, for it can come out of nowhere, a totally sleepless night that wipes out the next day. Old people live like this, around the good days and the bad days.

"Self-absorbed, self-preoccupied, inattentive to the needs of others"? "Passive, unconcerned, mentally and physically inactive"? You have to understand, we may be exhausted, our energies all bound up in getting through the day. "Internalize psychological disturbances rather than acting them out"? Since when is "acting out" such a great thing to do? But it's true, I take things to heart; in my better moods I call this *sensitive,* in my worse moods, just plain *dumb.* "Toughen up, sweetie," my Aunt Sady used to say, in that raspy old-lady-smoker's voice and Brooklyn accent that I loved. I had just started teaching, I was twenty-three, not much older than my students. It was good advice then; it is good advice now. I do try. But lots of people take things to heart and sleep fine.

Insomniacs have a "desire to avoid stimulation, preferring routine to excessive thrills and excitement"; they're "sensation avoiders," says Peter Hauri. Now *that's* a shoe that fits, and it's easy to see why. We don't need "thrills and excitement": negotiating each night's sleep is adventure enough. As filmmaker Alan Berliner says in *Wide Awake,* his documentary about living with insomnia, "My head hits the pillow and it's an adventure."

"Oversensitive to minor discomforts and unable to relax easily"? Okay, yes, I'm ridiculously sensitive to temperature, noise, light, air; if the room is too hot, too stuffy, too light, I don't sleep. The princess and the pea. If you sleep well, I'm sure this looks neurotic, but when your sleep is as fragile as mine is, you do get this way. When I used to fly around and give papers at conferences in Tokyo, Dubrovnik, London, and Stratford, I did it by taking pills, and I got badly addicted. These days I make a great effort not to get addicted, but I've had to cut back on what I do. "Come to Rome for spring break," says my friend Rena, who sleeps well. The two of us fantasize over dinner about what fun it would be; after dinner, I come to my senses and think, *No way.* I'd come home exhausted and addicted and it would take weeks to recover.

Does this make me "not sufficiently active or involved in outside interests"? You see the problem here. What is cause and what is consequence?

"Paying undue attention to our insomnia rather than work, hobbies, or outside interests"? How can we not? There is *never* a time when we're not dealing with this. *It's awful when you're never just worried about the task at hand, but [about] getting enough sleep to do it—I feel that way all the time,* wrote an insomniac friend, commiserating with me as I was about to take off for a four-day trip to England, leaving and returning in the middle of a teaching week, to speak at the memorial of Alice Stewart, whose biography I wrote. The trip, the talk, the memorial, the teaching were challenging, but possible. But what is impossible is that, at times like this, I stop sleeping.

Preoccupied with sleep? You bet. I've probably logged in more time thinking about it than most sleep researchers have. I certainly have more investment in finding out what's gone wrong.

"Somatically preoccupied, hypochondriac"? It's true, lying awake in the dead of night, you register every little ache and pain, and a twinge in the abdomen looms large. On sleepstarved days, everything hurts. The softest sweatshirt feels like a hair shirt; I keep squirming around looking for a label that might be scratchy, but there are no labels, just the feeling that I have no skin. Studies are finding that sleep deprivation increases pain sensitivity, as we've seen. Studies are also finding that sleep deprivation makes you more vulnerable to infection. If I've had a run of bad sleep and a student comes up to tell me she doesn't have her paper because she, *cough,* has a bad cold (they always stand six inches away when they tell you this), I get a cold, too. I choke down wads of vitamins—I figure my immune system needs all the help it can get. Probably I'd score high on the hypochondriasis scale of the MMPI. Probably I look like a health nut (luckily I live in northern California, where it doesn't much show).

Charles Morin, examining the beliefs and attitudes about sleep of 145 older adults, found that insomniacs had more anxiety about sleep and had stronger beliefs about the negative consequences of insomnia, more fear of losing control of their sleep and more hopelessness about its unpredictability, than other people do. He concluded that it's not the stress in their lives that keeps them awake; it's their *appraisal* of events, their "*perceived* lack of control over stressful events," their "dysfunctional beliefs and attitudes about sleep" (DBAS). What insomniacs need, he concludes, are "more effective stress appraisal and coping skills." But,

but, I want to protest, when I slog through days on three, four, or five hours of sleep, feeling like I'm on the edge of tears or tantrum, with a raging appetite and a mind skittery as oil on a hot skillet, this is not "*perceived* lack of control": this *is* lack of control, of my mental and physical faculties, of my energy, my mood. Our beliefs and attitudes may be "dysfunctional" in that they do not help, but they are not delusional. Besides, what Morin doesn't say is that sleep disturbance is itself a stressor, raising levels of stress hormones and ratcheting the stress system up in a way that makes us *physiologically* keyed to overreact.

"Maladaptive coping mechanisms"? You might say we have rather good coping mechanisms, considering what we're coping with. "Chronic complainers"? And yet seven out of ten insomniacs never even discuss their problem with a professional. The insomniacs I know, the insomniacs I met working on this book, are on the whole awfully good sports about accepting their condition: *I always put a smile on and went to work and did whatever for my family, no matter how miserable I felt.* Sometimes I think we're stoical to a fault. Ilene tells me that her patients "never bring up sleep," she has "to dig it out" of them: "'Tell me, exactly how much are you sleeping a night?' I say. 'Well, maybe two hours.' This woman does not mention this, unless I ask: *she does not mention it, even to her therapist.* I see incredible suffering like this all the time. What it is about our culture that doesn't give people the sense they have the right to talk about their sleep?"

When I suggest that this woman might not want to come across as a complainer, Ilene shakes her head: "I don't know where that stereotype comes from. *I* certainly don't see insomniacs as complainers—they don't even bring the problem up—and I've seen hundreds of people over the years. I'm the one who has to bring it up":

> "How much sleep did you get last night?"
> "Oh, well, I'm up and down a lot."
> "How much sleep would you say?"
> "Oh, maybe four hours."

"I'm not even sure it's about stigmatization—it's more like trivialization," says Ilene. "It's like people don't feel they even have a right to bring sleep up!"

Maybe it would be better if we ranted and raved, chained ourselves to the gates of the sleep clinics, stormed the National Institutes of

Health, demanding more and better research, howling out our pain and rage—if we *acted out* our emotions rather than *internalized* them. But that really would show the world we're a bunch of crazies.

Another stereotype we encounter—not stated in the literature but apparent in physicians' attitudes—is that we're a bunch of drug addicts or potential addicts. I'll come back to drugs in a later chapter, but here, while I'm talking about the inside view, I'll say this: What nobody sees is the nightly struggle many of us go through *not* to take a pill. *I go to bed thinking, Well, maybe, maybe tonight I can make it on my own. I lie there as long as I think there's a chance of getting to sleep, then at some point I just give up and take a pill. I have such a feeling of failure.* Yes. Always, these same questions: How long should I give it before I take a pill? What's the lowest possible dose I can get by with? What's going on tomorrow that I can afford to screw up or miss? And always that feeling of failure when we give in. We take medications because it's so much worse when we don't. We take them knowing there's a price to pay—*sleep now, pay later.* Many people refuse to take them at all. I talk to insomniacs who are housebound from exhaustion, their lives ground to a halt, who insist, *Oh, no, I'd never take a pill.* "I hear this all the time," says Ilene. "I have a client who sleeps two hours a night but won't take anything because she's afraid of getting addicted. What are the horrors of addiction that they could be worse than what she's going through?"

Carts and Horses, Causes and Consequences

So, which comes first, the personality that makes poor sleep or the poor sleep that shapes the personality?

One thing I know about myself: I do not have that natural pressure to fall asleep I see in other people. That curtain that drops nightly on others just doesn't come down on me. I can be dead on my feet and I won't drop off the way Bob does, and even if I fall asleep easily, I'm wide awake in a few hours. Things that disturb Bob's sleep a little—like eating too late or eating the wrong thing—wreck mine entirely. If something wakes me up just as I'm drifting off, I'm awake for the rest of the night—it's as though the pressure to sleep that has built up in the course of the day goes poof, up in smoke, and there's not enough left to put me under again. I read that "about 70% of persons suffering from chronic pain report poor sleep patterns"—and I'm amazed: that means 30 percent of people with chronic pain sleep through it! I read that when Theodore Spagna took photographs of people sleeping, "every time the sleeper was 'shot,' his bedroom was ablaze with light and the camera motor cranked up the next frame with a grinding whoosh"—and many of his subjects slept through it! That's what good sleep pressure does for you, the curtain comes down, the tide comes in and sweeps you away.

What is it about my sleep that's so fragile that a dream or a creaking floorboard or a snore or a body movement can kick me into consciousness? Sleep pressure is highly variable and probably heritable, as we'll see. But whatever the reason for such fragile sleep, whether it's *psycho* or *physiological,* it sets into motion processes that *do* become *psycho,* in the sense that they are crazy-making—and that are *physiological* as well, since they set the stress hormones flowing. You lose energy; you get cranky and dispirited; you fall behind; you get anxious about falling behind; you cut yourself off from people and get depressed about being cut off—and whatever neurotic tendencies lie dormant in you find fertile soil and bloom. And since you never do get that rejuvenating sleep that others get, and since sleep affects everything, everything gets sucked into the maelstrom, mood, energy, frame of mind, and there's this *spiraling down.* You go to the doctor and get told you're depressed or have "bad coping strategies," but she or he may be looking at the *effect* of the process and mistaking it for the *cause.* And I'm not talking only about next-day effects, which anyone who's lost a night's sleep is familiar with, but the changes engraved in a personality over time.

"Am I 'depressed'?" I asked a psychotherapist I used to see. One thing I always liked about this therapist was that she didn't give me a lot of dumb advice about sleep, confessed that she frankly didn't know what my insomnia was about. I'd seen her, on and off, in my late thirties and early forties; then, after my mother and aunt died, I went back to her for a few months. That was when I summoned the nerve to ask this question, steeling myself because I knew her answer would be honest and, since she knew me better than anyone, I'd have to take it seriously. She thought for a moment, then said, "I don't think we know *what* you are, Gayle—apart from this. I don't think we know how things would be for you, if you could sleep."

I think she's right—insomnia has shaped me in ways I can barely begin to imagine.

My point here is that many of the personality traits that researchers point to as the *cause* of chronic insomnia are as likely to be the *consequences* of living with insomnia as the cause. If you were to take normal sleepers and deprive them of sleep, randomly and unpredictably deprive them, over long periods of time—an experiment that would not be approved by any "human subjects committee"—you could make them concerned about their sleep, somatically preoccupied, socially withdrawn, mentally and physically inactive, indifferent and listless, and all the rest.

You could make them depressed, as studies now show. Recent *longitudinal studies,* studies that follow people through time (one of which followed subjects for more than forty years), have confirmed that insomnia is a risk factor for and predictor of depression. (Anecdotal evidence would have got you here sooner: *I don't see how they can say it's depression, when it seems so obvious it's the other way around,* says Roberta. *I think they've really got the cart before the horse on this one. No wonder they're not getting anywhere.*) In fact, in a study of eighty-six patients who suffered chronic insomnia, 70 percent of whom were depressed, the depression significantly improved when they started to sleep better. And you can put people in a foul mood. *I'm like Jekyll morphing into Hyde,* said a woman I talked to. *I didn't used to be like this, on edge all the time, about to explode, like a raw nerve, like a venomous creature, snapping, snarling. I wouldn't blame my husband for leaving me. I'd like to leave me too.* A 1946 paper showed that rats allowed to sleep only four hours a day became so aggressive that, after thirteen days, they could be handled only with heavy gloves; they became, after forty days, "almost vicious in their behavior."

Does the personality make the insomnia or the insomnia make the personality? "The causal web is not likely to be untangled easily," says Allan Rechtschaffen. I can only tell you how it works for me. I sleep two, three, four, or five hours and I'm awake, so wide awake that the return to sleep is highly unlikely, unless there's absolutely nothing going on the next day, a rare occurrence in my life—and even then it's not likely. That's the central fact of my existence, the fact I live around. It's just been there always, the tail that wags the dog.

Only once did it change—when I was pregnant. I slept wonderfully, though I had no reason to be sleeping at all—I was in no position to carry the pregnancy to term. It was extraordinary that during that most painful, confusing, and stressful of times, when I was anguishing the decision to terminate a pregnancy, I was sleeping better than I have before or since. I felt, for the first time, what it was to have the pressure to sleep that most people enjoy normally, only it took a flood of hormones to get me there. After that, I could never believe that my insomnia is *fundamentally* a matter of my psychological condition or what's going on in my life.

Moral Fables

When I see my friend Rick's hand trembling with Parkinson's, I wouldn't dream of suggesting he's bringing it on himself. Since 1959, when post-mortem examinations of the brains of Parkinson's sufferers turned up deficiencies in the dopamine-producing centers, nobody has been able to say that "the Parkinson's personality" is the problem. But insomniacs do get told such things.

I don't mean to imply that psychological factors—depression, anxiety, worry, and stress—play no part in disturbing sleep. Of course, they may have a powerful effect. But there's a huge leap from saying this to saying that *any* insomnia that can't be explained in physiological terms *as they are currently understood* (i.e., as apnea, RLS, chronic pain, or medical conditions such as Parkinson's) must have a psychological cause or origin. Nor do I mean to bash psychology; some of my best friends are psychologists and psychiatrists (truly), and I'd have probably majored in psychology if I hadn't loved literature more. If I seem to be coming down hard on psychological explanations of insomnia, I am reacting against centuries and centuries of assigning solely psychological explanations to this condition about which so little is known. I'm saying it's premature to toss insomnia into what Robert Sapolsky terms "the psychogenic bucket."

What if, in the not too distant future, we're hearing, "We used to believe that insomnia was . . . but we now know that there are . . ." too few neurons in an area critical to generating sleep, or too little of a crucial neurotransmitter, or some somnogen that's not being produced, or some receptors that aren't receptive—some glitch in the brain's extraordinary circuitry that leaves insomniacs without the neurological wherewithal to transition to or maintain normal sleep? Many researchers think that they will find some such explanation someday.

So why the high moral tone that gets taken with insomnia? I think that people's attitudes toward sleep are bound up with the deepest and murkiest parts of themselves, with unstated and often unexamined terms they've made with life, investments in positions they barely know they have. Sleep is so close to home, nothing is closer—in fact *home* is sometimes defined as the place where we sleep. Sleep is woven into the fabric of our daily lives, into the most intimate regions of our beings, who we are, the way we see the world, the things we need to believe.

We all have stories we tell ourselves, myths, rituals, propitiatory rites, some that serve us well, some ill, some that are totally off the wall. One story people often tell themselves is that, when things go well for them, it's because they're clever, good, virtuous, or otherwise deserving. Thin people take credit for being thin, and rich people assume they're superior because they have money, and successful people often forget how much blind luck it took to get them where they are. Good sleepers often assume that they sleep well because they're doing something right. But if they're doing something right, this means that I or anyone who has a sleep problem must be doing something wrong: I'm just not trying hard enough, or I get too worked up, or there's something on my mind or conscience—there are many forms blame can take, as we've seen.

But here's another possibility. Maybe people really suspect deep down that it's not about anything they're doing right or I'm doing wrong. Maybe they sense that sleeping well is not about anything anybody does, but that the gift for sleep is just that, a gift, as inexplicable and as unfair as extraordinary beauty or off-the-scale intelligence or athletic prowess. Maybe even the best of sleepers is not above feeling some insecurity, some fear that whatever it is about sleep that works its miracles and reconstitutes us from a tattered rag to our customary composure is actually fragile, incomprehensible, and beyond our control—that it is, like all natural endowments, a kind of grace. Because if my insomnia is not something I'm doing wrong, and your good sleep is not something you're doing right, then what's to keep the sleep fairy from deserting you as mysteriously as she has me? Too terrifying.

So I think a lot of the intolerance we encounter with regard to sleep is about control issues, as we say, ways of telling ourselves we're in control of something that is frighteningly unsusceptible to control. I think this may explain the obtuseness and intolerance of otherwise empathic people, and why problems sleeping, whether from insomnia or other sleep disorders, tend not to draw forth the understanding and compassion that other afflictions do. Muscular dystrophy wouldn't get you a lot of dumb advice about changing your attitude or taking a hot bath, but most people don't have to deal with muscular dystrophy on a daily basis, whereas every person, every night, negotiates a relationship with sleep.

I think control issues also explain some of the totally irrational practices and beliefs I come across in intelligent people. I know a man who takes a Benadryl every night when he goes to bed; for two decades he's done this. This man is a well-known cellular biologist at a major university; he knows perfectly well that this drug has long ago lost whatever effect it once had; but he takes it anyway. To propitiate the sleep fairy. When I hear things like this, I think of what my dog Nellie used to do each night as she bedded down. Nellie was a ninety-pound sheepdog. She'd begin pawing her blanket, dig at it as though it held a bone, pick it up in her jaws and shake it furiously, then hurl it across the room and plotz down on the bare floor, hitting it with a thunk and a sigh, and fall instantly to sleep. If I forgot to bring her blanket, she'd prowl unhappily around the room until I tossed her a towel. I sometimes think people are about that rational when it comes to attitudes and rituals around sleep. Not me, of course, just everyone else.

I wonder, also, if the stigma against insomniacs might have to do with suspicion of night people. "The status of night people," says Douglas Colligan, in *Creative Insomnia*, "is slightly higher than typhoid Mary's." Colligan did an informal survey and found the following attitudes: "'No normal person lives like that,' . . . 'They're all running away from something, they're probably loners or losers or both, they just don't want to be part of the life the rest of us follow.' . . . It is hard to find anyone who will say anything complimentary about someone whose day begins when everyone else's is ending." "Early to bed, early to rise, makes a man healthy, wealthy, and wise"—we all grew up hearing this. ("Early to bed, early to rise, anyone not like me is wacko and unwise" is what it really says.) Now it turns out that people who say such things may be taking credit for something that's no more a moral virtue than the color of their eyes or hair. But the prejudice runs deep, a legacy, perhaps, of our agrarian past when the common good depended on everyone being out in the field tilling the soil from sunup to sundown, and a late sleeper was a drag on the rest.

The stigma may go back to time immemorial, when the night held horrors. It's hard for us to imagine how terrifying the night was for our ancestors, how absolute the darkness. As A. Alvarez wrote in *Night*, "Until about one hundred years ago, the only source of artificial light was fire: millennia of fire, scraps of flame in the darkness of prehistory, fragile, easily extinguished." "Murderers and thieves, terrible calamities, and satanic spirits lurked everywhere," wrote E. Roger Ekirch in his history of night, *At Day's Close*. Towns during the Middle Ages and Renaissance had strict curfews, with penalties for anyone who violated them.

Anybody up and about at night was thought to be up to no good, a thief in the night, a lady of the night. "Good people love the day, and the bad the night," said a French proverb. "When it was said of any man, he keeps BAD HOURS, it was in effect stamping on him a mark of disgrace," said an eighteenth-century writer. "Why can't you go to bed at a *decent* hour?"—I can still hear my mother say this, as though the hours I kept were *indecent*. Electricity may have dispelled the darkness, sent the ghosts and ghouls scattering, but there's still this suspicion, at the beginning of the twenty-first century, that if you're a creature of the night you're up to no good.

I hate to hear the sufferers themselves buy into the blame, but this is what I hear:

I know it's something I've created because there's nothing wrong with me physically. I know I have brought this upon myself. I am a very anxious person and live a lot inside my head.

I know I'm neurotic about this, I'm sure I think too much about my sleep.

I'm not as disciplined as I ought to be—I ought to be better about keeping to a schedule.

If I was better about expressing my emotions . . .

I'm sure it's true what they say about secondary gains—I'm not sure what they are in my case, but I know they are there—why else would I be doing this to myself?

I am definitely a . . . high-strung, nervous type and come from a family . . . who also tend to somatize stress (irritable bowel syndrome runs in the family).

"Quit apologizing," I want to shout. "You can't sleep! It's a miserable way to be—don't make it worse by heaping blame on yourself!" We can always find something we've done wrong, and maybe it's more reassuring, in a way, to assume that we're bringing this on ourselves than to admit that nobody really knows what's gone wrong with our sleep—because, if it is something we're doing wrong, there might be something we can do to make it right.

But there is one thing well known about insomnia: it's a pain in the ass to be around. It's hard on friends, lovers, spouses, children, parents, relatives, roommates, and doctors. It's the cause of more divorces than

anybody knows. It requires infinite patience, but it's more likely to provoke irritation.

> *Over time it seems that the people around us get fed up. . . . I know that
> most of the people in my life who have left me because of this are very lov-
> ing people. I know that they meant well . . . but in the end they didn't
> know how to "fix" me so they gave up. I also know that I put a lot of
> people through hell, because I was (am) often tired and can be very mad
> at everyone.*

Because it's not well understood, and because it's not fun to be around,
insomnia gets moralized. "There's no rest for the wicked"—we've all
heard that; or, as a German proverb states, "The best pillow is a clear conscience." (I find this proverb quoted in a Freudian article on insomnia.)

When blame is encoded in our proverbial expressions, when it's enshrined in our cultural myths and in our literary and medical lore, it's
impossible not to internalize it. Maybe this is why we haven't organized
on our own behalf. Imagine—a support foundation for insomniacs?
"Chronic complainers," "All in their heads," "Bringing it on themselves," "Why don't they just shut up and take a pill?" And in our heart
of hearts, we probably agree, or part of us agrees—I know it's in me, this
voice—if I were more *sane* or more *normal,* I'd "sleep the sleep of the
just."

CHAPTER 4

Sleepless in Seattle

The Conferences

You know the story of the guy who's looking for his wallet
under the lamppost. "Are you sure this is where you lost it?"
says his friend. "No," says the guy, "but this is where the light
is best."

Peter Hauri, interview

My first introduction to the world of sleep research was in Seattle, at the
2002 meeting of the Association of Professional Sleep Societies (APSS).
Every June since then, I've gone to these annual APSS conferences. Just
after I've dug out from under final exams and said good-bye to the grad-
uating seniors, just as I'd like to be kicking loose and going somewhere
with Bob, who reminds me we haven't had a vacation in so long that neither of us can remember, I descend into the subterranean, dimly lit vaults
of hotel conference rooms in Seattle, Chicago, Philadelphia, Denver, Salt
Lake City, Minneapolis, caverns the temperature of a crypt, cold dead
air blown about by fierce air-conditioning, where I spend six days shiv-
ering, starved for light, processing information. These are meetings
where scientists, physicians, psychotherapists, health care workers, sleep
clinic technicians gather from all over the world to share the latest in research and treatments. They began in 1960, when Allan Rechtschaffen
"called all the world's sleep researchers that he knew to Chicago for a
sleep conference," and "all twelve of them" came. "A year later, at the
second conference," as Peter Hauri recounts, "there were about twenty-
five of us, and five years later there were close to three hundred." The
conferences I go to have five thousand or more in attendance. They are
high power, high quality, and huge.

Negotiating this scene on three to five hours' sleep and a drug hangover is surreal. The lighting is kept dim for the PowerPoint presentations.

The speakers are all adept at this technology, waving wands of light nimbly over charts and graphs projected on to the screens above, often over-relying on PowerPoint to make *the* point ("Just *say* what you mean!" I want to say, feeling alone and unscientific in my partiality for the spoken word). Plenary lectures are held in football-field-size ballrooms, the speakers so far away that they're tiny dots, their images projected huge onto screens around the room. Each afternoon there are sessions where work in progress is tacked up on, well, posters; these are called—"poster sessions." The abstracts of these studies are published in a volume the size of a phone book, free to members of the Sleep Research Society, twenty-five dollars to nonmembers.

I apply to the Sleep Research Society, explaining that I am a professor and an insomniac writing a book on insomnia, and I'd like to be a member. I am turned down, a terse form letter. The next year, armed with a glowing recommendation from an eminent sleep researcher and a more detailed description of my project, I apply again; again, I am turned down, the same terse letter. At the suggestion of the sleep researcher, I query this decision; I hear nothing back. At his suggestion, I query again—again, no response.

This is not a field that welcomes outsiders.

❁

I steel myself for the reception the first night, a dressy affair in a grand ballroom. It's a lavish spread, ham, roast beef, champagne freely flowing. Well, at least you get something for the price of admission, I am thinking as I snarf down my fifth piece of smoked salmon, one of several elegant hors d'oeuvres that keep appearing at my elbow on a silver tray. (I'm reeling from the cost of this conference, but, I have to admit, this beats the mousetrap cheddar that gets served up at the Modern Language Association meetings.) I know no one. Everyone's huddled together in small groups, intensely conversing, no entering wedges anywhere. I can't even recognize anybody from the photos I've found on the Web. I walk around the room, making the widest possible circle so as to take the maximum time; then I walk around again. I get a few curious stares as I pass by the fourth time, but I keep walking, around and around. Sitting alone seems too pitiful; besides, I came to mingle.

Finally I see a man standing alone, white-haired, gentle-looking, gazing out over the room. Something about this man seems approachable. I summon my nerve and walk up to him and say, "You look like you don't know anyone here, either." He smiles and says, "What makes you say that?" Something about his amusement tells me I've called it wrong, and sure enough, he turns out to be a famous researcher who's done pioneer work on REM, as I learn at the plenary session the next morning, where I watch him receive a major award. But I did call it right about the gentleness; I learn, in subsequent years, that Adrian Morrison is not only one of the most distinguished of sleep researchers but one of the best liked. He earned my everlasting gratitude that night.

He finds it intriguing that I'm an insomniac writing on insomnia, and as we chat, he introduces me to various people who come up to talk to him, explaining that I'm an insomniac writing on insomnia—and these *are* names I recognize. *Great,* I think, an entering wedge, except that nobody but him finds it interesting that I'm an insomniac writing on insomnia. A few look at me like they haven't heard right. One looks down his nose and says, appraisingly, "You should perhaps get your face x rayed; you have a facial structure that"—his eyes move critically down my face—"may be impeding your breathing." Mostly eyes flicker, guarded, glance away. I feel like one of the laboratory animals, loose in the banquet hall.

I vow that I will be very careful from now on about telling anyone I'm an insomniac. To identify myself as an insomniac is to put myself in a relationship with this world I don't want to be in—it's to identify myself as a *patient, not* a professional, and not a popular kind of patient, at that. I think of other things I might say as I move through these meetings: I'm a journalist, covering the conference; I'm a science writer, writing a book about where insomnia research is today; I'm a sociologist, trying to get a sense of the sociology of the meeting; I'm an anthropologist, studying you all as a strange, exotic tribe. Any of these has enough truth to it that I might pull it off. But who am I kidding? I have "outsider" written all over me, my gypsy skirts, my unruly hair, my language itself bears the stamp of thirty years in a classroom with California undergraduates. This is SO NOT FUN.

I tell myself I'm lucky to be an outsider. There's nobody here who can turn me down for an article I submit, or a grant proposal, or a job. I'm exempt from the fiercely competitive struggle to get ahead in this world; the sources of my funding are elsewhere. I get to be an independent. I get to ask why the emperor has no clothes. I tell myself this is a good position to be in.

It just doesn't *feel* good.

I am glad there are no more unstructured social events. From now on, the dinners all center on lectures. Each night there's a dinner presentation that goes on till 9 P.M., and each morning starts off with a breakfast meeting at 7 A.M., a time of day that's totally trippy when you go to bed at 3 A.M. "Going to a sleep conference, are you?" joked a friend as I took off for Seattle for my first of these conferences—"Well, at least you'll get some sleep." Har, har, har.

Where Are the Women?

And all this has come about in fifty years, I think, with amazement, wandering the halls the next morning, looking for my meeting room, only fifty years since that breakthrough discovery of REM: the field is still in its infancy. "Plenty of research opportunities here," I hear, more than once. "This area is wide open." Lots of areas are said to be "wide open."

Women's sleep is one. In fact it's so wide open that there are hardly any papers on it.

There's a lunchtime event, fifty dollars extra, where I hear Margaret Moline of the Sleep-Wake Disorders Center (New York Presbyterian Hospital, Cornell) talk about women and sleep. Moline is a tall, dark, thin, intense woman who takes the subject seriously, covering as many aspects of women's sleep—premenstrual, pregnancy, menopausal, and postpartum—as the hour allows. "There's not as much published as one would expect for this many years of sleep research," she says. "Studies of women's sleep across the reproductive cycle have been few and far between. Of these, sample sizes are small, and there are differences in study design and data collection procedures that make it difficult to get a sense of what's going on. There is very little known."

"Is this because the researchers are mainly male?" I ask her after her presentation. I have noticed that there do seem to be more men on the podiums, though there are about equal numbers of men and women in the audiences.

"Oh, I have a lot to say about *that* . . . ," she replies, rolling her eyes. "They didn't even start looking at women till the nineties, when NIH mandated it." Seventy-five percent of sleep research, according to a 2003 report for the National Institutes of Health, has been conducted on men.

There are many reasons researchers don't want to use women subjects. If women's sleep really is different at different times of the month, data would have to be collected at different times, which gets costly. Besides, there's the risk of pregnancy or the complicating factor of birth control pills to be considered. Given how scarce funding is, you can understand why researchers go for the least problematic kind of subject—and that's young, healthy males. But this means that they're not looking for differences between women's and men's sleep, which means that they're not finding differences, which gives them the sense that there are no differences, so they don't *have* to look—and the subject goes on being ignored.

There is only one presentation on women besides Moline's. The speaker starts out by saying, "There is so little known about sleep disorders in women, so little research, that in some ways it's an embarrassment." I find it kind of embarrassing that a guy's giving this presentation. I'm hoping he'll say something about the doubling of women's sleep complaints at menopause, and he does: he attributes it to hot flashes, to increased rates of apnea (apnea becomes more frequent in women after menopause, on account of weight gain and perhaps also the decline of progesterone, since progesterone has a protective effect on breathing)—but he explains it mainly in terms of the "psychic distress" women experience at midlife, their depression about aging, empty nests, divorce, loss of parents. So the reason women experience sleep disturbance at menopause is, again, psychological upset.

But, but, I am sputtering, menopause is a biological as well as a psychosocial event, a time of major hormonal upheaval when our bodies are adjusting to radically declining levels of hormones. As a woman who's felt the grip of hormones not only at menopause (which was like one long, excruciatingly drawn-out spell of premenstrual tension) but also in my turbulent adolescence and during my brief pregnancy, I can tell you that these were *not* psychosocial events, especially the pregnancy, which so blissfully knocked me out at a time of high anxiety. I have high hopes of something more informative, as I head off, at the conference the following year, to a session called "Psychological and Physiological Correlates of Sleep Quality during Menopause and Beyond," where the speakers are all women. But three out of four of these speakers attribute menopausal sleep problems primarily to depression and anxiety and "dysfunctional beliefs and attitudes about sleep" (DBAS). They find that the women with the worst sleep also have the worst attitudes. Well, sure, I'm thinking, attitude can mess you up: if you lie there with clenched teeth, furious because you're awake, you'll never get back to sleep. But just as surely, if you're waking up repeatedly and are unable to get back to sleep, you're going to *develop* an attitude—so even if the women with the worst sleep have the worst attitudes, that doesn't tell you what's causing what.

The fourth paper in this session, "Endogenous Sex Hormones and Sleep in Older Women," by Patricia Murphy of Cornell University Medical

School, is as brilliant as the others are dull. Murphy, who begins by apologizing for her chattering teeth (it's that cold in this ballroom), finds a strong relationship between wakefulness and levels of *luteinizing hormone* (LH), the hormone that causes the ovaries to release the egg. Levels of LH are higher in the older women than the younger women she looked at, and LH pulses are associated with awakenings, perhaps because LH raises temperature, and elevated temperature is disruptive of sleep. Also interesting is that in older women, LH levels are highest at 5:08 A.M., about the time we lie there buzzily awake, whereas in younger women levels peak some time in the afternoon. Murphy finds, further, that the ratio of estrogen to LH is a strong predictor of sleep quality: in young women, estrogen levels are higher in relation to LH, but as estrogen declines, LH pulses "may be breaking through the protective barrier of estrogen, resulting in unrestrained release of LH." Finally, I think! A study that looks at menopausal sleep problems as though they have something to do with our bodies rather than our psychic upsets.

Another study, this at a poster session, catches my attention, "Orexin A and B Levels Change in the Hypothalamus during the Estrus Cycle and Aging in Female Rats." A blond with a Lauren Bacall voice and an accent I place as Finnish when I get close enough to read her nametag (it says Helsinki) stands by the poster; she is the lead author, Tarja Porkka-Heiskanen, and she looks friendly, so I stop and chat. She explains that just preceding ovulation, the orexin, or hypocretin, system, the wake-up neurotransmitter that's deficient in narcoleptics, is stimulated and the rat's sleep is disrupted.

"Why?" I ask. "Why the increased vigilance?"

"The females are getting ready to mate," she explains patiently.

Oh. Right.

These two studies are tremendously exciting. Porkka-Heiskanen's investigation explains a way the reproductive cycle disrupts sleep, and Murphy's offers an explanation for that temperature havoc and wiredness many menopausal women experience, even apart from hot flashes. But then, when I get to the insomnia sessions . . .

Nonpharmacological Management of Insomnia

The insomnia sessions are of two kinds, *nonpharmacological management of insomnia* (behavioral modification) and *pharmacological management of insomnia* (drugs). I attend session after session called "Behavioral Insomnia Therapy," "Use of Cognitive Behavioral Therapy for Chronic Insomnia," and "Current Studies of CBT." I hear: "B is for behavior change, C is for cognition, altering beliefs and attitudes." I hear: "Adhere to a regular time getting up, get out of bed when you can't sleep, decrease time in bed." These phrases are repeated like mantras. The air is thick with acronyms—CBT (cognitive behavioral therapy), SR (sleep restriction), SH (sleep hygiene)—and with terms like *cognitive distortion, cognitive restructuring, cognitive modulation,* and, of course, *DBAS* (dysfunctional beliefs and attitudes about sleep). Dysfunctional beliefs include: "Insomnia is necessarily detrimental to physical and mental health," "If I can't sleep, I won't be able to function tomorrow," "I'll be irritable," "My immune system will be compromised," and "There is something wrong with my sleep system." Functional beliefs include: "You don't need as much sleep as you think you do" and "There is nothing wrong with your sleep system—it's not that your sleep system is broken, but that your arousal system is working too well."

One speaker says, "I tell them they sleep more than they think they do—that can be very soothing. I tell them that sleep changes with age— that too is reassuring. I tell them to get rid of that 'illusion' that 'if I could only sleep, all the rest of my problems will be solved.'" "Sleep," says a speaker, "is the back door to getting help: complaining about sleep is safer than saying, I'm psychologically distressed." (Where have I heard this before? Ah yes, "Paraphiliac Preoccupations and Guilt in the Etiology of Insomnia," Dr. B. Karpman, 1950: "Insomnia is a mask for anxiety, depression," a cover for "a type of mental conflict which is not acceptable socially.") Freud lives in these sessions, combined weirdly with the power of positive thinking.

I keep looking around at the audience, trying to gauge how people are reacting. I seem to be the only one taking notes, fingers clattering madly across laptop keys. I get some pretty weird stares, like what *can* she find so fascinating? Questions from the floor indicate that not everyone's convinced.

> *Question:* But I have patients who wake up early and they're not depressed.
> *Answer:* I'd restrict time in bed.
> *Question:* But what do you do with a patient who just doesn't improve? What *do* you do . . . ?
> *Answer:* Restrict time in bed.

> *Question:* But what about the patient who's tried everything? [These are
> physicians asking these questions, and there is real concern in their voices.]
> *Answer:* Most insomniacs tell you they've tried everything, but they
> haven't taken their problem seriously enough to follow this regimen.
> They have to restrict time in bed and regularize wake-up time, seven
> days a week for several weeks.

So, the method works—for everyone, it is implied—it's just the *patients*
who don't work, who don't stick to it. The problem is *noncompliance,* a
term I hear a lot in these sessions. The problem is also, according to these
speakers, getting the message out, since most physicians don't have training in CBT or time for it. So, says a speaker, "we made a package that includes a tape and a pamphlet explaining about CBT and DBAS and SH
and SR and suggestions about relaxation techniques." Instructed in these
principles, patients can now teach themselves how to sleep. Oh, great, I
think, the HMOs are going to love this—no need for a physician or a psychotherapist anymore, only the cost of printing and postage.

I think these researchers vastly underestimate the extent to which
word is out. You'd have to live in a cave not to hear it. You can read
about CBT and SR and SH in the hundreds of self-help books that crowd
bookstore shelves, in women's magazines, in the in-flight magazine of
Southwest Airlines, in leaflets given out at health food stores, on dozens
of sleep-advice Websites. Word is certainly out at my HMO—though I
come across one survey of physicians' attitudes that suggests that physicians don't take time with these methods because they don't actually
think they work.

To rain on this parade would be like flashing a Communist Party
membership card at a Fourth of July picnic in the 1950s. Dissent could
only come from the outside—and it does, from a Frenchman.

> *Question from the floor:* I've been coming to these conferences for fifteen
> years, and what we hear hasn't really changed in all that time. We know
> that CBT has some success, but you're still not addressing sleep
> specifically. So, I ask myself and I want to ask you, what are we doing
> in this field?
> *From a panelist:* No one begrudges a good wine its age—if it works, it
> works.
> *From another panelist:* No, no, there are new studies that show
> efficaciousness. . . .
> *From another panelist:* You may be frustrated because the sleep system is
> left unaddressed; but science shows it's the arousal system that's the
> problem.

What *science* is he talking about? I wonder. The science I've read says that the sleep system is barely understood.

After the session is over, I make a beeline for the Frenchman, Michel Lecendreux, a physician who works with children. When he understands what I am asking, he rolls his eyes and says, "It's so depressing, really, I've been hearing this for so long."

"So, do you have success with behavioral modification in your practice?" I ask.

"Some," he says. "But what all this is, is a *coping* mechanism—they're just telling people they should cope with their problem; they're not really addressing it. Besides, there are so many different types of insomnia—they're not addressing this."

I'm glad somebody besides me feels there are more types of insomnia than these speakers allow for, and that what this approach does is manipulate rather than understand the sleep system. "Feeling sleepy is *good*," says a speaker on one of these panels. "It shows that the sleep pressure, the homeostatic drive, is building up." No, feeling sleepy is *not* good, not when you need to be awake. As someone who has spent half my life trying to stay awake and the other half trying to get to sleep, I can tell you, it's not good; in fact, it's not tolerable in the work I do.

I'll have more to say about behavioral modification in a later chapter. Here I want only to give the sense I take away from these meetings. One impression I get is that these researchers are genuinely trying to help people gain control of their insomnia without drugs; they bring considerable energy and conviction to what they're doing, and they do help a lot of people. But they're also invested in what they're doing (aren't we all?): behavioral modification is what they know how to do, what they've been trained to do. They have made careers off this approach, gained the respect of their colleagues—they get to be here, giving these talks. As one speaker said, to a question from the floor, "I make my living doing behavioral therapy—*and* I think it's highly efficacious." There's not a lot of incentive to go looking for the limits of a practice one is invested in, to launch studies that probe the weak spots—to ask, for example, what kinds of insomniacs these methods do and do not work for.

"How long does the efficacy of behavioral modification last?" comes a question from the floor.

"How long does a drug remain efficacious?" the speaker shoots back, visibly irritated. These two know one another, and the questioner works for a drug company (I later learn), my first hint that not all in this room are in perfect accord.

Pharmacological Management of Insomnia

When I get to the sessions on pharmacological approaches to insomnia, I feel the speakers are more in touch with the realities of insomniacs' lives. Rather than airbrushing the problem away, they acknowledge that insomnia makes a serious impact on quality of life and health. I want to cheer when I hear Tom Roth, a sleep researcher at Henry Ford Hospital, Detroit, say, "Today we know insomnia may not be secondary to anything. Where once we thought it was a symptom, today we see it as a disorder in its own right, with a significant impact on daily functioning." I want to give him a standing ovation when he says, "This is a chronic condition, a long-term disorder, so the idea you can use medication short-term is perplexing. Drugs are not recommended for more than twenty-eight days, but in fact many people take them for years. In the real world this is common."

The "real world" seems much closer in these sessions, the world I know, where people take drugs more or less indefinitely and where we face, every night of our lives, agonizing questions about what kind of drug to take and how much and whether we can get by with none at all. At these sessions, speakers are not so enthusiastic about behavioral modification. When asked if a certain drug is more effective when combined with cognitive behavioral therapy, one speaker replies, "I'm not convinced we have as much proof about behavioral therapy as some would argue. CBT hasn't been proven so effective. Those studies are written by psychologists; they don't demonstrate improvement in total sleep time, and in fact, with sleep restriction, total sleep time goes down." Another speaker adds, "Then, too, they're very highly selected patients: a criterion for selection is their refusal to take medication."

But I'm wondering why everyone's so keen on zaleplon, a drug that doesn't do a thing for me (zaleplon is the generic name, Sonata is the brand name). "Zaleplon is the only hypnotic that can be taken in the middle of the night, that doesn't affect recall or reaction time," I hear; "with zaleplon, you don't have to increase dosage, and there's some suggestion of improvement in nights it's not taken." Wait a minute, I think, at the evening session where these claims are being made—isn't that who's paying for dinner? I reach for my program, and sure enough, the session is underwritten by Elan, the maker of Sonata, though not a word of this connection is breathed in the session or on the program. (At subsequent conferences, these evening presentations are identified as "industry-sponsored," but in Seattle, my first conference, they are innocuously termed "Satellite

Symposia.") Quite a lavish dinner, too: succulent sirloin, an array of exquisite hors d'oeuvres, tasty dessert canapés, unlimited wine. I've never been so wined and dined at a conference.

"Drug money—ah, well, might as well enjoy it," says the young man sitting next to me, tucking into his chocolate mousse.

Another evening event is paid for by Sanofi-Synthelabo, the giant pharmaceutical company that at that time made Ambien, and at this session I hear similarly enthusiastic claims made for zolpidem (Ambien). All these sessions give Continuing Medical Education (CME) credit, which makes me uneasy. Health care professionals are required to take a certain number of hours of continuing medical education each year to keep their licenses current. In 2001, drug companies paid over 60 percent of the costs of these programs and seminars, as Marcia Angell, former editor of the *New England Journal of Medicine,* reports in *The Truth about the Drug Companies.* This means that doctors get their information about drugs from the producers of the drugs, a system that has its disadvantages: it's a bit like going to a used car salesman for advice about buying a used car, only the stakes are much higher. Ambien, at three dollars a pill, is a blockbuster, a drug that generates a billion or more a year in sales (or did until it went off patent—at its peak it generated more than $2 billion). *Patents* give drug makers exclusive marketing rights and the right to charge what they want for twenty years; when the patent expires, competitors are allowed to sell unbranded versions, or *generics,* for a fraction of the original price.

This is a different kind of "investment" than I was sensing with the nonpharmacological proponents. Many of these speakers have long "disclosure" lists, acknowledgments that they've received research support from or acted as consultants to Upjohn (Xanax), Sanofi-Synthelabo (Ambien), Cephalon (Provigil, the new wake-up drug), Pfizer, Abbott, American Cyanamid, Bristol-Myers. Researchers today routinely supplement their incomes with consulting fees, honoraria, and stock options from drug companies; they are required to disclose that they have such relations, but not to disclose *how much* they are paid. I do not mean to impugn the integrity of these speakers. Given how tight funding is, where else are researchers supposed to turn for support? And just because a study is funded by a pharmaceutical company, it's not necessarily a bad study. But there is truth to the old adage "Who pays the piper calls the tune." There is incontrovertible evidence, and lots of it, that researchers with financial ties to pharmaceutical manufacturers are more likely to report findings that support the sponsors' drugs and less likely to report risks and side effects than independents are. Drug companies wouldn't spend this kind of money if they didn't get a return.

Everyone in the medical world knows that this sort of thing goes on, and more of us who are not in that world know it too, as exposé after exposé is published (a half dozen books came out in the years I spent writing this book), and as drug after drug that has been aggressively marketed turns out to be so dangerous that it's pulled off the market. Cynicism crackles through these audiences. "Here comes the sales pitch," mutters a man sitting next to me. "I wonder how much he got paid to say *that!*" says someone else. But I hear no outrage, only resignation that this is the way things are. Nor do I find anybody who wants to talk about it. "You might talk to Dr. X," says a researcher I ask about this. "Of course, he may not want to talk to you; his research is pretty heavily dependent . . ."; and sure enough, he does not want to talk to me. (More than one researcher refused to talk to me at all about this issue or any other: "I don't speak without an honorarium," I was told, more than once.)

I become really uneasy when I hear, from a speaker with a particularly long list of disclosures, that tolerance to current drugs does not develop, that users don't have to increase the dose to get the same effect. He flashes slide after slide, refers to study after study, to support his case. Others are uneasy, too.

> *Question:* This is all wonderful data, but in contrast to being in the trenches, well—we have patients who come in and say, no matter what they're on, they say it's stopped working, and it's very difficult to get them off.
>
> *Answer:* Clinical experience is going to give you certain evidence that doesn't relate well to lab data, but it is my belief that when a person who starts on a medication finds it doesn't work—it's because they never found an effective dose. If you get them on an effective dose, they don't need to increase it.

My own experience tells me that these drugs build tolerance, and rapidly, too: within days, not weeks, I need a larger dose to produce the same effect. Two minutes on the Web tells you this is the way it works for many of us.

"Is there any reason hypnotics shouldn't be taken for life?" asks Wallace Mendelson, recently retired from the University of Chicago. "If a patient is hypertensive and you put him on beta blocker, the reaction is, isn't it wonderful we have such a drug; if an insulin receptor is deficient, you say, isn't it wonderful we have insulin. But people cry 'drug abuse' when you give a drug to an insomniac, who is perhaps a person with an altered GABA-receptor function." I perk up my ears at this: it's the only time I've heard it suggested at these sessions that insomniacs might have a neurochemical deficiency that would explain why they need these drugs. Sleep medications, or *hypnotics,* as they're called—which include benzodiazepines, such as Xanax and Restoril, and so-called nonbenzodiazepines, Sonata, Ambien, Lunesta—all work on the GABA (gamma-aminobutyric acid) receptor sites. GABA is the major braking system of the brain, the system that inhibits the firing of excitatory neurons: these drugs accentuate its action. I corner Mendelson after the session and ask, "What makes you say insomniacs have altered GABA-receptor function?"

"By inference, we know it," he says. "That's where the drugs have their effect."

"Is anybody looking at this?" I ask. He backs off a bit.

"Well, it's probably only a small subset, most insomnia is probably conditioned, a learned behavior."

"But what if this sort of dysfunction explains why one person gets conditioned to insomnia and another does not?"

"That could be," he says. "Sure, what a great idea." (Actually, it's a blindingly obvious idea; he just wants to get rid of me.)

I ask, "Is there any literature?"

He replies, "Well, there's Michael Bonnet." But I've talked to Bonnet, and I know that's not the lamppost he's groping under, to use Hauri's image for where everyone pretty much is in this enterprise.

"Nobody else?" Nobody he can think of. (Oddly enough, I later discovered that that he himself had written about this.)

Some excellent reasons not to take sleep medications for life are given by other speakers. "You take the pills enough and you develop another problem, hypnotic-dependent disorder, with daytime impairment issues, such as falls," says Kenneth Lichstein. Daniel Kripke, professor of psychiatry at the University of California, San Diego, flashes a slide of the Grim Reaper, death with his hood and scythe, to illustrate "the dark side of sleeping pills." Kripke starts out by saying, "I do not accept support or honoraria from hypnotics companies or from tort lawyers. I realized I could not offer an objective view of sleeping pills if I took money from manufacturers. I think the issue of support is important." He worked on the 1960s American Cancer Society survey that turned up the connection between cigarettes and cancer and heart disease. That study also turned up a connection between the use of hypnotics and increased mortality, as did a follow-up study done in the 1980s: those who reported taking sleeping pills thirty or more times per month had a 25 percent higher chance of dying in the six-year follow-up period than those who said they took none, which puts this habit right up there with a pack of cigarettes a day in terms of risk. (And these were huge studies, involving a million or more people, which gives them weight.) The correlation does not, Kripke cautions, prove causation; there might be some underlying condition that's increasing the mortality. But it is cause for concern. Besides, Kripke claims, sleeping pills stop working after a few weeks; people continue to take them only because they feel so bad when they stop.

The whole picture is confusing, what with some researchers saying that hypnotics build tolerance and others saying that they do not, with some implying that they're as safe and as necessary as insulin for a diabetic and others suggesting that they may be killing us. I should say here that there are sleeping pills and sleeping pills. The benzos and nonbenzos all work on the GABA neurotransmitter system, but they work on different receptor subtypes and have slightly different effects; and the nonbenzos are shorter-acting. There are also antidepressants that were not developed for sleep but which can have sedating side effects that make them useful for sleep: doxepin (Sinequan) and trazodone (Desyrel) have been around a long time, while the SSRIs (selective serotonin reuptake inhibitors, which include Prozac, Paxil, Zoloft) are newer. Most of the conference speakers are keen on the nonbenzodiazepines and down on the antidepressants, especially the older antidepressants, and yet when I ask a doctor at my HMO for something to help me sleep, I'm always offered trazodone, the drug most frequently prescribed for insomnia in the United States today. (I'll try to make sense of this picture in the chapter on drugs.)

And there are no long-term studies to support any one of these drugs over any others. There are, as Kripke points out, a hundred million benzo prescriptions written yearly in the United States, and yet there are no long-term studies. "If people are going to be taking these drugs for years," says Kripke, "we need large long-term studies—these should be high priority. You can see why the drug companies don't want to do such studies, because they know that the drugs build tolerance, and there are concerns with addiction that might open them to litigation. But *why* hasn't the NIH looked into them? The lack of government curiosity about them is extraordinary—these are controlled substances, with a high potential for abuse."

I am torn so many ways, listening to these discussions. I am, as I sit here, experiencing a massive drug hangover myself, but I wouldn't be here at all if it weren't for these drugs they're talking about. I wouldn't, for that matter, be functional enough to keep a full-time job. I'd have long ago taken early retirement, assuming I'd have even got tenure in the first place. But I don't want to hear how bad these drugs are for me—I know they are—and I want even less to hear hype about them. What I would like to learn from these meetings is something about the neurobiological, neurochemical, neuroanatomic, and genetic underpinnings of insomnia. Are our GABA systems underactive? Are our hypocretin or histamine systems overactive? Or what?

Controversial and Unresolved?

Late from a breakfast meeting, I dash to an 8 A.M. session, "Controversial and Unresolved Issues in the Treatment of Insomnia." I have high hopes for this session, for there are many controversial and unresolved issues I'd like to hear discussed. There's a line outside the room; I elbow my way in, braving dirty looks, thinking, whoever did the room assignments sure underestimated interest in this subject. I lean against the wall and concentrate on not passing out.

Charles Morin, who is chairing this session, is a nice-looking young man with a Quebec French accent. He strikes me as high-minded and principled: "Do we want to do research to enlarge the clinical field, or to make money?" he shoots back to a question. But the session fizzles into the minutiae of treatments and ways of measuring their effectiveness. Not much "controversy" here: there's hardly even any disagreement. It's a small world, this world of insomnia researchers, disproportionately small for the enormity of the problem. They all seem to know each other, to have known each other a long time. They strike me as too young to be old boys, but what I'm seeing here looks like old boy networks, the bantering, the schmoozing: "Great study," "Really exciting" (this to a talk that inspired no questions). I see that it works in this world pretty much the way it works in the world I used to be a part of: you need to get along, need the good will of others to be invited to speak at conferences, to review books and articles, to have your papers accepted for publication, to get grant proposals funded. In the audience, there may be someone who decides whether your work goes on. In the audience is almost certainly a competitor for your next grant. Image is important. Success is important. There's more than a little public relations gloss in many of these presentations.

The most interesting thing said at this session is by Daniel Buysse of the Department of Psychiatry, University of Pittsburgh School of Medicine: "We need to talk about the explosion of knowledge in neurobiology. There's a whole world out there, there are new findings about hypocretin, about the hypothalamic system—it's a big mistake to ignore it." (Buysse is a psychiatrist—"the only MD on the panel," as he pointedly remarks—who comments provocatively, "Psychology is just biology and physiology we don't understand yet; it's just neurology we haven't found the pathways for.") But that's the last I hear of neurobiology at this session.

I am about to faint, what with the sleep deprivation and an unfortunate mixture of drugs coursing through my system, and with terminal boredom, when they start up with the DBAS and the SH and the SR again. People begin to leave and I find a seat. I plop down next to a guy who is sighing loudly; I roll my eyes at him, he rolls his eyes back. He mutters, "That's not how it works, that's not how it is, it's not like that at all—it's a problem like diabetes." I encourage him to go on, and he says, under his breath, "These guys are all PhDs, they were all brought up on Freud, but you have to unlearn traditional psychotherapy, you have to think outside the DSM box—the whole problem is the DSM, it took us in the wrong direction, it generated a major problem conceptualizing insomnia. The only guy who made sense on this panel is Buysse. There was a *Wall Street Journal* article a few years ago that said the psychotherapist who doesn't learn neurobiology in the twenty-first century should be called a social worker."

After the session, we continue to talk. A.L. has a clinic in the southwest which has, he told me, a very good success rate and a waiting list. "Fifteen years ago, when I was just starting out, I just assumed, like everyone else, insomniacs are all crazy, so I hired a psychologist to deal with them. Well, that didn't do a thing, so I asked, *Why?* and began reading neurology and began unlearning most everything I'd been taught. Insomnia is a neurobiological problem to which a person is genetically predisposed, a problem of neurotransmitters and hormones—and I don't just mean estrogen and progesterone, but growth hormone and the hypothalamic-pituitary-adrenal system. Getting hold of it is neurotransmitter management. You can do this with current drugs—and I don't mean benzos, they're horrible, there's amnesia capacity, people get addicted." He claims success with low-dose doxepin, an idea he got from a poster at a conference years ago, a study by Wallace Mendelson. "Hardly anybody's studying the older antidepressants—once a drug goes off patent, it doesn't yield the profits anymore, so nobody's interested. But I've had success with a dose so low that you wouldn't think it would have any effect; yet it does."

I am fascinated, and I urge him to go on. "Yeah," he says, "but I can't get anyone to listen. I come to these meetings, and I can't find any data that suggests I'm wrong, but when you treat in a nonstandard fashion, there's not a lot of welcome for it. There's an entrenched conservatism in health science. But there's new data coming out all the time, better technologies for looking at the brain. This is a good time for you to be writing," he says encouragingly. "There's a lot coming out. There wasn't for a long time, but there is now."

Later that same conference, I hear other interesting ideas. I talk to a Canadian physician who similarly complains that the people working with insomnia are psychologists who don't understand the biomedical underpinnings of the problem. He thinks that some insomnia may be a mild form of bipolar depression, *subclinical,* that is, not fully manifested. "Insomnia comes on around fourteen, which is when bipolar comes on. If you look at family histories, which Americans do not, you'll find insomnia and suicide and drug abuse in the families of most insomniacs. Bipolar is one of the most inheritable of disorders: if you have a parent who's bipolar, you have about a 30 percent chance of inheriting it." Bipolar is what used to be called manic depression, wild mood swings between highs and lows. This doctor associates the hyperarousal that researchers find in insomniacs with the manic stage (which might explain the mysterious fluctuations some insomniacs experience, when their insomnia gets worse for no apparent reason—some insomniacs, that is; for many of us, insomnia is pretty constant). He treats insomnia with antiepileptic and mood-stabilizing drugs, valproate, lamotrigine, topiramate, nothing I'd want to go near. But the idea is kind of fascinating. It strikes me that a wealth of information is being missed because nobody's asking insomniacs about family histories—and that information may also be missed because doctors and clinicians aren't being asked what they know.

"Why don't you present this theory at one of these conferences?" I ask.

"That would be scientifically irresponsible," he huffs. "I haven't done the studies, I don't have the data. There are a lot of quacks in this field—and there's a 40 percent response to placebo."

"Well, why couldn't there be a panel about things doctors have found that worked? What's wrong with some speculation?" He is not interested.

The more I think about it, the more I realize how little of the speculative or theoretical there is in these presentations. Apart from that passing reference to GABA dysfunction, I hear hardly any speculation about what might be wrong with the sleep-wake mechanisms of insomniacs. A well-known sleep researcher I talked to told me that the proposal he submitted to this conference had been turned down on the grounds that it was "only theoretical."

Why should the speculative be ruled out like this? And where are the sessions on the neurobiology, the neuroendocrinology, the genetics of insomnia? I think, thumbing through my program for the dozenth time. Who is trying to understand insomnia—not just manage it, but understand it? "Most insomnia researchers are doing the behavioral stuff as opposed to trying to find the physiology," as Michael Bonnet told me. "The rest of the research is pharmaceutical. The behaviorist consensus blocks research on one side and the pharmaceutical research blocks it on the other. Almost nobody's looking for the cause."

Still Searching . . .

The poster sessions are the lifeblood of these conferences. These are studies in progress, open for critique, posted on—yes, posters. The setup is engagingly funky, like a junior high school science fair: the posters are fastened with pushpins on corkboards propped up by metal stands that I keep tripping over as I try to read and walk. Bulletin boards line up in rows, facing one another. Through the narrow passage between them swarms a crowd.

There's a vitality at these sessions, the sense that things are being discovered. I hear accents and read nametags from Brazil, Chile, Australia, Poland, Germany, France, Sweden, Japan, Russia, the United Kingdom. All around me, the buzz and hum of conversation—"Elegant study," "Excellent methodology," "Very nicely done," "What did you find when you doubled the dose of . . . ?" "Did you find that the New Zealand mouse was the best model for . . . ?" *Elegant* is the term of highest praise, and I see what is meant by it, not the cut of a skirt or the turn of a phrase but an exactitude that controls for complex variables, that does a delicate balancing act, keeping all these balls in the air, then bringing them down, one by one, with a finely tuned, carefully sequenced precision, each piece fitting into place. There are a lot of very impressive people walking around. The variety is staggering: researchers who are working on guinea pigs, fruit flies, cats, rats, mice mingle with psychologists and geriatricians and epidemiologists and representatives of pharmaceutical companies. Huddled around one speaker is a group of sleep technicians interested in CPAP (*continuous positive airway pressure*, the machine used to force air through the upper airways in apnea). Around another speaker is a group animatedly discussing the "Co-localization of G-Aminobutyric Acid and Acetylcholine in the Somas of Neurons in the Latero-Dorsal and Pedunculo-Pontine Tegmental Nuclei in the Cat."

The program says that authors of posters with odd numbers will be there between 1:30 and 2:15, and authors of posters with even numbers will be there between 2:15 and 3, and, based on this information, I chart a course through the maze. But in fact it's not nearly so well organized. Some authors are standing by their posters, some are not; it's catch as catch can. Sometimes the crush of people forces me to move on before I can take in what I'm reading or formulate a question; sometimes the author's so surrounded that I can't find a way of breaking in. Some posters are swarmed, others have a wide berth around them and the author stands looking forlorn. I feel bad, I would ask a question if I could, but "Neostigmine-Induced REM Sleep Enhancement in C57BL/6J (B6) Mouse Is Concentration-Dependent and Blocked by Atropine" strikes me dumb.

There are many titles that give me only the barest inkling of what's at stake, though I have a sense that it's important: "Serotonin Modulation Reveals Two Types of GABAergic Sleep Promoting Neurons in the Ventrolateral Preoptic Nucleus (VLPO)"; "Actions of Both Orexin A and Orexin B in the Myenteric Plexus of the Guinea-Pig Small Intestine"—this from Tokyo. Hypocretin (orexin) is getting a lot of attention. The discovery of this arousal system that's defective in narcoleptics is turning out to have relevance way beyond narcolepsy.

But what of the insomnia posters? There are nine hundred posters at the 2003 Chicago conference, a particularly exciting conference, since 2003 was the fiftieth anniversary of the discovery of REM—but only seventy-eight are on insomnia, though insomnia is the sleep disorder that affects more people than all the others combined. Most of the insomnia studies are about behavioral modification and drugs, or about methods of measuring sleep or assessing methods of measuring sleep: "a new ambulatory tool for insomnia evaluation"; "an evaluation of CPAP therapy." There are studies of the efficacy of this drug over that, of whether CBT is more or less effective combined with this drug or that. Some of these studies seem amazingly obvious. Insomniacs have "significantly lower rating in alertness and mood." Well, yeah. "Sleep and Daytime Consequences in Partners of Patients with Obstructive Sleep Apnea"—people who sleep with people who snore have difficulty sleeping and staying awake the next day. Maybe the terminology for this disorder is even looser than I thought, but I wouldn't have said someone kept awake by someone else's snoring was an insomniac.

When you see this sort of thing placed side by side with sophisticated attempts to understand the sleep-wake system, you see what Buysse meant: there is a world of neurobiology out there that insomnia researchers might do well to heed.

On the third day of the Seattle conference, I haul myself out of bed for a 6 A.M. meeting of the American Insomnia Association Committee, which I'd seen a brief mention of in the program. I find room 424 in the Sheraton, where there's a sign that says, "American Insomnia Association Committee, June 12, 6 A.M." There's not a soul in sight. I do a reality check. Yes, this is June 12, yes, this is 6 A.M., yes, this is room 424, and yes, I am in the Sheraton. I go down to the front desk, where there's a schedule for the day, but there's no mention of it; I go over to convention headquarters, but it's not open yet. I find a worker who has a copy of the master schedule, but he finds no mention of it. "Maybe they all slept in," he cracks. Then, to my pained expression, he says, "Well, I'm sorry, I can't help you—it's just nowhere."

No, not *nowhere*, I wouldn't go so far as to say that, but neither does it seem to be anywhere. The entire field of insomnia research is squeezed down into this narrow funnel of behavioral modification and drugs, and a very limited selection of drugs, at that, most of them working on the same GABA system. There is next to nothing at any of the conferences I attend about diet or nutrition. "It's surprising how little is known in the area of vitamins and minerals," wrote Ernest Hartmann, director of the Sleep Clinic at Boston State Hospital, in 1978; it's as true today. And though millions of people make use of alternative approaches to insomnia, I hear only one paper that partly addresses alternative treatments, where I learn that valerian, hops, and chamomile may have small benefits after a few weeks, and that they, like the benzos and nonbenzos, work on the GABA system.

And there are other approaches that are pushed to the margins. A question comes from the audience to a panel of insomnia researchers: "Some years ago Peter Hauri presented some fascinating results from a study on biofeedback—was anything ever done with that?" The speakers all look around at each other to see if anyone has a response, and finally one replies, "No, I don't think so. Biofeedback takes thirty to ninety sessions—that's quite an investment." The question refers to a 1981 study by Hauri that found that insomniacs with muscle tension responded to one kind of biofeedback and insomniacs prone to rumination responded to another kind, a finding that pointed to crucial differences among insomniacs. But distinctions of this sort aren't being made at these conferences: the treatments offered us are one-size-fits-all, and anything that's too time-consuming or labor-intensive, even if it's shown to be effective, falls by the way. If it can't be packaged, tied up in a tidy cost-effective bundle, there's no time, no room. I feel like Alice in Wonderland at the Mad Hatter's tea party: no room, no time, move down.

I hear acknowledgment that there are things not known about insomnia, but that's not what the speakers dwell on. I guess nobody wants to draw attention to what they don't know. Nobody likes problems they can't solve—and in fact researchers can't *afford* problems they can't solve, since they need results in order to get the next grant. Every researcher I talk to complains about the drain of constantly applying for grants. Emmanuel Mignot estimates that younger researchers spend as much as 40 percent of their time writing grant applications. U.C. Davis sleep researcher Irwin Feinberg tells me, "No sooner do you get a grant than you have to worry about where the next grant is coming from." "To be a working scientist," says medical anthropologist T. M. Luhrmann, "you must be funded. Not only must you be funded once, but you must work on projects that can be reliably funded year after year until you retire. . . . Most scientists, then, cannot indulge themselves in good but speculative ideas. The peer review system that awards the grants tends to be conservative, and speculative projects often fail."

So the funding system fosters caution. No wonder that, as Bonnet told me, early on in this book project, "insomnia research has been stalemated for ten, no, twenty years."

I go to every "meet the professor" session I can fit in, looking for someone who has what Evelyn Fox Keller calls "a feeling for the organism." These are breakfast and lunch meetings, fifty dollars a plate, where we sit around tables of eight to ten to hear an expert talk about some aspect of sleep, "Women and Sleep," "Sleep and Genes," and so on. In the ten minutes or so we're given to eat, before the speaker begins, I swing into my heartiest let's-get-this-group-talking mode and ask, "So, where are you from, and what do you do?" I want to know what drew them to this field.

Here's what I hear:

"Because there was an opening and I needed a job."
"Because my husband was director of the sleep lab."
"Because I wanted to do obstetrics but I didn't like the hours.
    There's less burnout in sleep."
"Because I'm in pulmonary and that's where the field was going."

(There are quite a few in pulmonary, and most of them, not surprisingly,
are more interested in apnea than in insomnia.)

"Because I fell in love with sleep."
"Because I'm fascinated by sleep and everything about it."
"Because you can make an improvement in peoples' lives with
    procedures that aren't invasive."

I talk to people who radiate concern when I tell them I'm insomniac, and
rush in with advice (which makes me feel awkward, since I'm here not
as a patient, seeking therapy or sympathy, but as a researcher, seeking
information—which makes *them* the "subjects," not me). But my sense
is that most people go into this field for the reasons people go into any
field—"by chance, like everybody else," as one says.

At a breakfast meeting with about twenty-five people in attendance, the
speaker asks, "How many of you believe problems with sleep cause depression?" Four hands shoot up, one of them mine. I am dumbfounded:
in a group of two dozen people who treat insomnia, only three think insomnia makes you depressed? Have they never had a bad night's sleep
themselves? But they've been told depression causes insomnia; they
haven't been told insomnia may cause depression: therefore, they do not
believe that it does. (Again, I'm not talking about major depression, which
is a whole other issue.) The speaker then tells them that studies have been
finding that insomnia can be a risk factor for depression, and they write
it down. I guess now that they believe it, they'll see it.

I look around and I think well, maybe they never did have a bad
night's sleep. They look fine, they're not in crisis, while I am barely holding it together. A 7 A.M. breakfast when I'm in Philadelphia is 4 A.M.
California time, an hour I often see, but not at the beginning of the day.
An odiferous plate of bacon and fried bread is plunked down in front of
me, and my stomach shrinks; as I watch my tablemates ladle on syrup
and butter and tuck in, I think, maybe we really *are* different species.

At this same breakfast meeting, the speaker tells us, "If they're sleepy, they probably don't have primary psychophysiological insomnia. If they're sleepy, they have fatigue and listlessness, and that means depression, and you should treat it with an antidepressant." I see people writing this down, and I want to shout, "Wait, that's not true!" Some of us do get sleepy (I for one could happily curl up under the table at this moment); and some of us get sleepy sometimes but not other times. It is true that when insomniacs are tested for sleepiness, they're often surprisingly alert; they tend not to fall asleep easily the next day, or even the next night— but you can't conclude, as this speaker does, that "anyone who is sleepy has fatigue, low energy, lethargy and wants to sleep to escape their lives." There are insomniacs and insomniacs, and even one and the same insomniac is not always, well, one and the same. Distinctions are being shaved off here, lost sight of, lost completely. All cats are gray in the dark, as the adage goes, and, as Hauri's parable of the man under the lamppost says, the dark is where we are.

Later the same day, I plotz down on a bench, trying to summon the energy to get myself to the exhibits. My feet have gone numb and the strap of my computer case is severing my arm from my shoulder. I'm too old for this, I think, relieved to find a place to sit.

There's a fresh-faced young woman sitting alone, and we begin to chat. I am very glad to have someone to talk to, and I tell her as much. "Oh, this is a hard conference," she says, "very unfriendly. I've been coming a few years, and I thought I'd know someone. But you're the first person who's spoken to me." Katie is a psychologist who does family practice in Southern California. I ask her what she thinks causes insomnia. She says she thinks insomnia reflects relationship issues. "Problems arise," says Katie, "when there's a mismatch: what matters is how well the parent and child mesh, which determines if the child feels accepted. If the mother perceives the child as difficult, there's a problem." She believes there are fewer problems in cultures where children sleep with parents; issues arise, she says, when the child is sent off to sleep alone in the dark. "When my daughter was having trouble sleeping, I took her into bed with me and nursed her when she cried—and the problem went away. Much of what parents see as a behavioral problem is simply behavior that's not convenient."

I tell her about the cache of letters I found in an old steamer trunk after my father died, letters my mother wrote him while he was overseas during World War II and I was an infant. "She kept saying how hard it was to get me to sleep, how she'd come in hours after putting me down and I'd still be wide awake. 'It must be your energy she has, because it's not mine,' she wrote in one."

"Sounds like a mismatch to me," says Katie. "Maybe her response turned your energy into hyperreactivity." I file this away, to think about later. I resolve to sit down and read these letters all the way through. There are things I need to know.

I realize that this is the first time I've heard this kind of talk at these conferences. The psychological approaches I've been hearing about are almost entirely behavioral, about conditioning and DBAS, as though everybody's given up on the kind of psychotherapy where you try to get to the root of a problem and talk it through. I'm actually more at home with Katie's language, which makes some attempt to differentiate us as individuals, than with the talk I've been hearing, which treats us all like Pavlov's dogs. Yet behavioral modification has been shown to be more effective with insomnia than "talk therapy"; also, it pathologizes us less, calling us "dysfunctional" rather than "psychopathological"—though it still posits worry and upset as the source of the problem.

Exhibits

After I've rested my aching feet, I decide it's time to get myself to the exhibition hall, which, in my zomboid state, is totally trippy. "Win a Teddy Bear," it says at one booth. "It's midnight. Do you know what your mice are doing?" Sales representatives flash me toothy smiles and catch my eye as I wander by, which is startling after days when nobody's met my eyes or cracked a smile. It's carnivalesque, hawkers at booths giving away free T-shirts, mugs, umbrellas, ballpoint pens. Dishes filled with chocolate candies invite me to stop by and chat.

There are booths for light boxes, diagnostic equipment, sleep scoring systems, software programs, systems for data management and networking, devices to measure breathing problems and keep upper airways open. Blond-haired, blue-eyed models mill around, plastic tubing wound around their necks and stuck up their noses; people wear CPAP masks that make them look like Darth Vader. Someone is walking around in what looks like a wet suit cross-hatched by plastic tubing, monitoring devices stuck to it like barnacles. On a counter, a rubber leg sits twitching. A restless leg, I presume.

There's money to be made in sleep disorders, that's clear. We millions of sufferers are a marketer's dream.

Ambien has a very posh display, a sort of carpeted arbor, deep, plush couches I have a hard time resisting, but I know if I sit down I will never get up, so I stand talking with a sales rep who hands me a glossy brochure and boasts, "We have 64 percent of the market." Yeah, I know, I'm part of your market, and I am at this moment massively hungover from your product (my fault—I should never have taken seven milligrams at 3:30 . . .).

But it's the Sonata booth that is truly over the top, a "virtual" 3-D theater. A generically pretty blond hands me a pair of 3-D glasses and leads me into a sort of horse trailer, only bigger; the door shuts behind me, and I'm locked into the virtual theater. "A day in the life of an insomniac," flashes on the screen. "Uh, oh," I think, "this might cut too close to the bone," not sure I can deal with more of what I've been going through all morning: wavy lines, uncertain depth perception, mind basically nonfunctional though I'm walking around. But no, this "day in the life of an insomniac" is nothing like my own. It begins, "This is Tom, who tosses and turns for hours"—on the screen is a picture of Tom, tossing and turning—then, "This is Kathy, who has chronic insomnia"—picture of Kathy, having chronic insomnia—"and here's Doug, who takes a drug for an anxiety disorder, but still can't sleep"— picture of Doug, etcetera. "Which would you like to discuss? Push the button on the panel in front of you." My hand gropes around in the dark, can't find the panel, *buzz* goes the buzzer. "Time's up," chirps the voice. "We're discussing Tom." Tom, we are told, has transient insomnia— "better treat it or it might become chronic; untreated insomnia may lead to auto accidents or depression." Then there's an image hovering midair, like in those 3-D horror movies I remember from when I was a kid, except that these are not screaming skulls but graphs and charts. Then a scientist in a white coat appears on the screen, come to tell us what it all means—oops, it's the speaker from last night's dinner, talking about Sonata again.

As I leave, the generic blond hands me a sleep mask and a pair of earplugs in a velveteen sack marked "Sonata" and a sheet with six questions to ask patients—"We hope this helps you identify insomnia." Christ, I think, these people must think doctors are idiots. I add the sleep mask and earplugs to the rest of my booty. By now, I have four pens, two umbrellas, two flashlights, a mug, and several notepads, all with drug company logos, all stuffed into the canvas bag handed out at registration, which has a drug company logo on it, too. Cute, I think, except that this nonsense is why Ambien costs $3 a pop. Your drug dollars at work.

There are booths for the Restless Legs Syndrome Foundation and the Narcolepsy Network. I stop by the RLS Foundation and learn that it was begun in the late 1980s by a group of eight people with RLS, all of them quite elderly. It now has 120,000 members, eighty-five support groups, and representatives that work with NIH. I have a long talk with a woman from the Narcolepsy Network, another advocacy group that came from humble beginnings. Begun in the mid-1980s by three or four women, it now boasts more than 1,200 members, including families, physicians, and researchers. It maintains dozens of patient support groups, distributes a quarterly newsletter, hosts a Website, participates in clinical trials, and advises members about disability laws and other matters. There's a feeling of optimism at both these booths, a sense that things are moving—and they are, and these groups are part of the reason why (as we'll see).

Everybody I talk to thinks a patient advocacy group for insomniacs is a terrific idea. The woman at the Narcolepsy Network suggests I go talk to the National Center for Sleep Disorders, the sleep center at NIH. I walk across to their booth and ask the guy sitting there what he thinks of an insomnia advocacy group.

"Great idea," he says. "Why don't you talk to the people at the Narcolepsy Network?"

"But they—that is, they're the ones who sent me over here."

Why do I get the feeling that nobody wants to deal with us?

There Is Nothing Like Sleep...

"Tell them to restrict sleep," say the behavioral modification people. "Restrict sleep, restrict time in bed." "Tell them they don't need as much sleep as they think they need." But when I go to the sleep-deprivation sessions, I hear that sleep deprivation does worse things than anyone imagined. When I wander into these sessions from the behavioral modification sessions, I feel like I've stepped into another conference. The talk here is not about self-soothing skills and coping mechanisms, but hormones, peptides, cytokines, neuroimaging. There's a buzz of excitement, the sense that things are being discovered, though what is being discovered is as alarming as it is fascinating.

David Dinges is a portly dynamo of a man who has done extensive work on sleep deprivation and whose enthusiasm is irresistible. He and his colleagues at the University of Pennsylvania have been studying partial sleep deprivation—*partial,* the kind most people experience, as opposed to *total,* which is the kind that's been mainly looked at. "I have spent twenty-seven years of my life sleep-depriving people, hundreds and hundreds of them," says Dinges, drawing a laugh from the audience; "I've taken away 24,924 hours of sleep time." He talks about how difficult it's been to get sleep loss taken seriously, how deeply entrenched the tough-it-out attitude is, how stubbornly the myth has persisted that we don't actually need sleep, how "the lack of understanding about the function of sleep led to the popular view that sleep was unwanted and useless." He and British sleep researcher James Horne have locked horns on this issue, as it were, had some very lively debates. Horne says that we need no more than five hours' sleep a night, that what sleep loss affects is mainly motivation; people are still basically functional, they just need to try harder. Not so, says Dinges: "People only appear to be functional because they're in social situations, interacting with others, but if you remove the props, leave them alone, put them behind the wheel, they become dangerous. They take longer to react and their reactions become unreliable: even when they think they've adjusted to sleepiness, there are severe cognitive impairments. There are lapses in attention, microsleeps, involuntary sleep attacks. A four-second lapse is all you need to drift out of lane."

"There is some cognitive price for any amount of sleep you reduce," says Dinges; "there are neurobehavioral deficits, and the more sleep you lose, the more impaired you are. Learning and acquisition of new information is reduced, problem solving erodes . . . alertness, energy, and vigor decrease, confusion increases and motivation declines." Sleep loss affects any activity that calls for sustained attention, and since attention is fundamental to all cognitive performance, sleep loss affects all cognitive performance. And Dinges has found that people do not adjust, cannot overcompensate, no matter how motivated they are. "Sleepiness is relentless," he says, "no matter how cleverly humans disguise the impairment. . . . The sleep system is monumentally resistant to tampering with. You need what you need, and it's more than five hours' sleep for benefit, more than six for further benefit: with eight hours you get better at a task, with six you hold your own, with four you actually get worse."

Dinges and his colleagues have found individual differences in the way people respond to sleep deprivation, "by an order of magnitude" (meaning, *huge*). Hans Van Dongen, one of Dinges's colleagues, reports, "Some people are resilient, and some are vulnerable. You bring them in again and they show the same thing, and the next time you bring them in they show the same thing again. If you're vulnerable, you're vulnerable." The difference is so replicable that these researchers are talking about it as a *trait,* a quality that's inborn and lifelong, like height or eye color (as opposed to a *state,* which is transient and changing in response to environmental influences). "We haven't a clue what makes the difference," says Dinges, "but since it's traitlike, it may be something in the genes."

I ask "the woman question"—I ask the woman question whenever I get the chance—"Did you find any differences between the way men and women respond to sleep loss?" A long pause, then one of the other speakers on Dinges's panel responds, "These studies are very expensive; the least problematic subjects are young, healthy men—so that's who we look at." Dinges says, "We haven't looked at it systematically, but it seems that as far as *performance* is affected, men and women are comparable, though women do rate themselves as *feeling* more fatigued for longer after sleep loss." This point flies by, nobody seems much interested in it, but I file it away, to think about later: it could be important that women experience sleep loss more extremely than men do. Dinges adds another revealing bit of information: "We have difficulty getting women to stay in the lab for twenty-five days—they don't seem to have that kind of discretionary time." Aha, so it's not only that women are more difficult to study—it's that they have less *time* to be studied.

So much for the effects of sleep deprivation on the brain. What does it do to the body?

I hear several talks by Eve Van Cauter and Karine Spiegel, the University of Chicago researchers who, together with Rachel Leproult, did the landmark study discussed earlier, which subjected young, healthy men to four hours of sleep a night for six nights and produced in them the hormonal profiles of much older people. (They are impressive women—mostly women researchers on their team—Belgian, with interestingly accented English, dynamic speakers, formidably self-possessed, they never miss a beat—and wouldn't you know it, it took women to notice that hormones play a part in the story.) Their sleep-deprived subjects had elevated levels of cortisol and decreased levels of growth hormone. Growth hormone, as we saw, is necessary to cell repair and the restoration of tissue. Lose it, and you lose muscle and build fat, especially around the abdomen (which is more of a problem for men than for women, actually, since men past the age of thirty get all their growth hormone from one big pulse that occurs during deep sleep, and they lose most of their deep sleep as they age, whereas women have spurts of growth

hormone dispersed throughout the twenty-four-hour cycle). These researchers produced, after only six nights of reduced sleep, signs of insulin
resistance in young, healthy subjects. They then looked at people who restrict their sleep voluntarily over months and even years, to see how they
adapt, comparing young, healthy men who regularly slept less than six
and a half hours a night to those who slept an hour or two longer—and
they found signs of insulin resistance in short sleepers, too. "It would
seem that they do not adapt," reports Spiegel; "These young, healthy
subjects were, by curtailing their sleep, making themselves insulin
resistant."

Insulin resistance is a feature of *adult-onset diabetes,* a type of diabetes
not usually seen until age forty or older, where the fat cells, overtaxed by
too much eating and too much insulin signal, become unresponsive to insulin. In the decade since 1996, there's been an 80 percent increase in
Americans with diabetes, most of it, adult-onset. Figures from the Centers for Disease Control say that nearly 21 million Americans are diabetic and another 41 million have elevated blood sugar that could reach
diabetic level. One in three children born in the United States in 2000 will
develop "adult onset" diabetes, so many that, in 1997, the American Diabetes Association and the World Health Organization recommended
changing the name to "type 2 diabetes." Adult-onset diabetes is different from *childhood-onset diabetes,* an autoimmune disorder that destroys the insulin-releasing parts of the pancreas. But both types involve
high blood sugar, unabsorbed glucose and fatty acids that accumulate in
the bloodstream and get into places they don't belong, gumming up arteries, damaging kidneys and eyes, increasing the risk of cardiovascular
problems—and promoting weight gain.

Diabetes and weight gain loom as enormous health crises in the world
today, and researchers see both as related to the reduction of hours that
we sleep. In the last half of the last century, the incidence of obesity
nearly doubled (deaths due to obesity may soon overtake tobacco as the
leading preventable cause of death); and in the last century, average sleep
duration in the United States decreased by two hours.

Van Cauter calls sleep deprivation "the royal route to obesity." Insulin resistance moves us down this route, reduced levels of growth hormone push us along, but what really speeds us there is that sleep deprivation lowers levels of *leptin,* a hormone that signals the body when it
has had enough to eat, and raises levels of *ghrelin,* a substance that stimulates us to eat more. Subjects who slept four hours a night for two days
had an 18 percent decrease in leptin levels, a drop that signals the brain

that there's been a reduction of caloric intake comparable to being underfed by nine hundred calories a day for three days. "The body is screaming famine in the midst of plenty," says Van Cauter. And maybe it makes sense, as Spiegel says, since "if animals are in a situation of having to stay awake, it means there's something really wrong; there may be a need to increase food to remain stronger." These researchers also found a 28 percent increase in levels of ghrelin, the substance secreted by the stomach in anticipation of a meal. "Young, healthy subjects rated their hunger significantly higher, and they wanted junk—sweet foods, salty foods, foods high in fats, carbohydrates, and calories," says Van Cauter. "Subjects who had the most disrupted levels of leptin and ghrelin were the ones who felt the hungriest. Their appetite for cakes, candy, ice cream, potato chips, pasta, and bread increased, though their appetite for fruits, vegetables, and high-protein nutrients did not. We don't know why food choice would shift, but since the brain is fueled by glucose, we suspect it seeks simple carbohydrates when distressed by lack of sleep." The upshot of all this is that—as Van Cauter says—"trying to lose weight while being in a sleep-deprived state is like Rollerblading uphill."

Researchers are also finding that sleep deprivation, even partial sleep deprivation, undermines immune resistance. Spiegel found that subjects whose sleep had been restricted to four hours a night for six nights had, when immunized against influenza, less than half the immune response of those who had slept well. "If you get flu shots, get sleep first, or you won't get as much immunization," reports Van Cauter. One study found that those who got a good night's sleep after being vaccinated against hepatitis A showed *twice* the immune response after four weeks time than subjects who'd stayed awake on that night.

The sleep-deprived have fewer *natural killer cells* (NK), white blood cells that are a crucial line of defense against infections and cancer. When a virus or bacteria enters the body, natural killer cells rush to the affected area to destroy or inactivate the intruding organism and repair the damaged tissue. Even modest sleep loss—only one night of sleep deprivation, between 3 and 7 A.M.—results in a 30 percent reduction of NK cell activity. Sleep loss not only lowers the level of white blood cells, but raises levels of *cytokines*, proteins that appear when the organism is under threat. (Cytokines include *interleukin-1, interleukin-6 [Il-6],* and *tumor necrosis factor.*) These are a necessary response to challenge in that they activate immune responses, but when they hang around the system, they assail the body's tissues. These so-called *inflammatory markers* can become a source of inflammation associated with problems as diverse as heart disease, stroke, diabetes, arthritis, gum disease, cancer, allergies, and autoimmune conditions; some researchers think they may even be associated with the buildup of plaque found in Alzheimer's. Levels of cytokines go up in the natural course of aging, as the immune system loses the ability to regulate itself, but even one night of disrupted sleep leaves Il-6 elevated the next day. Inflammatory markers may also account for the pain and bodily discomfort that sleep loss produces. Subjects whose sleep was restricted to four hours a night for ten days reported more headache, backache, stomach pain, and generalized body pain; researchers cited their elevated Il-6 levels to explain the physical discomfort.

Inflammatory markers, especially *C-reactive protein (CRP)*, are associated with heart attack. CRP is as powerful a predictor of heart attack and stroke as cholesterol levels. Levels are low in the young and healthy, but rise with age, obesity, diabetes, smoking, a sedentary life—and sleep loss. This may explain the strong association between poor sleep or short sleep and increased cardiovascular risk that epidemiological studies have been turning up: sleep deprivation activates the inflammatory response and inflammation raises cardiovascular risk.

Sleep-deprived is not a condition you want to be in for very long.

What's an Insomniac to Do?

So what message should I take from these conferences? I hear from the behavioral modification people, "Restrict sleep, restrict sleep," "A little sleep loss won't hurt you," "You don't need as much sleep as you think you do." Of course, they're not suggesting that we starve ourselves of sleep forever, but they are telling us to go through a period of drastic sleep reduction for however long it takes to consolidate sleep, without regard for our age, gender, or state of health, and then, once our sleep has been consolidated, to keep sleep on the short side. Meanwhile, the researchers who study sleep deprivation are finding that even one night of restricted sleep may compromise the immune system, that less than a week of it creates insulin resistance and metabolic dysregulation, that short sleep may be putting us at higher risk of heart attack, diabetes, and disease.

What to think?

My body says, go with the sleep-deprivation people. My body tells me things are not right when I lose sleep, and they're not-right all the way through: my heart's working overtime, I'm metabolically deranged, cold all the time, hollow at the core. I eat like I'm stoking a dying fire, not for the pleasure but the energy, and my mood hits the wall. (There's not much discussion at these conferences about what sleep deprivation does to mood. Maybe it's not supposed to matter. It matters to me.) My body makes no bones about it, tells me loud and clear how much sleep it needs: seven hours is great, six is okay, five sucks; with three, I can stumble through a day, but with less than three, life's not worth living; and after a few days of being starved for sleep, if I get on a plane or swim too long I get a cold. My body needles me with a whole host of ailments—arthritis, gum disease, autoimmune problems (Hashimoto's, persistent rashes, allergies)—that make me suspect some inflammatory responses have gone awry. My body tells me that Dinges is correct: "You can't cheat the system": there is "something that neurologically keeps track. . . . There's nothing like sleep, normal, healthy sleep. You get a tremendous benefit from sleep." It tells me Hobson is correct: "Sleep is the body's own best state of defense."

And where are the insomniacs in these discussions? What do *we* have to say about where we think the problem comes from, which treatment works best, what other treatments might help? We are as invisible, as voiceless, at these conferences as we are in the world outside. "Do you think there might be something to learn by talking to insomniacs?" I ask a researcher standing by a poster. "Oh, that's another kind of research. You won't find that here."

*

But in the years since my first conference, in 2002, there are signs of change. In 2005, Donna Arand, Michael Bonnet's coauthor (and wife), invited me to be on the board of the American Insomnia Association, the organization I wandered around in search of that morning in Seattle. She and Bonnet are looking for patient input into this organization—which is a step in the right direction.

The scene shifts rapidly in this world. The drug exhibits get wilder, zanier, with different players taking center stage. At the 2006 meetings, Sonata was not much in evidence, but from the Takeda booth, maker of Rozerem, wafted the aroma of fresh-baked cookies, which drew us all like flies. Sepracor, maker of Lunesta, took us for a ride (literally—we lay back on recliners, eight or ten of us in a circle, toes pointed toward the center, and were whirled round and round, while video monitors mounted on the chairs advertised the virtues of Lunesta). The industry dinners are as lavish, and they still give Continuing Medical Education credit, but the conference program now states loud and clear that they are not part of the conference.

Each year I sense change. Things are "moving so fast scientifically," the field "is growing so fast that few researchers can even take the time to write a book," as Dinges says. There seems to be more speculation, at each conference, about physiological etiologies for insomnia, new ways of understanding insomnia that are opening up.

I turn now to these developments.

CHAPTER 5

The Brain of an Insomniac

Insomnia may not be in their head—it may be in their brain
and in their body as well.

Daniel Buysse, University of Pittsburgh School of Medicine

*It's like my sleep thing is broken. I have a cousin who I'd
never met, she said the exact same thing*—my sleep thing is
broken.

It took a long time for anybody to recognize that there really is "a sleep
thing," that sleep is an active, dynamic behavior and not just an absence
of activity in the brain and body. It took until 1953, to be exact, when, in
the lab of Nathaniel Kleitman, Eugene Aserinsky noticed the rapidly moving eyelids of his sleeping subject. Before this, it was assumed that nothing much went on when we slept—lights out, all systems down. But here,
suddenly, in the supposed stillness of sleep was all this activity, the eyelids
jumping back and forth, the blood pressure rising, the heart racing, the
breathing erratic, the penis erect. It's amazing that it took all those ages
for anyone to *see*, when those rapid eye movements were there on the surface, nothing hidden about them. Hadn't anybody ever watched a sleeping baby or a napping dog? Yes, Aserinsky had, and so had William Dement, also a student of Kleitman's at the time: they had, by Dement's
account, "spent . . . over 200 hours staring at the eyes of sleeping infants."
But they missed the eye movements—because "even when they are looking, people usually see only what they expect to find," and "the idea that
the brain is completely active during sleep, not turned off, flew in the face
of thousands of years of believing differently." It was not believed such
things happened, therefore it was not seen—and then when it was seen, it
was not believed: it was thought to be a glitch in the recording machinery.

The discovery of rapid eye movement (REM) revolutionized the understanding of sleep. Here was evidence that sleep is not just the cessation of brain activity but a behavior in its own right, actively generated and actively maintained. Here was evidence that there were two kinds of sleep, REM and so-called nonREM, as distinct from one another as each state is from wakefulness. Now it turned out that beneath the placid exterior of sleep was a world of complex activity, precisely timed, elaborately modulated, regulated by mechanisms about which nobody had a clue.

The mystery of sleep is the mystery of the brain, the most complicated three-pound object on earth. A lump of gray matter the consistency of cream cheese, it doesn't look all that different from a chimp's brain, yet it contains about a hundred billion *neurons* (nerve cells), as many as there are stars in the Milky Way. Each neuron connects to thousands of other neurons, and somehow this vast, ever-changing webwork, these hundreds of trillions of connections, give rise to all we are and all we know. More was learned about the brain in the 1990s, the so-called Decade of the Brain, than in all the decades before, but as neuroscientist Antonio Damasio summarizes,

> The current description of neurobiological phenomena is quite incomplete, any way you slice it. We have yet to resolve numerous details about the function of neurons and circuits at the molecular level; we do not yet grasp the behavior of populations of neurons within a local brain region; and our understanding of the large-scale systems made up of multiple brain regions is also incomplete.

In fact, not a single one of the brain's behaviors is entirely understood, including sleep.

"It's dark in there," as a medical student once said.

How to tease information out of this lump of gelatinous goo? Where in the brain would you look for sleep—and where would you look for insomnia, a subjective condition for which there are no objective measures? There is no single "sleep center": sleep is diffuse, all throughout, a process or an array of processes and interactions among various areas of the brain, an elaborate dance of *neurotransmitters,* some of which take center stage at some points, others at other points. (A neurotransmitter is a chemical messenger. When it's released by an electrochemical charge into the *synapse,* or gap, between neurons, it makes contact with the *receptor* of the next cell, and the contact elicits changes in the neighboring neuron, either stimulating or inhibiting its firing. About a hundred neurotransmitters have been identified, including *serotonin, norepinephrine,* and, most crucially for sleep, *gamma-aminobutyric acid* [GABA]; there are probably many more.)

The sleep system cannot be considered in isolation from the systems that keep us awake. As Peter Hauri says, "Whether one is awake or asleep depends on the relative dominance of either the arousal system or the sleep system." Sleep requires an activating of the mechanisms that quiet us down and a quieting of the mechanisms that keep us awake: the arousal system must be inhibited and the inhibitory system must be activated. It is, as Allan Hobson describes it, a "complex push-pull system of activation and inhibition."

Sleep and arousal signals are governed by two systems, the *homeostatic,* which refers to the buildup of sleep pressure, and the *circadian,* which is related to the time of day (*circadian* means "around a day"). Sleep pressure builds in proportion to the time we've been awake, according to the simple principle that the longer we stay awake, the sleepier we get. But if it were only the buildup of homeostatic pressure that makes us sleepy, we'd just wear down and down, and that's not what happens, because the circadian system, which is linked to the cycles of light and dark, kicks in at certain hours to perk us up—so that even when we've been up all night, we get a second wind around 6 A.M. (6 to 10 A.M. and 6 to 8 P.M. are peak times, and 3 to 4 A.M. and 3 to 5 P.M. are dips); and these peaks and troughs correlate with changes in body temperature. How sleepy we are at any given point, then, depends on how many hours we've been awake *and* what time of day it is.

To make matters more complex, the sleep system must render us insensible to the environment but not entirely insensible. It must shut us down, disconnect us from the world, but not entirely: sensations must be able to get through so that we can come quickly awake. Sleep, unlike coma or death, is readily reversible—it has to be, because sleep is risky, renders us vulnerable: we have to be able to come quickly out of it. The sleep system has evolved over many millions of years, and though we don't know what for, we know it's important: it must be important— why else would nature take such risks? "If sleep does not serve an absolutely vital function," as pioneer sleep researcher Allan Rechtschaffen famously said, "then it is the biggest mistake the evolutionary process ever made."

Sleep, as Rechtschaffen wrote, is a biological behavior that works best "under relatively narrow conditions of the internal and external environment." And there's the rub. Because such conditions are difficult to achieve, and because sleep is so readily reversed, sleep is fragile.

Of Mice and Men

Much of what is known about the brain comes from the study of animals. You can do things to animals that you can't do to humans, inject a substance into this or that part of the brain or lesion it or remove it, and see what happens. "Mice are so much easier to study than human beings," says sleep researcher Irwin Feinberg, who has been studying both for four decades. "You can use pharmaceutical probes to block receptors or make them respond, you can watch chemicals accumulate and dissipate, you can create mutant mice in which a receptor has been knocked out, you can study receptor function in a way you can't in human beings. But it's very difficult to study humans, difficult to control their conditions. Do you really think you could get an insomniac to stop taking sleeping pills for any length of time, or to cut out her nightcaps, or her naps?"

Mice (or rats) may be easier than men, but the day I visited Feinberg's sleep lab at U.C. Davis, they did not look all that easy to me. Feinberg and his coresearcher Ian Campbell drove me out to the edge of the vast, agricultural Davis campus, past barns and fields with grazing cows and horses, to a small wooden building where the rats were kept. There in their cages, in a room dark except for a dull red glow (red light doesn't interfere with circadian rhythms), were a dozen or so rats, sniffing and scratching and doing their rat things, except that these wore little helmets of implanted electrodes. Cables ran from their helmets through an amplifier to a computer screen in the next room, and on this screen appeared the squiggly lines of their EEGs. The researchers had injected them with a chemical to see how it would affect their sleep; they would then take their data through months and months of careful analysis to get one tiny piece of information: that this chemical injected at this point in the circadian cycle produces this effect—one piece of the vast puzzle of sleep that may someday add up to something, or not. I felt a rush of pity for the little animals, and pity for the researchers, too, to see how difficult it is to tease information out of the inside of a skull, a citadel that jealously guards its secrets. This painstaking work, so painfully dependent on these rats (and cats and dogs and monkeys) who give their all, and on these researchers, patiently watching, scrupulously recording, analyzing, tabulating, writing up their results, this is how we know most of what we know about the brain—mute, inglorious, underfunded, basic research. Any notions I still had of "why don't they just find the part that doesn't work in us, and fix it?" were laid permanently to rest that afternoon. I was filled with a feeling I can only describe as humility.

We owe our understanding of the inhibition of bodily movements during REM to the work of French researcher Michel Jouvet, one of the grand figures in this field, and one of the most fascinating. Jouvet, a member of the Resistance during World War II and the author of a novel, *The Castle of Dreams,* performed a series of elegant operations severing certain neural pathways in the *brainstem* of the cat, the area at the top of the spinal cord. When those pathways were severed, something extraordinary happened: the cat was asleep, insensible to external stimuli, yet it acted as though it were awake. It behaved, as Jouvet described it, "as if it could see a mouse, advancing slowly, its head held forward and downward as it pursues its imaginary prey"; or it pawed the air "with ears flattened backward and the mouth open, ready to bite," seeming to be fighting an imaginary enemy. Jouvet had destroyed the area of the brain that causes the body to be paralyzed during REM, the part that keeps signals from getting through to the muscles. The cat was, he surmised, acting out its dreams, attacking, stalking, pursuing, exploring.

It's not always easy to apply what is learned from animals to humans, but in the case of Jouvet's finding, later research documented that damage to this part of the brainstem could have the same effect in humans— as happens in REM behavior disorder, where the brain's signals get through to the body, and men (mainly men) try to act out their dreams. But there's a problem using animals to study insomnia: if insomnia is defined as a *complaint* (as we saw that it is), then only humans can get it. Researchers have long lamented the lack of an animal model for studying insomnia, but they have recently been widening their definitions on the basis of animal behavior. A study headed by Larry Sanford found that certain strains of mice and rats are more susceptible to "fear conditioning" than other strains, and more susceptible to disrupted sleep. Researchers have bred fruit flies that behave like insomniacs. Fruit flies seem an unlikely model for human beings, but in fact their sleep has many features of ours. It gets worse with age; it responds to stimulants and hypnotics, as does ours; there are long sleepers and short sleepers, and they rebound after sleep deprivation by sleeping longer the next night. Researchers have taken short-sleeping fruit flies and crossed them through ninety generations, producing extremely short-sleeping flies. These flies don't "complain a lot," reports Washington University sleep researcher Paul Shaw, but their sleep occurs in short bouts through the day and night; when the lights are turned on, they wake up and stay up, while their normal siblings go back to sleep. They withstand stress pretty well: when you starve them or desiccate them (things you're not allowed to do

to animals, Shaw comments wryly), they are hardy. But they "fall a lot—
their balance is disturbed." And "they cannot learn, though their normally sleeping siblings can; and their lifespan is considerably reduced."

Fruit flies are not human beings, of course, but these experiments suggest that sleep behaviors that resemble insomnia in humans may be genetically produced and may occur in the absence of stress or psychological upset.

Since you can't do the sorts of things to humans that you can to animals or flies, researchers have had to depend on accidents and disease to
learn about the human brain. One of the earliest breakthroughs in sleep
came from Dr. Constantin Von Economo, a Viennese baron and doctor
in the early twentieth century. In 1917, Von Economo saw his first of thousands of cases of the disease he would name *Encephalitis lethargica,* or
sleeping sickness, a variant of the influenza epidemic that swept Europe
and America during and after the First World War, claiming the lives of
more people than had died on both sides of the war. Victims of sleeping
sickness had radically disrupted sleep, some suffering from an inability
to sleep at all that ended in death, others falling into "a state of most intense stupor or even a comatose condition," as Von Economo describes
it, that also led to death. (Others sank into a stupor from which they neither revived nor died. Oliver Sacks came across some of these in an in-
stitution, years later, and treated them with L-dopa; it awakened them
miraculously, but with such dire side effects that he had to discontinue
the treatment. This was the basis of the film *Awakenings.*)

More than 5 million people died of encephalitis before the epidemic
ebbed ten years later. During these years, Von Economo observed, analyzed, and autopsied thousands of cases. He found that damage to the pos-
terior (rear) of the *hypothalamus,* a small structure at the base of the brain,
caused excessive somnolence, and that damage to the anterior (front) area
of the hypothalamus caused sleeplessness. The hypothalamus is anatom-
ically and functionally very complex, having within it many specialized
cell groups, or *nuclei,* and exerting an influence way out of proportion
to its size (it's about the size of a grape). It keeps the internal environment
of the body constant, regulating not only heart rate and hunger but also
water balance, blood sugar, and temperature; it also regulates the release
of growth hormone, thyroid hormone, and stress hormones. Von
Economo was able to report, in 1929, that it regulates sleep and wakefulness as well.

Only in the past decade have Von Economo's observations come to
be fully appreciated. "A few years ago," recounted Clifford Saper at the

2005 sleep meetings, "I and some colleagues at Harvard stumbled on a tiny bunch of neurons just behind the optic nerve that has the ability to turn off all the awake systems." Whereas most neuronal systems in the brain are active when we're awake and become quiescent with the onset of sleep, these neurons, located in the part of the hypothalamus Von Economo described as the generator of sleep, fire about twice as fast during sleep. "It looks as if this cluster of neurons inhibits all the neurotransmitters involved in wakefulness, arousal and consciousness," says Saper, who, with Thomas Chou and Thomas Scammell, published these groundbreaking findings in 2001, terming this small cluster (the *ventrolateral preoptic nucleus*) the *sleep switch* (and small it is—a thousand, maybe a few thousand neurons—for the enormous influence it exerts). Animal studies also confirm that when this area is lesioned, the animal loses its ability to sleep deeply or to maintain sleep: it may get to sleep, but it won't stay asleep. "You can actually correlate sleep loss with loss of neurons in this area," says Saper, who adds the fascinating information that "elderly people have been found to have 50% fewer neurons in this area, which might account for their problem maintaining sleep."

Here's how they think it works. (This next part gets technical, but bear with me—it's only a few pages.) Neurons in the sleep switch generate GABA, gamma-aminobutyric acid, the major inhibitory neurotransmitter of the brain; it "sends outputs to," as Saper says, "all the major cell groups in the hypothalamus and brainstem that participate in arousal," turning down vigilance, tension, muscle tone, anxiety. In the complex push-and-pull interaction of sleep and wakefulness, the arousal and inhibition systems are in close proximity, with wake-promoting signals ascending from the brainstem through the hypothalamus and the thalamus (just above the hypothalamus) on their way to the cerebral cortex, the seat of the all-important executive functions. These wake-up signals are relayed through clusters of neurons that generate the wake-up neurotransmitters histamine and hypocretin, neurons that fire rapidly during arousal but are quiet during sleep. *Histamine* is what's damped down by *antihistamine*, the ingredient in cold medicines and over-the-counter sleep remedies that makes you sleepy. *Hypocretin* is the neurotransmitter that Emmanuel Mignot discovered was deficient in narcoleptics. The hypothalamus contains *all* the hypocretin-producing neurons in the brain, all ten thousand of them, not very many—and this is the *only* part of the brain that contains these crucial wake-up neurotransmitters, without which the person is unable to maintain wakefulness. We see again and again, with the brain, how such tiny losses have huge effects.

What are the mechanisms by which the system shuts down consciousness and renders us insensible to the outside world? The *thalamus* is key. A bundle of nerve cells in the center of the brain, it relays information from the eyes and ears and all parts of the body and passes information among various parts of the brain. When we're awake and attentive, signals cycle back and forth between the thalamus and the frontal cortex, information looping to and fro—this *thalamocortical looping,* as it's called, is what keeps us buzzing, what we experience as consciousness. In order for sleep to occur, for the brain to shift from an aroused state that's open to stimuli from the outside world to the closed state of somnolence, these neurons must cease their rapid firing and the looping must slow down. The GABA-generating neurons of the sleep switch initiate this transformation, causing neurons to fire more slowly and to fire together (the synchronization is picked up by the EEG as "waves"; this is what the EEG registers as sleep). The thalamus is said to perform an *intermittent gating mechanism,* "intermittent" because some signals can get through the gate and alert us—bright lights, loud noises, the sound of a child's cry, our own name.

Something else that's interesting about falling asleep: it usually happens suddenly, when (or if) it happens. While we're awake, the firing of the wake-promoting neurons inhibits the activity of the sleep switch, keeps it buttoned down. As we transition from wakefulness to sleep, this inhibition is lifted. The transition is at first gradual, like the slow movement of a hand across a dial, and we get sleepier and sleepier; but then, suddenly, we fall asleep—and the transition is abrupt, like a switch that flips from on to off. Or, we come awake, also abruptly, for the switch works both ways—when the inhibition on the sleep system is lifted, the switch flips us awake. Saper likens the process to a "flip flop switch," an electrical circuit or mechanical device designed to go decisively in one direction and stay there, until it flips in the opposite direction, and stays there. This sudden shifting assures that we spend most of our time "in either a clearly waking or sleeping state, with relatively brief times spent in transitions"; for, as Saper says, "an animal that walked about while half asleep would be in considerable danger."

The trigger that presses the switch into the wakeful position is thought to be hypocretin: if you have too few hypocretin neurons, the switch doesn't fully flip you into wakefulness, and you're neither quite awake nor quite asleep—which is what happens with narcoleptics. But insomniacs inhabit this intermediate zone, too. "When you're an insomniac, you're never really asleep and you're never really awake," says a character in the film *Fight Club.* When you spend nights hovering just beneath the surface of consciousness, not sure whether you're asleep or awake (or, sure that you're awake, while the EEG says you're asleep), you feel like the switch hasn't fully flipped—which raises the question, which crucial neurons or neurotransmitters might be missing or malfunctioning in us?

But if hypocretin turns the sleep switch off, what turns it on? The search for a "sleep substance" is as old as Aristotle. It feels, intuitively, as if some sleep substance accumulates, "as if a chemical factor builds up and the longer one stays awake the more this chemical accumulates," as Jerome Siegel says. A hundred years ago, experimenters extracted the cerebrospinal fluid of a sleep-deprived dog and injected it into a wakeful dog to see if it got sleepy—and it did. It's just that nobody has been able to figure out what the key substance is. "That's what I've spent most of my life trying to find out," says James Krueger of Washington State University, a foremost authority in this area. "We thought it would be simple, and it's not."

The neurotransmitter *adenosine,* which accumulates during our waking hours and dissipates during deep sleep, is known to be crucial in the buildup of sleep pressure. The longer we're awake, the more of this chemical builds up in our brains, until "at certain levels of adenosine, sleep becomes irresistible," says Robert McCarley of Harvard Medical School. Caffeine interferes with the action of adenosine, which is how it prevents drowsiness. But there are other sleep-inducing substances, including the inflammatory markers interleukin-1 and tumor necrosis factor, which, as we saw in the last chapter, are a part of the immune system; their presence explains why we get sleepy when we have a bacterial or viral infection. *Growth-hormone-releasing hormone* induces sleep, as does *prolactin,* a hormone released with sleep and also with lactation. But as far as anybody can tell right now, there is no one sleep substance, no single neurotransmitter or neuromodulator that is solely or exclusively responsible for initiating and maintaining sleep; there are multiple substances that interact complexly. "There are a lot of substances put forth, and a lot have good stories, but we don't really understand," says Tom Scammell.

More is known about the circadian system than the homeostatic system, but that's still not a lot. It is known that there's a master clock, a cluster of neurons in the hypothalamus (the *suprachiasmic nucleus*) that regulates the timing of sleep and waking, synchronizing sleep and wakefulness with the cycles of light and dark. It instructs the nearby pineal gland to produce melatonin, which makes body temperature decline and causes sleepiness. If you lesion this nucleus, sleep becomes randomly dispersed throughout the twenty-four-hour period. But exactly how it works and how it interacts with the homeostatic system remain mysterious.

So this is what researchers think the sleep-inducing mechanisms look like and how they work, more or less, as of 2007. Every few months, a new piece of the puzzle is found that helps fill in the picture and bring us closer to understanding how the system works—and closer, we hope, to understanding what goes wrong when it doesn't work. Saper speculates, "What we might be seeing in insomniacs is a loss of neurons in the sleep switch, or neurons that aren't firing." Other researchers speculate about "weak thalamic gating mechanisms," excessive hypocretin or overly active hypocretin, or a failure of adenosine or some other sleep-inducing substance to do its work. But there are too many missing pieces for these to be more than guesses at the present time.

It's still very dark in there.

Sleepless Babies

One thing that's known is that human beings are born with different sleep propensities. "Parents have long observed marked differences in the arousal level of newborns," says Allan Hobson. "Whereas some are 'good' sleepers, others are hyperalert"; the fact that such differences "tend to be lifelong" suggests that they're "genetically defined." "It seems likely that in such a complex 'push-pull' system, not every human being is equally endowed," says Peter Hauri. "Some may tend more toward sleep, others toward wakefulness." "Just as there are various levels of intelligence without . . . abnormalities, so there are various balances between sleeping and waking."

There is variability in the timing of sleep and the pressure to sleep—that is, in both homeostatic and circadian systems. Some people are born night owls, some morning larks. Some people wake up and conk out at the same time every day and night, like clockwork, while others seem barely affected by the time of day; some are extremely sensitive to changes in light, others hardly affected at all. Some have such strong sleep pressure that sleep hits them "like a mallet" (as a friend says) and they fade out in midsentence or at the wheel; in others, the pressure and prompts are so slight that sleep must be artfully wooed. Such variability makes evolutionary sense, assuring that someone is always awake to stand guard. Or perhaps, as Hauri suggests, the tendency to vigilance may be not the extreme end of a continuum of natural variability but a defect in the system, some "yet-to-be identified neuroanatomical, neurophysiological, or neurochemical weakness in the sleep system, or excessive strength in the arousal system."

I come across lots of insomniacs who say that they've had insomnia *just always.*

> *I can't remember* EVER *being able to sleep! My parents told me I didn't sleep as a baby. As a child I remember being the* ONLY *one awake at slumber parties. I don't know how I made it in college on such little sleep.*

> *Insomnia has affected me since I was a five-year-old girl. Old movies,* The Twilight Zone, *and Alfred Hitchcock films kept me company till morning.*

> *I would get up in the night, when everyone else was asleep, and wander quietly about our home. I learned where the noisy boards were in the floors and how to avoid them. . . . I am now seventy-three.*

> *Remember many nights crying at 3* A.M. *as a child cause I knew it was going to be time for school soon and I was so lonely being the only one in the house awake.*

> *I am an insomniac and have been all my life. When I was a child it just seemed normal; . . . it was all I knew, and I just thought that is how things were. It was only when I started sleeping over at other people's houses that I realized that not everyone lay awake for hours.*

Many of these people had, like Jacqueline, the Frenchwoman whose story we heard earlier, happy childhoods and loving parents and cannot point to a stressful event or period that triggered the problem.

And yet the DSM-IV says that childhood-onset insomnia, also called *idiopathic insomnia* (*idiopathic* means "origins unknown"), is rare: "Primary Insomnia typically begins in young adulthood or middle age and is rare in childhood or adolescence." Childhood-onset insomnia was declared "rare" by two Stanford researchers, Christian Guilleminault and Thomas Anders, who claimed, in 1976, that insomnia "is the exception rather than the rule in young children," and where it is present, it is "a familial psychologic problem, . . . indicative of family problems rather than a physiological sleep disorder." "A sleepless baby is a reproach to his guardians," they say, citing as their authority a study from 1957, a decade when, as we saw, mothers were being blamed for anything that went wrong with their children, from autism to schizophrenia. Researchers today avoid words like "reproach"; they use the less stigmatizing term *limit-setting disorder,* defined as "a childhood disorder characterized by inadequate enforcement of bedtime by a caretaker, with resultant stalling or refusal to go to bed at an appropriate time." But it comes to the same thing.

One of the few researchers who has taken childhood-onset insomnia seriously is Peter Hauri. I interview Hauri, in the spring of 2003, on the eighth floor of the Methodist Hospital, part of the Mayo Clinic, Rochester, a vast complex of glass and steel towers that rises imposingly out of the Minnesota plains; Hauri heads a sleep clinic there. I had determined, after my experience at the sleep meetings that year, never again to reveal to a researcher that I'm an insomniac, but when I asked him what had drawn him to the subject, he told me, "My mother suffered from it, and I—I have a touch of it myself."

"Really?" I blurted out. "So do I!"

Hauri told me how his study of childhood-onset insomnia came about:

> Back in 1979, I argued that logically there should be some people who have weaker and stronger sleep systems—it's not logical to think that in everyone sleep works the same way. My colleagues couldn't be talked into it: the only thing they'd acknowledge was that some people have insomnia since very early; they called it childhood-onset insomnia and challenged me to document this new disease. So I did that study.

"That study" is "Childhood-Onset Insomnia," which he did with Elaine Olmstead in 1980; it was, as he says, "the *only* study of the polysomnographs of idiopathic insomniacs till that time" (a *polysomnograph,* or *polysomnogram,* includes the EEG and devices that measure eye movements, muscle activity, heart rate and rhythm). The researchers compared a group of people who had childhood-onset insomnia with a group whose insomnia came on when they were adults. They found that most of the adult-onset insomniacs could name a specific psychological stress that occurred around the time their insomnia started, but most of the childhood-onset insomniacs could not; in fact, half said their insomnia remained stable over time, through bad and good periods, whereas at least three-quarters of adult-onset insomniacs felt their insomnia fluctuated with mood or psychiatric conditions. Finding that the childhood-onset insomnia "did not seem to be caused by conditioning or psychopathological factors," Hauri and Olmstead hypothesized that there may be "a less psychological and a more neurophysiological/neurochemical basis" for it, may in fact be "some neurological impairment in structures relating to the sleep-wake balance." They made the further discovery that 55 percent of those studied with childhood-onset insomnia had at least one family member with sleep difficulties, whereas only 39 percent of those with adult-onset insomnia did, suggesting that those with childhood-onset insomnia were more likely to have come by their insomnia by way of their genes.

The researchers did in fact find evidence of neurological impairment: "significantly more childhood-onset insomniacs gave some suggestions of possible 'soft' neurological involvement such as histories of dyslexia or hyperkinesis, a diagnosis of 'minimal brain damage.'" (*Hyperkinesis* is an older term for ADD, attention deficit disorder, which is itself an older term for ADHD, attention deficit hyperactivity disorder. It's associated with restlessness, distractibility, and the inability to sit still or concentrate.) They also discovered abnormalities on the EEG, "abnormally long periods of REM sleep that are totally devoid of any eye movements." These findings were confirmed in a study Hauri did three years later, which found that five out of eight of the childhood insomniacs had, again, signs of "dyslexia, hyperkinesis, or minimal brain damage" and EEG waves of unknown significance. Psychologically, he noted, these five insomniacs seemed "surprisingly normal in view of their severe sleep disturbances."

Something else was intriguing: the childhood-onset insomniacs had extreme reactions to food, drink, and drugs, such that a cup of tea or some chocolate drink hours before bedtime would seriously interfere with their sleep. Hauri found they had "exquisite" sensitivity to stimulants and noise, and atypical reactions to medications, both hypersensitivity and insensitivity. I hear about extreme sensitivities from many insomniacs I talk to:

> *A piece of chocolate in the morning, I can't sleep at night; any sugar in the evenings and I can't sleep, or [I] wake up at dawn and can't go back to sleep.*

> *I react so strongly to caffeine, I'm afraid to breathe deep when I walk by Starbucks. Lots of things set me off—sugar is a definite no-no, so is a lot of salt late in the evenings, and, oh yes, I have a problem with peanuts. When I eat these things, I wake up with my heart pounding and I don't get back to sleep. And it's gotten worse with age.*

It's a fascinating question, whether childhood-onset insomniacs are more prone to such sensitivities than other types of insomniacs, but as far as I know, no one's followed it up.

When I asked Hauri if anyone had followed up on this work, he said, "Nobody works on childhood-onset insomnia today." I did a search and found only four studies besides his. The first of these, published in 1981, the same year as Hauri's study, argues, as he does, that childhood insomnia had been "prematurely discounted." Katharine Dixon and her team screened 186 children, using a questionnaire given to the parents and interviews with the children. They identified 16 insomniac children and found that "the mean length of the children's insomnia was over five years. It was not unusual for a parent to report the child's having a lifelong problem initiating and maintaining sleep." They concluded that these findings "warrant further, more rigorous investigation into childhood insomnia." Of the "further investigations" I found, one looked at two patients, and another was only an abstract. The abstract, by Swiss researcher Jean-Michel Gaillard, compared seventeen patients who had idiopathic insomnia with seventeen who had psychophysiological insomnia, and found that the "idiopaths" had less tenseness and anxiety, less "night to night variability" in their insomnia, and that "significantly fewer" of them "had depressive rumination." This conclusion was consistent with Hauri's observation of a "relative absence of . . . psychopathological factors" in childhood-onset insomniacs.

The final investigation, which seems to have had the last word on the subject, was done in 1996 by the same researcher who had the first word twenty years before, Christian Guilleminault, working with Pierre Philip, also at Stanford. "Only a small percentage of insomnia patients report childhood-onset of the problem," they say, yet as I read this study, fourteen of their sixty-five subjects reported it—over 20 percent! They found that the childhood-onset insomniacs did not actually have worse sleep, only that they had a *perception* of worse sleep, a perception not confirmed by their EEGs. (Yet the EEG is a notoriously problematic measure of insomnia—as we'll see—so much so that researchers today tend to credit the subjective account of the sufferer over the "objective" measurement when the two come into conflict, as they often do.) Guilleminault and Philip say they found no evidence of soft neurological impairment, and yet I can't see that they were looking, for their questionnaires asked about feelings of nonrestorative sleep, daytime fatigue, nightmares, night terrors, and sleep or psychiatric disorders in the immediate family.

And this is the sum total of research on idiopathic or childhood-onset insomnia. Childhood-onset insomnia is said to be rare, but it seems nobody's really looking for it. The best way not to find something, as my old

mentor Alice Stewart used to say (referring to the effects of low-dose radiation she was finding but nobody else was) is not to look. Idiopathic
or childhood onset insomnia does not have a category of its own in the
DSM-IV: it is subsumed by *primary* insomnia, which is conflated with
conditioned insomnia—even though Hauri's work suggests that
childhood-onset insomnia is not conditioned and does not require an
episode of stress to trigger it. Childhood-onset insomnia *does* exist as a
separate category in the more nuanced *International Classification of
Sleep Disorders* (ICSD), but, not existing in the DSM, it might as well not
exist at all. It was not discussed at any of the conferences I went to. Children's sleep problems were discussed, but this is different from childhood-
onset insomnia, where an adult remembers a condition that's been there
"just always." (Childhood sleep problems are said, by every speaker I've
heard and every study I've read, to be a learned behavior, a response to
stresses in the family, which I'm sure they often are—but *always?*) With
the disappearance of the category of childhood-onset insomnia goes an
important distinction, between the kind of insomnia that is more likely to
be in the genes and the kind more likely to be conditioned.

With the disappearance of childhood-onset insomnia also goes the
category of *idiopathic insomnia,* insomnia of origins unknown, since
the two terms are used interchangeably. Idiopathic insomnia is defined
in the *International Classification of Sleep Disorders* as "a long-standing
complaint of insomnia" with "onset occurring during infancy or early
childhood," which is not explained by "psychosocial stressors, other
sleep and medical disorders, or medications"; it is said to be rare. When
I've asked researchers why nobody uses the term anymore, I've been told,
"There's no reason—it just happened. The term has fallen out of use."
But if you eliminate "origin unknown" as a category or describe this type
of insomnia as "rare," you imply that the causes of most insomnia, are,
well, known. Premature closure, again.

When I've asked researchers why nobody's looking at childhood-onset
insomnia, I've been told it's difficult to study because you can't trust
people to remember how they slept as children. *Recall bias* is the bane of
retrospective scientific studies, that is, studies that depend on subjects' recollection of something that happened in the past. Alice Stewart came up
against this prejudice in her work: her critics argued that the mothers of
children who'd died of cancer could not be counted on to remember accurately what had gone on (as we saw in chapter 1). But when the mothers' memories were checked against hospital records, they'd remembered
the x rays perfectly well. Of course, there are other kinds of memories that

cannot be so easily checked out, and human beings are notoriously untrustworthy narrators of their own pasts. Yet it's a fundamental precept of psychotherapy that we can access our early experiences at least enough that a therapist can work with us to repair the damage they've wrought: memory is assumed to be at least this reliable. Why, then, the disinterest in what people remember about the way they slept as children?

What do you do with details like these: *I learned where the noisy boards were. My mother would leave my play things around the bed.* Invented? Perhaps. But then why are people so readily believed when they say things like, *It was my divorce that brought it on,* or *It was when I was studying for the bar.* Researchers accept these accounts without question, yet here, too, the person is looking back from the present and assigning a cause after the fact. Granted, getting a divorce or studying for the bar are events that would have occurred more recently than anything in childhood, but if you're going to be consistent in your distrust of people's memories, why not question these memories as well? (I wonder if these kinds of memories are so readily believed because they confirm the received wisdom that insomnia is caused by stress.) I'm not saying that such memories aren't true, only that they might not be the entire truth, that there might be other causes, earlier and more fundamental, buried in the past, lost in time.

I have no memory of how I slept as an infant; even my mother was hazy on the details, except to say that she could never get me to bed. But she left records. I was born in June 1943; my father was drafted when I was six months old, late in the war, part of the medical corps called up in anticipation of the invasion of Japan. During the year and a half he was gone, most of which he spent in New Guinea, treating General MacArthur's casualties, Mother wrote him two and three times a week. I didn't know these letters existed. I found them after my parents died, mildewed and bug-chewed, in an old steamer trunk my father had hauled with him on his every move since the war. I couldn't bring myself to read them, even when I was writing a memoir. It was too sad, all that love and hope and looking forward to a future, crumbled to a dead past. When I did finally get myself to read them—for this chapter—I got an earful.

"There is no sleep in that baby," she writes (March 4, 1944). And again:

> June 1, 1944: She hates to give in and go to sleep. She understands when we speak of going to bed and shakes her head vigorously in the negative.
> September 1, 1944: She has had a busy day, but this is one of those nights when she simply won't give up. . . . It is hard to understand why she

goes on these nocturnal escapades. Last night's lasted till 2 o'clock. And it was a particularly active one.

September 21, 1944: She is shaking the screws out of her crib, on hands and knees, butting her head against the panel, and alas showing no signs of weariness, although it is 10 o'clock.

October 22, 1944: It's 10:20 and G is trying to find every excuse not to sleep. She called me and when I went in she threw both arms around my neck pretending to hug me, while she climbed up the side of the crib and out over the side in a jiffy.

October 23, 1944: It is 10:30 and the little imp is still grunting and struggling.

October 30, 1944: I put her down at 9 and went in to check on her at 10:30, and there she was, still awake, not crying, just awake.

November 13, 1944: G's nap is not coming easily today. She lies there cooing, playing with her wooden toys. . . . Now she's on all fours, rocking the crib. She just isn't sleepy.

November 15, 1944: For two days she has had no naps at all. To bed early on those nights? Not at all. She stayed up till 10:30 on both of them.

My father's letters describe long periods of idleness between the times when the casualties pour in, when he's bored to tears, but for my mother, "there's no let up at this end," caring for "the world's most active baby," and no peace. He, at war, gets to sleep; she, at home, gets me:

November 23, 1944: G has had a couple of bad nights, last night till 3:15. No naps for two days.

November 29, 1944: It's 11:30 and G is still bouncing about her crib. She had no nap today. . . .

January 18, 1945: G is in bed every night by nine o'clock, but that doesn't mean she goes to sleep then. It is now 10:30, and the poor old crib is shaking violently.

That crib met a bad end:

Feb. 10, 1945: Well, the other night the inevitable happened. I heard a crash, and then a howl. G's crib broke down about 4 A.M.

There's a thing I did that she describes again and again: "When G awakens from a nap she lies there in her crib rehearsing her whole vocabulary: dada, mama, nana, goda, bow-wow, didi, tick-tock, big doll. Goes right through the group of words without a mistake" (Oct. 20, 1944). "It's now 11:30 and I put her to bed at 8:30. I still hear 'da-da car, mama car, didi, hot, hand, doll, bowwow, ticktock'" (Feb. 23, 1945). My friends who've raised children tell me their kids never did this sort of thing. Some kind of self-soothing device? An early fascination with words? Ever since I can remember, I've loved words: it's what drew me to Shakespeare, the shapes and sounds, the feel and texture, of words. (I'll have more to say later about sleep and words.)

And on, and on. . . .

Oct. 13, 1945: I've gotten up at six to practice the piano, about seven o'clock I hear an unusual noise, and there she stands, with all her nocturnal trappings, standing demurely behind me. How she climbs out of the crib with all her rigging I don't know. There is no putting her back to bed then. "I don't want to go in crib," she insists.

Oct. 15, 1945: I don't expect her to climb out of bed by herself this morning because I put the crib away from the big bed . . . .

Oh no, here she comes. How the little rascal did it I don't know.

The sleep of newborns is classically the bane of their parents' existence; there's nothing unusual about that. Babies have irregular sleep patterns, distributed around the clock, "very much like what we see in experiments in which people are isolated from external time cues," says Dement. Gradually those patterns become regular and shift to the night. At the end of the first year, the infant is usually sleeping fourteen to fifteen hours, mostly at night, with one or two daytime naps; by eighteen months, there's usually one nap, and by the end of twenty-four months, most babies are sleeping about half the time. My mother did not keep systematic records, but on the basis of her descriptions, it does not sound like this two-year-old was anywhere near twelve hours of sleep. It does not sound like she wants to sleep at all. Mother never mentions night terrors or fears of the dark or any kind of trouble other than a fierce desire not to let go of the day. She describes "a peppy and happy baby," "bursting with health," "mischievous," "sparkling," "the type of baby that gives one many laughs, so full of personality and joy is she," "everything is a game to her"—"these cloudy days can't dampen that baby's spirits." She may have been too enchanted with this baby—"How the little rascal did it [got out of the crib] I don't know," she says, adding, "I congratulate her for it!" "Limit setting disorder"? Perhaps. But she was dealing with a baby whose system was tilted toward wakefulness, and toward nighttime wakefulness, at that.

What if it's an underlying tilt, a predisposition toward fragile sleep, broken sleep, or sleep that occurs at the wrong times—what if it's this inborn disposition that explains *why* one person who goes through a stressful period becomes conditioned to insomnia, while another returns easily to normal sleep? When I ran this idea by Hauri, when I asked, "Do you think some sort of underlying predisposition may explain why one person gets conditioned insomnia and the other does not?" his reply was unhesitating: "No doubt." "With what percentage would you guess this would be the case? Fifty percent? Seventy-five percent?" He thought for a moment, then gave me an answer that blew me away: "Probably 100 percent." "Relatively mild psychological stressors," Hauri writes, "may push this sort of patient [the childhood-onset insomniac] to develop insomnia." Then, having chronic insomnia would lead anyone to maladaptive practices and attitudes and all the rest: "It seems almost impossible to lead the life of an individual with chronic, serious insomnia without developing other factors that are complicating the picture, such as poor sleep hygiene, learned maladaptive associations, psychiatric disturbances."

This means that when physicians and researchers see psychological disturbances in insomniacs, when they see maladaptive habits and attitudes and poor sleep hygiene, they may be looking at the consequences of a sleep problem rather than the *causes* (as we saw in chapter 3)—and may be altogether missing the underlying predisposition, the inborn vulnerability, that is the actual cause. If this sort of underlying vulnerability explains why some people are vulnerable to conditioning and others are not, then most insomnia is, strictly speaking, *idiopathic,* of origins unknown.

The kind nobody's looking at.

All in the Family

I met a woman on a plane who told me, in no uncertain terms, that her son was "born insomniac." When I told her that I was on my way to a conference in search of information about insomnia, she said, "Oh, you should talk to my son, he's always had problems sleeping."

"What do you think it's from?"

"The womb," she said, patting her stomach. "He came out that way. He never slept as a baby. I have five children, he's the middle, he's the only one like this."

I hear stories of restlessness that, mothers swear, began in the womb:

My mother used to say I kicked so much I kept her awake before I was even born, whereas my brother never gave her this kind of trouble; he slept before he was born and he's slept ever since. She said she could never get me to sleep for more than two hours at a time, and I still to this day can't sleep more than two hours at a time.

Is insomnia heritable? To hear people talk, you'd think it so. In *Sleep Demons: An Insomniac's Memoir,* Bill Hayes speculates about "an insomnia gene":

> I grew up in a family where the question "How'd you sleep?" was a topic of genuine reflection at the breakfast table. My five sisters and I each rated the last night's particular qualities. . . . If there's such a thing as an insomnia gene, Dad passed it on to me, along with his green eyes and Irish melancholy.

Anecdotal evidence suggests that insomniac parents have insomniac children, and insomniac children have insomniac parents. On the Web, I read things like this: *I've had it since I was a kid, and everyone in my family suffered from it: i.e., mother, grandmother, aunt, my children and great grandparents.* My student Tiffany told me, *I got it from my mother. She was always up at night, batting around the house. I guess I just got up, too.*

None of this tells us whether the problem is "in the genes" or in familial influences. But I come across fascinating accounts from people who did not grow up together, like Bonnie, the woman quoted in the epigraph of this chapter, who met her cousin late in life and discovered that her "sleep thing" was "broken," too. Or like this:

> *Everyone in my family has insomnia, mom, dad, two brothers and a sister. The funny thing is I have a brother I just found out about—my mother got pregnant while she and my dad were still students and they put him up for adoption—I just met him last year, and he has insomnia too.*

The DSM-IV acknowledges that "the predisposition to light and disrupted sleep has a familial association." I find only three familial studies of insomnia—and all three strongly suggest such an association. A 2000 study found that 35 percent of primary insomniacs (of the 285 evaluated) had a positive family history of sleep disturbances, "and the mother was the more frequently afflicted family member." A study done a few years later by some of the same researchers found a higher incidence, 72.7 percent of 77 primary insomniacs. In both studies, the mother is the family member most frequently affected, and in both studies, when the insomnia is familial, it tends to come on earlier and not to be "psychiatric." These findings are suggestive, though they still do not tell us whether the family influence is genetic or environmental. Genetic studies are needed to do that.

"The sleep disorders field is a bit late in doing genetic studies," says Emmanuel Mignot, the Stanford researcher who isolated the gene for canine narcolepsy. "Other fields have done much more." But it is moving fast. Mignot traced canine narcolepsy to a single mutation that renders the receptor for hypocretin nonfunctional. Narcolepsy in humans is not so simple. It may run in families, but it usually does not; it doesn't come on until the second or third decade of a person's life, and even when an identical twin is affected, the other twin, in 75 percent of the cases, is not. Researchers think that several genes may contribute to susceptibility, but the disorder also needs an environmental trigger. Researchers speculate that an autoimmune process may cause degeneration of the hypocretin-containing neurons in the hypothalamus, mimicking alterations caused by mutations.

Fatal familial insomnia is the first sleep disorder for which a gene was identified. This is a rare neurodegenerative disease (about sixty cases worldwide) which is, as the name says, familial, and is also, as the name says, fatal. With other sleep disorders, like sleepwalking and sleep-talking, familial evidence is arrived at by family histories. "If you have two parents who sleepwalk, there's a 60 percent chance that you will too," says Clete Kushida, director of the Stanford University Center for Human Sleep Research. Between a third and a half of all cases of restless legs syndrome, the creepy-crawly feeling that creates a desire to move the legs, "are of the hereditary type," reports Mignot; there is "a high concordance in identical twins, though research is only just beginning to establish a genetic pathway for the disease." Even apnea has a hereditary component, through obesity and bone anatomy.

Normal sleep patterns also turn out to be heritable, so much so that researchers refer to them as *traits,* inborn and consistent across time (like height or eye color), rather than *states,* which change in response to environmental influences. The first recordings of twins' EEGs, in 1966, found that the sequence of sleep stages of identical twins was almost completely concordant. Large-scale studies of twins have found that identical twins, even when not raised together, have sleep patterns more similar to one another than do nonidentical twins or other sibling pairs, in terms of bedtime, length of sleep, and *quality* of sleep. (Identical twins are genetically indistinguishable, whereas fraternal twins are no more alike genetically than other pairs of siblings.) A study of all adult twins enrolled in the Australian Twin Registry, nearly four thousand pairs, discovered that "the time at which an individual chooses to go to bed or to sleep, how frequently he or she takes naps during the day, and how long the individual sleeps at night are all influenced by that individual's genotype." Andrew Heath, lead researcher on the study, found that genetic influences even have a major impact on how well people *think* they sleep, "accounting for between 33–46% of the variance" in subjective sleep quality.

Belgian researcher Paul Linkowski studied twenty-six pairs of twins who did not live together, both identical and fraternal, and concluded that "genetic influences substantially determine" the variances and intensity of deep sleep, as well as "total waking time during the night." Linkowski estimates that the heritability of deep sleep is around 50 percent, "higher than for most human traits." This is important, since deep sleep is thought to be key to the homeostatic sleep drive—to sleep pressure—which is crucial to how well we sleep. These findings suggest that the curtain that comes down on Bob but not on me may be "in the genes." In fact, Bob's father was a very good sleeper who slept long and well through his late eighties. Neither of my parents, nobody in my family, slept like that; they weren't insomniacs, but they weren't gifted sleepers.

What are the molecular mechanisms, the genetic pathways, for this heritability? Work on this is in its infancy, but caffeine sensitivity may hold some clues. Caffeine sensitivity is highly variable: some people can drink a double espresso after dinner and fall soundly asleep, while others are kept awake if they eat one too many chocolate chip cookies. Family studies have found that caffeine response is more similar in identical than fraternal twins, and a study published by Swiss researchers in 2005 may tell us why. Caffeine works, as we saw, by blocking the action of adenosine, a neurotransmitter associated with the buildup of sleep pressure. The longer we're awake, the more adenosine accumulates, and the sleepier we get: then, during the course of sleep, it dissipates, and we wake up. Adenosine dissipates because an enzyme called *adenosine deaminase* (ADA) breaks it down. A team of researchers in Zurich compared subjects who had a normal gene encoding the ADA enzyme with those who had a variant gene that processes adenosine more slowly. They found that those who had the variant which made them less effective at breaking down adenosine had more deep sleep and fewer awakenings than those with the normal gene. "It seems that when this enzyme is inhibited, people have more deep and intense sleep," says Hans-Peter Landolt, a researcher on this study. "About ten percent of people have inherited the genetic variation from one of their parents," he explains. These are the genetically favored, the gifted sleepers, the people who can drink a double espresso and fall soundly asleep.

This study is tremendously exciting, the first to demonstrate the way a genetic variability may be linked to quality and depth of sleep. It's a discovery that could lead to therapeutic intervention: "For certain sleep disorders such as insomnia," says Landolt, "it may be possible to manipulate the adenosine system and inhibit the enzyme to enable people to have more deep and intense sleep."

It is likely that there are genes related to the processing of other sleep substances that are similarly involved in the amount and intensity of deep sleep. A 2002 study that found a mutation in the structure of a GABAa receptor (protein beta3) in a chronic insomniac points to this possibility. "It is very tempting to hypothesize the existence of a link" between the mutation and the insomnia, concludes the study. This could be exciting, as exciting as the discovery about hypocretin and narcolepsy, but when I asked one of the researchers if they'd followed it up, he told me that the rest of the family had refused to be tested. "As a result, we abandoned this project."

Why isn't everybody all over this—finding other families, doing this kind of genetic analyses?

More is known about the genes that regulate the timing of sleep than about those that govern sleep pressure. Circadian genes (called *clock, tim,* and *per*) have been identified that regulate various aspects of our biological clocks. A 1998 study by Mignot and other Stanford researchers found a variant on the clock gene that is associated with a preference for morningness or eveningness. A team of researchers looked at three generations of a family, daughter, mother, and grandmother, who got up and went to bed extremely early *(advanced sleep phase syndrome)*, and found that their DNA had a mutation of the per gene similar to that associated with early waking in fruit flies and mice. The study is "convincing evidence that a circadian sleep disorder, previously thought to be a product of habits or environment, has a genetic basis," commented David White, director of the sleep disorders program at Brigham and Women's Hospital in Boston. Since this problem affects about a third of the elderly, it could be that the gene functioning is affected by the aging process, said Louis Ptacek, one of the study's authors, who thinks this gives us clues that might be important.

British researchers in 2003 found that night owls and early birds also carry different versions of the per gene. "We discovered that the shorter variant of the gene is significantly more common in people with an extreme evening preference. This is even more so in patients suffering from delayed sleep phase syndrome, a sleep disorder where people fall asleep at very late times and have difficulty waking up in the morning," says Simon Archer of the University of Surrey, one of the British researchers.

Researchers are coming to see that how well and deeply we sleep, how long we take to get to sleep, how often we wake during the night, the time of night we're inclined to sleep are all affected by heredity. Early risers and late sleepers, like long sleepers and short sleepers, like good sleepers—and bad sleepers—appear to be "born" as much as, perhaps even more than, "made." Even our dreams may be genetically influenced. A twin study found that "if one identical twin had frequent nightmares then the other twin had a 45 per cent chance of suffering too, whereas with nonidentical twins there was only a 20 per cent chance." Michel Jouvet tells an intriguing story of how, when he'd been speaking about dreams at a conference, a colleague came up to him and told him the following: " 'When I was a child . . . I often had the same dream: I was passing in front of a big house and I saw a lady dressed in black opening the door of a long corridor.' Just at that moment, his twin brother, his spitting image, came up to us and heard the last few words of the story, which he went on to complete spontaneously: 'The lady opened the door of the corridor and hundreds of cats ran out.' His brother . . . looked at him in great surprise. 'How could you have finished my dream? I never told you about it.' These twins had had the same dream."

One of the most fascinating interviews I had was with Mike Young, head of the Laboratory of Genetics at Rockefeller Institute, who has been studying the per and tim genes in fruit flies. What Young has seen of the influence of genetic mutations on sleep behavior has made him question his earlier beliefs about how much control we have over sleep behaviors. "I used to think, when I encountered someone who couldn't sleep through the night, well, you just need to learn to control your life a little better, drink less or something, and your sleep will improve. But now I see there could be a hereditary component to a lot of this." "If the overall shape of human sleep-wake behavior is so deeply carved by our genes," he writes, then sleep behaviors may not "prove to be a simple matter of self-discipline." Rather, "variations in human wake-sleep behaviour" may be as "genetically determined" as "differences in hair or eye color."

Will insomnia turn out to be a "genetic" disease? Not in the simple sense, of a mutation on a single gene, as in the case of Huntington's or cystic fibrosis. There is one kind of insomnia that might be this simple: when

a person with delayed sleep phase syndrome, who's genetically programmed to get up late, gets caught in an early-bird schedule—and it's
difficult not to, in a world where the early birds make the rules—the mismatch might result in full-blown insomnia, producing dysfunctional habits
and attitudes and all the rest. (*If only I could sleep when my body wanted
to, from 5 A.M. till noon,* is a lament heard from more than one insomniac.) Most people are able to adjust, without too much trouble, to earlier or later schedules, but for the 10 percent who are extreme owls and
the 10 percent who are extreme larks, changing sleep patterns may be
"like changing your height or eye color," says Minneapolis sleep researcher Mark Mahowald.

But sleep is a complex behavior governed by a multiplicity of genes,
each contributing some small part, some to the timing and some to the
sleep pressure, some that are known and many that remain undiscovered. A predisposition to insomnia might involve genes that influence,
say, the sensitivity of the GABA receptors or the action of adenosine, or
genes that set the speed of the metabolism or affect parts of the sleep-
wake system we know nothing about, each making its own contribution,
each interacting with and influenced by environmental factors. Insomnia
is—as we see again and again—multifactorial, created by a variety of factors. Patterns of genes are important, as is gene-gene interaction and the
interaction of genes with influences such as diet, family, society, culture,
stress, for genes take their cues from—are expressed in response to—
environments that determine which genes get switched off and which
come into play. The old dichotomy of nature versus nurture is, as Matt
Ridley says, "a false dichotomy. It's not nature versus nurture, but nature *via* nurture."

Some insomniacs are unhappy with *all this talk about genes. If it's all
in my genes, it makes me a victim. That's a fatalistic point of view, like
my father was an alcoholic so I'll be an alcoholic too. I have to hope I
can do something to change it.* But most sleep genes make a predisposition, a vulnerability, not a fated path. I myself find it reassuring to know
my vulnerabilities, to know that there may be a physiological explanation for something so basic to my behavior, something I've had to apol-
ogize for all my life. Knowing one's genetic disposition is not a license for
irresponsibility: in fact, the more genetically susceptible we are, the more
careful we have to be. But knowing what we are puts us in a better position to make choices, insofar as our circumstances allow us choices, to
work out a way of living that's in accord with who we are, not at war
with who we are.

Other Ways of Looking In: Brain Scans

"The field of sleep disorders medicine lags behind other areas of medical research in the utilization of neuroimaging," says Eric Nofzinger, head of the Sleep Neuroimaging Research Program, University of Pittsburgh School of Medicine. Brain scans are difficult to do with sleep, which is, as we saw, a process diffused throughout the brain. As Nofzinger explains, "Sleep is a moving target. You need to know what you're looking for. You need to know which structures are involved in sleep regulation and in sleep disorders, so you know where to look. You need to know when to image them, what time of day or night. And it's important to choose a method that maintains, as closely as possible, the integrity of sleep."

The technology best suited to scanning over time is the fMRI *(functional magnetic resonance imaging)*, which creates a picture of living brain tissue by detecting minute magnetic fields around the cells. Functional MRI differs from structural MRI in that it gives a quick succession of images, like the frames of a movie. Whereas a structural MRI gives a static picture and is used to find structural, anatomical problems such as tumors or strokes, the fMRI can show how brain activity changes over time and how it changes during tasks. It shows how things *function.* "You can scan serially across the nighttime, get a moving picture of what's happening in the brain, how things are evolving, or not evolving, in the case of insomniacs," says Nofzinger. "But just try to get an insomniac to sleep in a scanner; their heads have to be immobilized and the magnet makes a loud clanging sound like a jackhammer." So the method he and his colleagues prefer is a type of *PET scan* (positron-emission tomography), where subjects can sleep without having their heads immobilized. Subjects are hooked up to an EEG so you know what stage of sleep they're in; a radio isotope is injected, through an intravenous tube, when they're at the stage of sleep you want to look at; the isotope becomes irretrievably embedded in the cells. Then the sleeper is awakened, put in a scanner, and the image is taken, showing what was going on at the time of injection.

What neuroimaging measures is glucose metabolism: as neurons in an area of the brain become more active, blood flow increases to that area to supply it with blood sugar, or glucose, for energy. PET scans show that in normal sleep there is a general decrease of activity across the brain. "Whole-brain glucose metabolism declines significantly (about 20 percent) from waking to NREM sleep, with most [of the] decrease in frontal

cortex regions, as the executive functions that keep us awake and functioning go off line." Activity also slows down in the thalamus, the gate
to the outside world, and in the brainstem, as the arousal systems cen-
tered there quiet down. But with insomniacs, "there's a lot less deacti-
vation," says Nofzinger, not only over the brain as a whole but in sleep
and wake-promoting areas—the hypothalamus, the thalamus, and the
frontal cortex.

"Insomniacs complain that their brains don't shut down, and they're
right," says Nofzinger: their scans show brains "lit up like a Christmas
tree." What's especially interesting is that Nofzinger's subjects had EEGs
that showed "normal" sleep—which suggests that the EEG doesn't pick
up all that's going on (more on this later). As for next-day effects, "waking scans of insomniacs' brains show lower metabolic activity over the entire prefrontal cortex," the area linked with executive function—the part
that's been perking away all night. Decreased activity in the frontal cortex is a sign of fatigue, as James Horne has shown: when healthy subjects
are deprived of sleep, this is the area that's most affected. Brain scans,
then, confirm the subjective sense insomniacs have, that they're tired during the day and wired at night—there's an *on switch that doesn't switch
off, an off switch that doesn't switch on, something wrong with the wiring,
something that just doesn't go off line* (these are the terms I hear).

But the question always arises, where is this activity coming from?
You could read the hyperactivity as a consequence of conditioned anxiety about sleep, as the behavioral-modification proponents explain it. Or
you could hold off assigning causality at this time because, as Nofzinger
says, there may be "some complex neuronal pathway that has at its core
some alteration in a collection of neurons in a small brain structure that
cannot be detected by the imaging study." Perhaps, as he speculates,
"there's an abnormality at the level of the brainstem that's genetically
hardwired differently, which, if you had a higher resolution, you could
see. Our methods are still pretty gross."

One cluster of neurons that neuroimaging does not pick up is the *ventrolateral preoptic nucleus,* "the sleep switch." That's sort of important.

Where We Are

When I asked Allan Rechtschaffen if he thought insomnia might be a
defect in the sleep system, he said, "There probably is some defect in the
sleep mechanisms—we have defects in every other kind of system, so why

not this?" But, he cautioned, "these mechanisms are so fantastically complex and so deep within the brain, how would you go about establishing if there's a problem with this or that part, or a problem with the way the parts go together, the coordinating activity? How would you know?"

Might insomniacs have too few GABA-generating neurons to flip the sleep switch or to hold it in position once it's flipped? Might we have defective GABA receptors, or too few of them? Might we have too many hypocretin neurons or neurons that fire too rapidly, producing an overactivity in those arousal circuits? Might there be other neurotransmitter systems and neural circuits we know nothing about? Mignot thinks so: "The discovery of hypocretin was good," he told me, "but there are other systems in there waiting to be identified."

When I asked Mignot why nobody was doing postmortems of insomniacs' brains, he said, "We wouldn't know where to look or what to look for. Oh, maybe if you were looking in the right place, if you had thousands of brains, you might find something, but now, with our present state of knowledge—no, I would not put money into a brain bank." Yet it was the postmortem studies he did of the brains of narcoleptics that found the deficiency in their hypocretin-producing centers. It was postmortem studies of restless legs syndrome patients that revealed a decrease of iron in parts of their brains. It was postmortem examinations of brains of Parkinson's disease patients that revealed a deficiency in the dopamine-producing centers (here, too, we see how damage to a tiny part of the brain has consequences huge and devastating to the individual). "National, NIH-supported brain tissue banks are well established and have proven vital to the success of human brain research in neurodegenerative disorders such as Alzheimer's disease and genetic disorders such as Rett syndrome," says the 2003 *National Sleep Disorders Research Plan*. But "an informal survey of national brain tissue banks reveals virtually no accrual of brains from patients with primary sleep disorders."

"I'd donate mine, if I knew where to leave it," I told Michael Bonnet, who gave me an odd look, then said something like what Mignot had told me: "We wouldn't know where to look—so I wouldn't go volunteering yours just yet."

"Well, I don't mean *yet*. I meant when I'm finished with it."

It says something about the present state of knowledge that researchers not only lack the tools to look, they don't yet know *where* to look. "Basically," says Bonnet, "we're going in the dark. We need a new measure or way of looking at sleep. I don't think it will be soon—these shifts don't happen too often. Sleep science is still in its infancy. It's amazing how rapidly it's advanced; it's all happened within my lifetime. What we do is real, but it's still not enough. We need a paradigm shift."

When Hauri told me the parable of the man searching for his wallet under the lamppost not because that's where he'd lost it but because that's where the light was best, he added, "We can only look where there is light. At this point, we might not be able to look where we want to see. Until we get some new research tools, there is still much that is not known about the brain, or the human."

CHAPTER 6

Sleep, Stress, and Stages of Life

I feel like a car whose idling point is set too high, like the engine's revving, racing.

My doctors say, "It's stress related, you're such a busy person." Don't give me that! I am a busy person. I have a happy life. I have what I want. What I need is sleep!

In the last chapter, we considered that what goes wrong in the brain of an insomniac might be a weak or defective mechanism in the sleep system. In this chapter, we'll look at ways the problem might be on the other side of the push-pull mechanism, in a stress system that's overly active or on hyperalert.

When scientists speak of the *stress system,* they mean something different from what most of us mean when we speak of *stress.* We usually use the word to mean some worry or upset that's caused by a stressful event or situation, an external pressure that makes us *distressed* or *stressed out,* like the loss of a marriage or a job, or being trapped in a marriage or job. But in scientific terms, the stress system refers to the body's mechanisms for mobilizing us for exertion of any sort, whether it's sprinting from a mugger or getting out of bed mornings.

The stress system is strong. It had to be strong for us to survive. It works within seconds, sending its signals along our nerves and through our blood, speeding our metabolisms and hearts, raising temperature. Faster metabolism, higher temperature and blood pressure, elevated levels of stress hormones are sometimes seen in insomniacs. Therefore it's been concluded that insomnia is caused by an arousal system that's hyped up, and methods of "managing" insomnia—behavioral modification, pharmaceuticals, and psychotherapy—aim at damping this system down. This is where "the light is best."

Hyperarousal

I first come across the idea of *hyperarousal* in a 1967 paper by Lawrence Monroe, one of Nathaniel Kleitman's students at the University of Chicago, where sleep science began. Monroe's study, "Psychological and Physiological Differences between Good and Poor Sleepers," is a classic, referred to by many subsequent researchers. Monroe compares a group of good sleepers to a group of poor sleepers and finds that the poor sleepers are *physiologically* closer to a waking state than the good sleepers: they have more body movements, faster heart rates, and consistently higher temperatures. Temperature needs to decline in order for sleep to be initiated and maintained. Whereas with good sleepers, temperature declines at sleep onset, falls to a nadir in the early hours of the morning, and begins to rise a few hours before waking, with poor sleepers, it remains generally higher through the night, declines more slowly, and continues to fall even through the time the good sleepers are waking up. Poor sleepers rarely rise and shine.

The personality tests Monroe gave his subjects indicate that the poor sleepers are more anxious, introverted, and hypochondriac than the good sleepers, so he concludes that their physiological hyperarousal is caused by psychological upset—they are emotionally roiled up, they have "adjustment problems." Whether they might be troubled and anxious *because* they can't sleep, whether their temperature might be higher because some thermoregulatory mechanism is out of whack—dysregulated, perhaps, by their poor sleep, since frequent awakenings raise body temperature—are not questions Monroe asked. The mind-set of the time wouldn't have encouraged him to ask. As a psychologist at a time when Freudian ideas still held sway, he assumed that the physiological activation he found in poor sleepers was due to psychopathology.

Nearly everybody who comes after Monroe accepts this explanation. Insomniacs, it is said, have higher body temperature, faster heart rate and metabolism, because they are emotionally or cognitively aroused: they worry too much, they're upset, anxious or depressed, and/or they have poor coping mechanisms.

But Michael Bonnet, a sleep researcher at the Dayton Veterans' Administration facility, presents an opposing view. He and his coauthor (and wife) Donna Arand have done dozens of studies of hyperarousal and are convinced that "poor sleep . . . is a physiological (as opposed to a psychological) event." Their studies find that people with primary insomnia have higher body temperatures, faster heart rates, and elevated metabolic rates (oxygen consumption) throughout the night and day, which suggests that hyperarousal is a twenty-four-hour problem; but they feel that "physiological factors are equally or more important than behavioral factors." In one study, he and Arand reproduced the symptoms of hyperarousal in young healthy subjects merely by giving them the equivalent of a few cups of coffee three times a day, the last time just before sleep. Caffeine speeds the heart, raises blood pressure, respiratory rate, metabolic rate, and stimulates the secretion of stress hormones. After a week of "caffeine-degraded sleep," the researchers began to see personality changes, an increase in "fatigue, confusion, anger, and depression," as Minnesota Multiphasic Personality Inventory (MMPI) values "moved in the pathological direction." They concluded that "personality types common in insomnia can develop *as a function of hyperarousal rather than causing hyperarousal*" (my emphasis). Now when Bonnet finds "more pathological [MMPI] personality profiles" in insomniacs, he's inclined to see them as an effect rather than a cause of physiological arousal. Insomnia, he says, has been "treated behaviorally in part because it hasn't been possible to identify a clear physiological disease entity."

I interviewed Bonnet at the Dayton Veterans' Administration facility, an extraordinary complex of porticoed and columned buildings spread out over acres of rolling lawn (it was built, Bonnet told me, during the Civil War—"when they had land"). Bonnet, a tall, thin, nice-looking young man, boyish though slightly balding, showed me into a sleep lab filled with computers and pieces of equipment I couldn't begin to identify; in an office stacked high with books and papers, we sat and talked. When I asked if he really is the lone voice I sense he is, he nodded, and sighed. "The hyperarousal stuff is pretty well accepted, but the idea that hyperarousal indicates real physiological changes in the brain is less well accepted."

I asked him what drew him to study insomnia, if he had sleep problems himself, and he laughed.

No, far from it. Actually, I was interested in sleep deprivation. Early on, I did a study that looked at whether people with insomnia were sleep-deprived. I was amazed. You'd think insomniacs would show symptoms of sleep deprivation, but they don't. When you deprive normal sleepers of sleep by frequent awakenings, they become basically nonfunctional. Not so with insomniacs: they show less daytime sleepiness; they don't act or test sleep-deprived. The question is, why not? So I thought, there must be another dimension here. I think they're held together by this arousal system. They're geared up, compared to those without it.

The symptoms of hyperarousal that he and other researchers are finding in insomniacs—elevated body temperature and levels of stress hormones, faster metabolic rate—are signs of a stress system under duress. When a person is faced with challenge, the *sympathetic nervous system* goes into action: the hypothalamus sends signals to sympathetic nerve endings throughout the body, which secrete *epinephrine (adrenaline)*, which primes the body for fight or flight. This is the first line of defense, and it works within seconds, along the nerves, to step up heart rate and breathing and constrict the blood vessels in the skin (which is what makes the hair stand on end). The second line of defense works within minutes, through the blood: the hypothalamus alerts the pituitary, which alerts the adrenals, small glands that sit on top of each kidney, to pour out cortisol, in what is called the *hypothalamic-pituitary-adrenal axis* (the HPA). These chemical messengers, *corticosteroids* or *glucocorticoid*s (I'll call them stress hormones), remain in the bloodstream longer than adrenaline and have more lasting effects.

The HPA axis and the sympathetic nervous system are the twin limbs of the stress system, working in tandem to prime us for challenge. (Bear with me here—this is important.) The *sympathetic nervous system* powers us up, steps up heart rate and breathing, and the *parasympathetic* calms us down, restoring the heart rate to normal and slowing breathing back down. The *vagal brake,* a nerve that connects the brainstem with the heart, slows the heart rate when the stimulus has passed; when it loses tone or effectiveness, heart rate and blood pressure remain elevated, and we stay primed. As we grow older we become "more sympathetic," as Bonnet says, which does not, unfortunately, mean that we become more compassionate, but that the sympathetic nervous system becomes more activated, levels of stress hormones go up, and the parasympathetic nervous system becomes less effective at calming the activation down. "Old individuals of all sorts tend to have the stress response turned on even when nothing stressful is happening," says Robert Sapolsky, author of *Why Zebras Don't Get Ulcers,* one of the best books on stress (the other is Bruce McEwen's *The End of Stress*).

Sleep requires that sympathetic nervous tension be relaxed and the parasympathetic system become dominant: if this shift doesn't happen, neither does sleep. And the shift doesn't happen easily in insomniacs. "Insomniacs have both increased sympathetic nervous system activity and decreased parasympathetic nervous system activity throughout all stages of sleep," as Bonnet and others have found. When Alexandros Vgontzas and his colleagues measured the cortisol levels of chronic insomniacs, they found that "the activity of both limbs of the stress system . . . appears to be directly proportional to the degree of sleep disturbance," and that higher levels of cortisol persist through the day. Some insomniacs have stress systems that are as activated as those of patients with *Cushing's disease,* a condition in which tumors in the pituitary or adrenals cause excessive production of cortisol. If you expose an insomniac to stress, the heart rate takes longer to return to normal, evidence of a vagal brake that's less effective at slowing it back down. If you make insomniacs exercise, their heart rate and temperature are slower to decline than those of good sleepers. If you tell a group of insomniacs and a group of normal sleepers that they have to give a speech the next morning, the insomniacs have a greater increase in norepinephrine excretion for twenty-four hours—and even on the following night, they have significant sleep disturbance.

"The problem," says Bonnet, "is that none of this tells us where the arousal is coming from. Faster heart rate, higher metabolism, stress hormones, can be caused by lots of things." Bonnet and Arand think there's a physiological basis; behaviorists think the cause is conditioned behavior; Vgontzas says that what insomniacs need is a good psychiatrist. Edward Stepanski says we don't know enough to know: "Whether the increased arousal observed in insomnia patients originates as a physiologic, cognitive, or emotional abnormality, it cannot be determined from the current research."

"A further problem," says Bonnet, "is that hyperarousal is not at this point diagnostically useful. No one of these characteristics—rapid heart rate, elevated temperature—is present in each and every insomniac. So you can't use it as a marker, proof positive identification of an insomniac. You can't use it as a diagnostic tool. No, you need to go to the next step, to devise an objective test with meaningful norms that allows identification and treatment of patients. You need to find something measurable."

All we can say at this point is that some of these characteristics are present in some—many—most?—insomniacs.

Stress-Scarred

Hyperarousal looks and acts like a stress system that's lost its *resiliency,* that's stuck in the on position. When stress goes on too long, the system loses its ability to recover from stimulus and return to normal. (Picture a stretched-out old rubber band that's lost its ability to bounce back.)

Resiliency of the stress system is not something we want to lose: it determines how well we respond to challenge, how we weather the storms and vicissitudes of life. We lose it in the natural course of aging, in any case (women faster than men, according to one study). Levels of stress hormones go up and up, the sympathetic nervous system remains activated, and the parasympathetic system loses its ability to calm it back down, which leaves us more vulnerable to subsequent stressors, more reactive to even relatively mild stressors, physiologically and psychologically keyed to overreact. When the stress system loses its ability to bounce back, so do we. Stress is no longer simple and external, such that, when we remove the stressor, the problem goes away; it has taken up residence within our system, altered our neuroendocrinology, left us with what one researcher calls a "neurobiological scar."

Early abuse or neglect may leave such scars. Studies of women who've experienced childhood sexual abuse and people with posttraumatic stress disorder find that they have persistently activated HPA systems and high levels of cortisol (a condition called *hypercortisolism*). Such changes are found in rats who've experienced maternal neglect. They're even found in rats exposed to prenatal stress. They are also found in people with major depression, but there's an important difference between them and insomniacs: they have elevated levels of cortisol but not of norepinephrine (in fact they have depleted levels of norepinephrine), while insomniacs have elevated levels of both. "This suggests," as Bonnet says, "that there really is a difference between insomnia and depression—which not everyone is willing to grant."

Is this what's gone wrong with insomniacs, that we have more early or prolonged exposure to stress than other people? We've been psychologically or physically abused or neglected, or made to feel unsafe for extended periods of time, and this has put us on permanent alert? I find surprisingly few studies that ask the question whether insomniacs have more stress in their childhoods than other people do. It would be easy enough to ask us, but researchers shy away from studies that depend on subjects' memories. A more reliable study design would be to take a bunch of healthy people, find a way of objectively recording when they're being exposed to stressors, follow them for a few decades, and see what happens to their sleep. But *longitudinal* studies (as these are called) are costly and time-consuming, and have not been done with insomnia.

Anecdotal evidence suggests that some insomniacs have stress in their backgrounds and some do not. With some, the connection between early trauma and insomnia is all too clear.

He [an uncle] came into my room every night, or at least it seemed like every night, I must have been 6, 7, 8, I lay waiting for him to come, I was petrified. I have never slept since. I can't feel safe in a bed, I can't stand anyone to touch me. I've had fibromyalgia, Graves' disease, and bad bouts with depression, and have tried every sedative and antidepressant known to man.

And this from writer Aminatta Forner:

For as long as I can remember I had a strained and somewhat tenuous relationship with sleep. . . . I grew to be afraid of the dark. We lived in West Africa. My father was an opposition politician and sometime political prisoner. . . .

As an adult I dislike sleeping in a house on my own. I will sit in front of the fuzzy, comforting light of the television for as long as possible, just to avoid going upstairs into the dark.

On the other hand, Romanian writer E. M. Cioran, whose insomnia drove him to the brink of suicide, had an idyllic childhood. So did my friend Roberta. So did Jacqueline: *Absolutely nothing to account for it,* as she says, *except the genetic.*

I know two women who were sexually abused as children: one sleeps, the other doesn't. Of people who experience traumatic events, only 20 to 30 percent suffer long-term effects from them. Why are some people devastated by the sorts of experiences others sail through unscathed—what makes the difference? Why "different individuals respond differently to ostensibly the same stimulus" is, as a 1998 study says, "arguably the most important question in behavioral research."

We seem to be born with different susceptibilities to stress, with systems that make us more or less reactive to stressors, more or less vulnerable to the long-term ravages of stress, more or less "porous" to the arrows life slings our way. Some strains of mice and rats are more easily fear-conditioned by exposure to foot shocks than others are—and the strains which are more easily conditioned show greater sleep disturbances. "Different strains of mice, different strains of us," as Daniel Buysse says.

The genetic determinants for such differences in humans are not yet known, though a fascinating study published in 2003 suggests a possibility. Researchers followed 847 New Zealanders from birth to age twenty-six, some of whom carried two copies of the short variant of the 5-HTT gene, some of whom had two copies of the long variant, some of whom had one of each. (The long variant of this gene makes more serotonin available, the short variant, less. The 5-HTT gene, which determines how our cells manage serotonin, has been a focus of depression research since serotonin has been recognized as being key to depression.) The researchers tracked subjects' exposure to events such as sexual and physical abuse, long-term unemployment, money troubles, difficulties with relationships, over the course of twenty-six years. Those who had two copies of the long gene had the most emotional resilience: whether they'd been severely mistreated in early childhood or endured financial losses or ill health, they did not become depressed. Those with one long and one short version were "moderately vulnerable to depression." Those with two copies of the short variant were much more likely to develop depression. (This is what's known as getting "the short end" of the gene.) Depression is, of course, no more determined by one gene than insomnia is, but this finding may help explain why some people are so badly clobbered by events that barely faze others.

Bonnet speculates that hyperarousal "is genetic—and it's situational." He describes it as "a higher set point that could be genetic or induced." Metabolism and blood pressure are heritable; so are patterns of cortisol release (these are more similar in identical than fraternal twins); therefore, hyperarousal is likely to be heritable, so "insomnia might be a heritable trait." But genetic studies need to be done before this can be more than speculation.

"The set point of the HPA axis is genetically determined," write O. Van Reeth and colleagues, "but can be modulated and reset to other levels by early or later stressful experiences." But what about those insomniacs who have no stressful experiences in their childhoods that would reset the stress system, yet whose stress systems nevertheless seem to bear the scars of stress exposure, to be set on permanent alert?

What chronic insomniacs all have a lot of, in our past and present experience, is sleepless nights. Whatever else is going on in our lives, this is going on: we are dealing, on a daily basis, with broken, fragmented, barely adequate sleep. We are dealing on a daily basis with a powerful stressor. When sleep is disturbed, each awakening triggers a pulse of cortisol secretion, and the more sleep is disturbed, the more activated the stress system becomes, and the cortisol levels go up, up, up. Sleep disturbance not only raises the levels of stress hormones, it keeps them elevated even during the parts of sleep when the stress system is supposed to be quiet. Cortisol is timed by the circadian clock to be highest in the early morning and to decline throughout the day, to reach a low point in the late evening and be lowest in the early part of sleep, during deep sleep. But after a sleep-deprived night, cortisol levels remain high not only into the next day but into the next evening and into the first few hours of sleep.

Thus sleep deprivation not only stimulates the stress response, it impairs its resiliency, its ability to return to normal. Spiegel and her colleagues found, when they produced elevated cortisol levels in young, healthy males by curtailing their sleep for only six nights, that "sleep loss, even partial, appears to delay the normal return to evening quiescence" and to affect "the rate of recovery of the HPA axis in response to a challenge." They described "a feed-forward cascade of negative effects," a vicious circle wherein increased exposure to stress hormones impairs the resiliency of the stress response, stress hormones go up, and the resiliency of the system is further impaired. "These observations challenge the common belief that, on the day following a night of partial or total sleep deprivation, the primary effects of sleep loss are behavioral, rather than physiological," conclude Van Cauter and Spiegel. "It is possible," says Van Cauter, "that the elevated evening and nocturnal cortisol levels occurring in insomniacs reflect the impact of partial sleep loss." And these are young, healthy males the researchers are looking at, not your typical insomniac, who is more likely to be female and therefore more clobbered by sleep loss, more likely to be elderly and therefore more vulnerable to all types of stressors, and perhaps not at the peak of health and therefore more vulnerable generally—and who is almost certainly not going to get the good stretches of recuperative sleep necessary to quiet the system back down.

This is a vicious circle in which sleep disruption begets further sleep disruption. It's especially vicious when you realize that elevated levels of cortisol damage the part of the brain that regulates the delicate feedback loop that dampens down the cortisol release, the *hippocampus,* a part of the brain that's also crucial to certain kinds of memory. When the mechanism for countering the process is impaired, the process keeps accelerating, so the more cortisol we have, the more we'll keep on having more. No wonder that hyperarousal is "a twenty-four-hour condition," as Bonnet and others have found. Chronic insomnia is as potent a stressor as an unhappy job or a miserable marriage, as any of those pressure-cooker, no-exit, no-control-over situations that keep the stress hormones flowing and the system ratcheted up. Add to that the element of unpredictability that makes stressors more stressful, and insomniacs may not even need external stressors to keep us revved up: we carry with us our own built-in stress-producing mechanisms in our sleepless nights.

The DSM-IV describes the vicious circle of insomnia as a problem of attitudes, behavior, habits: "The more the individual strives to sleep, the more frustrated and distressed he or she becomes and the less . . . able to sleep." If you change the attitude, goes the thinking, you'll remove the stressor and the problem will go away. Hence that advice insomniacs often get: "Schedule time to relax. Calm down." But it's not just frustration and distress that's pushing the snowball these researchers are describing; it's physiological processes inscribed in our nerves and brains. As Bonnet says, "Your physiology changes and you're sort of trapped in it." Insomniacs may have trouble sleeping, then, not because we're upset or pressured or because we have bad attitudes and habits, but because we—well, because we sleep so badly. Chronic insomnia in itself may be sufficient to keep the system primed.

Even the racing minds that practically come with the territory of insomnia may be a function of altered physiology. In *Sleep Demons*, Bill Hayes describes lying awake when he was a boy, *my mind racing like the spell-check function on a computer, scanning all data, lighting on images, moments, fragments of conversation, impossible to turn off.* We are told our minds go racing because we have ruminative, obsessive, inward-looking personalities, or because there's too much stress in our lives. But what if our minds race because there's too much cortisol coursing through our systems? Caffeine, which sets the stress hormones flowing, can make this happen, as any of us knows who's crawled into bed at the end of an overcaffeinated day and laid there listening to the sound of our own wheels spinning. (In fact Hayes grew up in a family where Coke—which is full of caffeine—ran freely as water; his father headed a Coca-Cola bottling factory.)

The cortisol connection was driven home to me by Josh, a student who's had raging insomnia since he was put on the synthetic cortisol prednisone to keep his body from rejecting a transplanted kidney. (Cortisol is so effective an immune suppressor that a synthetic version, a steroid, is given to patients with organ transplants to keep their immune systems from rejecting the foreign body.) The one time I took prednisone, to damp down an overreaction to poison oak, it gave me insomnia a pill couldn't touch. I'd been told to take it for a week; I quit after a few days, deciding that I'd rather live with the rash than without sleep. Josh, who was going to have to be on this drug for life, pointed out philosophically that it was better to lose the sleep than lose the kidney, which he'd likely do without the drug. He described a sleep pattern like mine: *I get two hours of good sleep and then an additional two to four of just rolling around.* He described a racing mind: *When I get into bed I have [a] racing mind, not constructive thinking, just racing.* But Josh's mind hadn't gone racing before he had all this cortisol pumping through his system: *Nothing like this happened before the operation. I was never like this before.* It's true that he had gone through the traumatic event of a kidney transplant, but on the basis of what synthetic cortisol did to me, I'd say the drug alone was sufficient to bring on this response.

But you can't just say, "It's bad sleep that makes bad sleep," because it only seems to work that way with those of us who sleep badly. If you deprive normal sleepers of a good night's sleep, their sleep is usually better the next night. Something about our system is more reactive—and then the insomnia keeps on ratcheting it up. Maybe with some of us the reactivity is inborn, maybe with some it's been environmentally primed, and surely in all of us it's related to the cumulative effect of disturbed sleep. There are many routes to this place, and much that remains unknown.

When I hold up the idea of hyperarousal and look at it in relation to myself, I get a confusing picture. In ways it fits, in ways it does not. I'm not what you'd call "hyper." We all know people who have hummingbird metabolisms, who seem set to a higher register. I'm not one. Nor am I like the colleague I dine with who startles when a waiter across the room drops a tray, nor am I like the friend whose anxiety level is so wearing that I refuse to travel with her anymore. (Both these women sleep well.) I strike people as laid back. A friend tells me I have "great body calm" (we say things like this in California). Dentists tell me I'm a terrific patient (I see lots of dentists). I don't get particularly anxious about travel, except about morning flights. I don't get flapped about things other people get worked up about, though I'm sure I do get anxious about things others do not—I take things to heart, and I take on too much. My metabolism tends to be sluggish; I gain weight easily, and I'm always cold. I was the only kid on the block who didn't run around barefoot, my feet were too cold—and that was before Hashimoto's blitzed my thyroid. My body temperature is consistently low, and so is my blood pressure. Whenever somebody takes my blood pressure (it ranges between 109/71 and 98/58), they tell me how nice and relaxed I am. Actually on cold days, I feel barely alive.

When I took one of those tests where you spit into a wad of cotton four times a day and send the cotton off to a lab, it found that my cortisol levels are slightly elevated—though not as high as I expected—and interestingly skewed to the hours I keep, highest not at 6 A.M. but at 9 A.M. But my heart rate is faster than Bob's, and when I get up in the night to pee, my heart takes a long time to slow down. I can well believe that my vagal brake is stripped. And I do seem to be "held together" (Bonnet's term) by some sort of arousal system that kicks in on days I need to push myself through teaching, traveling, conferences on three to four hours' sleep. I seem to weather sleep loss better than Bob does, who wilts. I'm no better able than he is to do real mental work, days like this, and I'm usually in a lousy mood, but I seem to have this other gear to shift into, a kind of frenzied energy. I can't take the long naps he does to make up for lost sleep (though I can sometimes take a short pick-me-up nap); I can't imagine ever falling asleep at the wheel, though there are times I've dropped off in airport lounges—which suggests there's an element of will to it. Is it that I'm "held together" by this system, I wonder, or that I've learned to hold myself together with it? Sometimes it feels like I've learned to hold sleep loss the way a seasoned drinker holds booze.

But sleepstarved days, days I'm on overdrive, those are the days I feel like a bundle of nerves, when I really might startle if a waiter drops a tray. I sigh a lot, I mutter to myself, it all seems so overwhelming, my heart races and strains as though it has an appointment somewhere else. Those are the days Bob tells me, "Calm down." Those are the nights when I get into bed and the system keeps on whirring. If you met me on a day like this, you'd say, That's one hyperaroused insomniac. But I can tell you, sleep loss is a powerful element in this ratcheting up.

Stressful Times

Work, too, can be an element in the ratcheting up, when there's too much going on in my life. This is where the external stressors come in.

Everybody I know complains that they're working too hard, and most of us are. In the year 2000, Americans put in the equivalent of an extra forty-hour work week more than they did in 1990, contrary to the trend in Europe, where the work year has become shorter. Europeans shake their heads in wonder at the way we work. Whenever I hear Belgian researcher Eve Van Cauter speak at the conferences, she clucks her tongue. "It's extraordinary to be in a seminar like this and see people struggling to stay awake: the question is, why do we do it?" In Europe *burnout* is a medically recognized syndrome. It's a category in the *International Classification of Diseases,* where it's defined as "a state of vital exhaustion"; it's associated with disturbed sleep patterns, headaches, and hyperactivity of the stress system.

In the United States, burnout is not a medically recognized syndrome—even though 53 percent of American workers say that work leaves them "overtired and overwhelmed." The conditions of today's work world—the longer hours, the increased technological complexity of many kinds of work, the continual reorganization of workplaces, the mergers, acquisitions, downsizing, outsourcing—leave workers feeling barraged by forces over which they have no control. Twenty percent of American workers saw their jobs disappear during the 1980s, a trend that's been worsening each decade. "The hire-and-fire culture, rising unemployment, heavier workloads, more intense demands, generate a climate where people are feeling constantly under threat. . . . Companies today have become real stress-producing factories. It is no longer machines which break down. It is the workers themselves." "It used to be that as long as you did your work, you had a job," said a worker. "That's not for sure anymore. They expect the same production rates even though two guys are doing the work of three. . . . I swear I hear those machines humming in my sleep."

The work world is changing so rapidly that the conditions of my day, where you trained for one job and worked at it all your life, look as anachronistic as the typewriter I wrote my dissertation on. My students will not be able to count on becoming qualified for a single discipline that defines who they are and what they do their whole lives through. "We will need to reskill ourselves constantly every decade just to keep a job," says science writer James Burke. We can also expect to spend more time commuting to and from work, as the search for affordable housing pushes us into outlying areas and traffic snarls worsen.

As Barbara Ehrenreich learned when she went to work researching *Nickel and Dimed*—as a Wal-Mart sales clerk, waitress, cleaning woman, hotel maid, nursing home aide—these jobs are bone-achingly exhausting, and one is not enough: you can work "harder than you ever thought possible—and still find yourself sinking ever deeper into poverty and debt." Seventy percent of American women with children under eighteen currently work outside the home—and since women still bear most of the responsibility for children and family, they come home to a "second shift." "The reality of mid-life women's sleep is predominantly one of disruption," write University of Surrey sociologists Jenny Hislop and Sara Arber. Caught up in "the often unremarked tasks of organizing, managing, trouble-shooting, worrying, and anticipating and attending to the needs of others to ensure the well-being of the family unit, . . . a woman is always considered as 'being available' and 'on duty,' and responsive to the needs of her children at a time regarded by others as a period of rest and recuperating." I find the term *electronic leash* for the new technologies that allow work time to bleed into what used to be free time, the cell phones, pagers, laptops we never leave behind. But I find no term for the umbilical cord of responsibility that ties a mother to her children, whatever the age of the child, or the mother.

Feeling out of control is a recipe for stress. "The people who are under someone's thumb, who are low ranking and don't have any decision-making," says McEwen, "are the people who always experience more anxiety." They're taking orders from everyone; they're the first to be laid off. "You're all nerved up, you're stressed, you don't know what somebody's gonna pull on you next," says a woman interviewed by David Shipler in *The Working Poor.*

The lower your position in the pecking order, the higher your stress level. The few studies I find of ethnicity and sleep suggest that African Americans sleep worse than whites, as do Hispanics and other "others." In New Zealand, it's the Maoris who sleep worst. A study of insomnia in different occupations found less of it among physicians and managing directors and more among manual workers. The lower your income and education level, the higher your chances of insomnia—unless you're a woman, that is. "The better educated you are, the better you sleep, but only if you're a man. Men who make more money sleep better, but women who make more money don't sleep better," reported Tarja Porkka-Heiskanen, presenting the findings of a European Union research project, "Sleep in Ageing Women," at the 2006 sleep conference.

Hard as work can be on sleep, unemployment is harder. "Studies that distinguished between the different classes of nonworkers showed the highest risk . . . was in retirees, followed by homemakers." (I wouldn't call homemakers "nonworkers," but never mind.) The poor not only have less control over their circumstances but have fewer outlets that might alleviate stress, like a vacation, a psychotherapist, a sleeping pill at three dollars a pop. They have more health problems, more cardiovascular disease, respiratory disorders, and higher rates of cancer; they have more need of health care and less access to it. Today there are something like 45 million Americans who are uninsured and millions more whose coverage is so inadequate that they might as well be. There are millions besides who are within a hairsbreadth of becoming uninsured, who lose insurance when they change jobs, when they're laid off from a job, when they're too sick (or tired) to hold onto a job, when an employer decides to discontinue coverage.

A physician wrote me, describing a day in the life of her practice at a free clinic in Alabama:

> Most of my patients cried yesterday. That happens pretty regularly, but not most in a few hours. Goodyear is buying Dupont and closing the plant here; a woman who's worked there for 24 yrs, knows nothing else. A woman who has worked for a nursery since she was 19, 30 years, is being laid off. People aren't buying shrubs.

More and more people are living with these kinds of uncertainties, as wealth becomes concentrated into the hands of the 1 percent at the top and large chunks of the middle class slide down the slope to join the working poor. "All it takes is a bit of bad luck in employment or health to plunge a family that seems solidly middle-class into poverty," writes *New York Times* columnist Paul Krugman.

This kind of glaring inequality has been shown to be harmful to the health of individuals and society. No wonder people are sitting on powder kegs, about to wig out. I don't know if there's more road rage in California than other places, but I can't drive four blocks to the market without a huge, hiked-up vehicle appearing on my back bumper that seems to want to grind me into the ground. Now we also have expressions like *air rage, desk rage, phone rage, going postal* that have become a part of the language. I don't see how anybody sleeps, to tell you the truth. And yet they do. Even if insomnia rates are going up, as surveys suggest they are, most people sleep.

Five minutes in the lives of most people I know, and I'd stop sleeping. I don't know how anybody deals with the kinds of job insecurities I see all around: I've had tenure so long I can hardly remember a time when I didn't. I have summers off and a long Christmas break, and I can schedule the hours I teach. It's true that teaching generates anxiety—even after all these years, there's performance anxiety—but as long as I can control the hours I work, I can carry on without too much violence to my sleep. It's when I take on too much, when I feel I can't get it all done, when I lose a sense of control, that sleep goes out the window. I get like my friend Becky: *I have days scheduled down to every fifteen minutes, I can't focus on anything because of all the other things I need to be doing. When I get like this, it's bye-bye sleep.* But Becky lives like this all the time. She's a part-time instructor who drives two hundred miles a day to three different colleges to teach six courses a term and has no assurance of reappointment one year to the next. With this kind of pressure, I'd come unglued.

Put me in Joe's life, and I'd never sleep again. Joe is a San Francisco corporate lawyer who puts in seventy to eighty hours a week, whose work takes him to Tokyo, New York, London three and sometimes four times a month. Joe is a marvel to me. "It's a thrill," he tells me, "waking up in a hotel room in a new city. I never know what my job is going to throw my way, and I love it—I never get bored." The mastery he feels in his work, the high pay and sense of possibilities, makes a world of difference between him and Becky: he's riding the wave, she's barely keeping afloat. But Joe also has natural endowments Becky does not. He's a gifted sleeper, has been all his life; he drops off quickly, comes to just as fast, and never needs more than six hours. If you have a strong sleep pressure and a resilient stress system, you can sail through life's stresses with aplomb, whether you're climbing the corporate ladder or enduring the grinding conditions of poverty. It's like having an exceptionally strong digestive system: you can eat nails.

Stephanie is another marvel to me: an unhappy childhood, a life like a war zone, and she sleeps like a stone. When she was a kid, she'd sleep out back in the treehouse rather than risk coming home to the beatings she'd get from her father. A typical conversation with Stephanie goes something like this: "They're putting us in these crummy offices and I'm the only one who'll stand up to the boss about it. Nobody wants to be seen talking to me, they all know he hates me." After a sixty-five-mile drive home on a harrowing L.A. freeway and a day's work that starts at 8 A.M. and ends at 7 P.M., she watches a bit of TV, and "sleep comes down like a mallet," as she says. That's what good sleep pressure and an unflappable stress system do for you. I can tell you it's not about "attitude," because she's full of rage.

One of the most poignant responses I got when I went out looking for stories was this one.

Dear Professor,

Two years go I was having a terrible time with insomnia. I would go for days with no rest. . . . I went to see a doctor about the problem. I was expecting the same old run around, based on past experiences talking with doctors about insomnia. Instead she offered me an interesting speculation, one that I have thought about many times before, but was relieved to hear from a trained medical professional.

She said that we have dramatically changed our life styles. We have gone from being a hunting and gathering society, to a world where we can survive by being inactive. We can sit at a desk for 8 hours a day, go home, and watch TV. . . .

We have changed so quickly, but have we evolved?

At the time, continues this "San Francisco insomniac,"

> *I was working behind a computer. I quit my job, told my boss I could not sleep and it could be due to my work. I began to change my entire life for the sake of sleep. I work as a photographer now, no longer spending hours sitting, or in front of a computer, except for right now. I try to keep my life free from stress, and I live a very simple life. I am happy. Yet I still can't sleep.*
>
> *. . . I eat well. I exercise daily, but I don't work out close to bedtime. I don't take drugs. I try to keep a schedule. I get into bed by ten and get up by seven. In actuality, I get in bed, and after my girlfriend falls asleep, usually in less than 30 seconds, I lie in bed until the sun comes up. I'm aware of all that happens in between.*
>
> *I no longer get angry in the middle of the night. I think I have accepted my sleeplessness, in a way.*

This man rearranged his life and work according to the sane and sensible principles we all know should help. But he still can't sleep.

It is clear, from the high rates of insomnia among the unemployed and poor, that insomnia is related to stress. But it's also clear, from the wide variation in the ways people respond to stressful conditions, that it's too simple to say "insomnia is stress" or even that "insomnia is caused by stress." What you can say is that the stressful conditions of our lives may be pushing those of us who are vulnerable into more sleepless nights, may be putting us at risk of getting stuck on permanent alert.

What you can also say with certainty is that stress undermines health and longevity. "If you can't turn off the stress response at the end of a stressful event," explains Sapolsky, "the stress response can eventually become as damaging as some stressors themselves." Since cortisol is an immune suppressor, elevated levels put you at greater risk of infection and disease. Since prolonged exposure to cortisol leaches calcium and other minerals from bone, you're at greater risk for osteoporosis. Since cortisol in the early stages of sleep suppresses the release of growth hormone, you lose muscle and accumulate fat, and since stress makes fat cells more insulin-resistant, you're at greater risk for diabetes and cardiovascular problems. The effects of stress are, in fact, like those of sleep loss—no surprise, since sleep deprivation is a stressor.

But for some people, like the San Francisco insomniac who quit his job and still couldn't sleep, the external stressors are not the ultimate determinants of sleep quality. Nor are they with me: I can take a sabbatical that gives me fifteen months without teaching, I can strip my life of external pressures, and my sleep is only marginally improved. Stress can make it worse, but taking away the stress doesn't make it all that much better.

Teen Troubles

There are points in a life when insomnia is most likely to rear its ugly head, stages when people are particularly vulnerable to it: adolescence, menopause, and senescence. When insomnia makes an appearance at one of these points, the problem is usually ascribed to "stress." Each of these stages of life is said to be a "stressful time," and often it is (what age is not?). But each stage also happens to be a time when momentous biological changes are taking place, changes that may make the stress system more reactive, especially when hormones are involved. Let's follow the *psycho* and *physio* ways of accounting for insomnia through these points of greatest change.

Adolescent-onset insomnia has had, until recently, very little research attention. It is said by the DSM-IV to be "rare." And yet many people trace their insomnia to this time. *I've had insomnia since I was 11. I'm 17 and I've forgotten how to sleep. I don't think it's stress, because school's good, except I fall asleep at 4 A.M. and have to be up at 5:30—* I hear this sort of thing again and again, along with plaintive cries for help. A friend's son confided to me,

> My parents think I'm on drugs, but all I am is tired. I used to get straight A's, now I just can't wait till school is over and I can come home and sleep. I sleep a few hours, then I'm up all night again. That's when I do my homework, but my grades are going down. I really need some help.

The 2006 National Sleep Foundation sleep survey found that, of the adolescents surveyed, ages eleven through seventeen, 16 percent thought they might have a sleep disorder. Only 7 percent of their caretakers thought they did.

The usual response is to blame the teenager—such bad habits, coming home and sleeping, then staying up all night, what can you expect?

Also cited are the stresses and strains of teen lives, the new pressures and pleasures, social and academic, that adolescents are confronting. It's true, young people today are juggling a million activities; they spend more time working for wages than they did at any time in the past; they consume more caffeine-loaded sodas and junk foods than I have in a lifetime; and they live on the Web. They have computers and cell phones and television sets in their bedrooms—77 percent of sixth graders had TVs in their bedrooms in 1999, compared to 6 percent in 1970.

Many of their problems are, of course, behavioral and situational. And yet adolescence is a time when profound biological transformations are taking place, not just the obvious hormonal changes, but changes that are invisible. For reasons nobody understands, the circadian clock shifts, and it happens in rhesus monkeys, too, so it's not bad habits, it's biology. The melatonin release, which is a measure of circadian timing, shifts to a later hour. This shift seems to be associated with sexual development: in any group of pubescent girls, as Mary Carskadon says, you see a range of physical types, from the sticklike to the nubile, and it's the nubile whose clocks have swung to a later hour, according to melatonin in saliva tests.

Besides the time shift that occurs at adolescence, a major reorganization of brain function is taking place, "maturational changes greater in magnitude than those produced by aging over the next four decades," says pioneer sleep researcher Irwin Feinberg, who has been studying age-related changes in the sleep system for about that long. Adolescence is when we begin to sleep less and to lose deep sleep. Average sleep time drops from about ten hours before puberty to seven hours in late puberty. The loss of slow wave sleep, the deepest kind (so-called for the large, regular waves it makes on the EEG), is precipitous: between ages twelve and fifteen, there's a 40 percent decline in deep sleep. Adolescence is also when the brain loses a good deal of its plasticity, its ability to reconfigure itself in response to stimuli from the outside world. This loss is related to a huge reduction in the number of connections between neurons (synapses), as unused circuitry drops away, a process that continues through early adolescence. With this loss goes the remarkable resiliency children have, their ability to recover quickly after brain injury and to learn foreign languages easily and without accent. It is thought that this loss of synaptic density may also account for changes in sleep that occur at this time.

When the brain is changing so radically and so rapidly, there are lots of things that can go wrong—and there are lots of things that *do* go wrong. Several sleep disorders make their appearance at this time, not only insomnia, but narcolepsy and delayed sleep phase syndrome, where the circadian clock shifts even later than is normal in adolescence. A deranged synaptic pruning, the elimination of too many or too few synapses or the wrong kinds, speculates Irwin Feinberg, might be the cause of schizophrenia, which comes on in late adolescence.

Whatever the cause or causes, adolescents are at increased risk for insomnia. But it's the girls who are at greatest risk—*after* they begin to menstruate. A study based on interviews of a thousand adolescents found that there was no significant difference for insomnia risk between girls and boys before puberty, but that after the onset of menstruation, girls "were approximately 2.5 times more likely than boys to have insomnia." That seems so crucial, yet the study was done only in 2006; it's one of those questions where you have to wonder, why didn't anybody ask before? Adolescence is when I first became aware of the problem— and I was one of the nubile ones. I shot up, shot out, bursting out all over, spikes and surges of crazy energy, hormonally driven. My clock swung way late and never shifted back; then, just as I'd be drifting off to sleep, there was my mother calling my name, telling me if I didn't get up right then and there I'd miss the bus that picked me up at the end of the block at 7:30, depositing me in class at 8 A.M., where we'd stand, hand on heart, reciting the pledge of allegiance. High school was surreal. I'd spend the rest of the day fighting sleep, then come home and crash and begin again.

It may be the surge of estrogen that girls get at adolescence that accounts for their increased vulnerability to insomnia. Estrogen "primes the body's stress response," increasing the secretion of cortisol and promoting a stress response "that is not only more pronounced but also longer-lasting in women than in men." Women have been found to have longer-lasting cortisol responses during the phases of the menstrual cycle when estrogen and progesterone levels are highest. The hyperreactivity of the female stress system, according to one researcher, may be "an evolutionary adaptation to help mothers protect their young." But it may also explain why women are twice as likely as men to experience depression and significantly more prone to stress-related problems such as panic disorder, generalized anxiety disorder, posttraumatic stress disorder, and autoimmune disorders—and why many of these problems come on at adolescence. (Men are more prone to antisocial behaviors such as alcoholism, addiction, autism, schizophrenia, but women are more vulnerable to affective disorders—i.e., disorders affecting the emotions.) The difference arises at puberty, keeps on through the childbearing years, and declines after menopause to a rate that's equal to that of men of the same age—which suggests a link with estrogen.

Social and psychological factors play a part, too, of course, in the ratcheting up of the female stress system. Women are statistically more likely to be poor, to be subject to violence and abuse, to be caught in situations where neither fight nor flight is possible. Their role as the primary caretakers of children and the aging makes them conduits for the anxieties of others. They're conditioned to internalize conflicts rather than act them out. Any of these factors might make them more vulnerable to stress disorders. But there seems also to be something about the female stress system that's intrinsically more reactive, especially at points when the hormones are fluctuating, like adolescence and menopause. If you get an especially strong dose of hormones at adolescence, as I did, judging by my spurt of growth and the hormonal havoc it wrought, it may throw the system into high gear. Then, between adolescence and menopause, as you're exposed to cyclic fluctuations, to dips and surges in estrogen and progesterone, the system stays ratcheted up.

Or, do we only have this kind of sensitivity to our hormones if our stress system is already ratcheted up? Not all female insomniacs have this kind of reactivity to hormones, as I was surprised to learn when I started collecting stories (I'd assumed they were all like me). Is our reactivity to our hormones related to the state of our stress systems? A question to be asked, but not one I've seen asked.

Change of Life

It seems unfair that menarche, with its tide of hormones, brings on insomnia, and then the ebbing of tide at menopause brings it on more, but that's the way it works. At menopause, women's sleep complaints more than double. "Hot flashes" are the explanation given by most sleep experts—and no doubt, hot flashes may disrupt sleep; except that the sleep disruption often persists for years after the hot flashes have faded away. "Conditioning," say the experts: the hot flashes disrupt sleep, and then insomnia settles in like a bad habit. "We hypothesize that it could reflect a behaviorally conditioned insomnia which has been initially triggered by night sweats and persists after the night sweats and their directly associated sleep disruptions resolve," write Andrew Krystal and colleagues; "it does not appear to be directly related to hormonal changes." The other explanation given is psychic distress, "unresolved grief related to going through menopause," in the words of Krystal et al.

I don't buy the bit about psychic distress, because rates of depression in women actually *decline* after menopause. Contrary to popular conception, "midlife is not the predominant high-stress period for women." Depression rates go down, yet insomnia rates go up—this alone should unseat the simplistic equation of insomnia with depression. Many women I know (myself included, on my better days) are actually in better shape psychologically in their fifties and sixties than they were when they were younger, on a more even keel—except when they can't sleep. They will tell you that it's the disrupted sleep that wrecks their moods, not their moods that wreck their sleep. They will tell you that the disruption is physiological.

> *You are not necessarily worried about anything. You may have had a happy and productive day. But when you try to sleep, you feel "wired" and fatigued at the same time. Something will not turn off. If you do fall asleep, you may wake up several times, but not because of nightmares. You just wake up, feeling really hot and covered in sweat. . . . This kind of insomnia is primarily a physiological event.*

The effect is particularly dramatic when menopause is brought on rapidly, by hysterectomy or cancer drugs: *I had a hysterectomy several years ago, and I have not had a good night's sleep since*—I hear this again and again. Ilene was a good sleeper until chemotherapy plunged her into menopause and insomnia. After a few years, the insomnia went away, disappearing, mysteriously, at a time she was under the pressure of a book deadline—which gave her a strong sense that the problem had not been "about stress."

Menopause, though it affects every woman who lives long enough, is not well understood. What is known is that it is a time when our bodies are adjusting to declining levels of estrogen and progesterone. The changes may begin years before, in the so-called *perimenopause,* when hormone levels fluctuate widely. Some researchers think that it's the *fluctuations,* rather than the depletion of hormones, that create the problem, because the other trouble spots for women's sleep are also times when hormonal levels are fluctuating: at menarche; just before menstruation, when estrogen and progesterone levels plunge; and just after a woman gives birth, when estrogen levels plummet from the high point they were at during pregnancy. These are also the points when women are at greatest risk for depression.

One reason that hormonal fluctuations disrupt sleep is that they raise body temperature. Since temperature must decline for sleep to come on, anything that keeps it elevated—an electric blanket or a hot room—may inhibit sleep. Anything that facilitates a drop in temperature, such as a cool room or a hot bath, may facilitate it (a hot bath seems an odd way of cooling down, but if it's taken a sufficient time before bed—forty-five minutes, experts say, but I find I need twice that—the rapid dropping off of body temperature may trick the brain into thinking it's time for sleep). Ovulation raises body temperature so reliably that women use it as a guide when they're trying to conceive; and ovulation sometimes disrupts sleep. Women with PMS have higher body temperatures throughout the night, and so do women who take birth control pills, which may be why birth control pills interfere with deep sleep. Hot flashes, of course, raise temperature in a big way, but even without them, postmenopausal women have temperature fluctuations more extreme than men's, more volatile changes from highs to lows throughout the night. *I get into bed cold, and I wake up hot and throw off the bedclothes; then I get cold and squirrel around and reassemble the covers*—this is a recurrent refrain: *It drives my husband nuts, but I can't help it—my temperature's all over the place.* This temperature dysregulation then sets in motion another vicious cycle: raised temperature disrupts sleep and disrupted sleep further raises temperature.

My menopause was pretty much a nonevent. I experienced nothing I'd even describe as a hot flash, more like a warm suffusion, which I never much minded since I'm always so cold. But what was intolerable was that premenstrual tension would descend on me, as it always had, just before my period was due, bringing with it insomnia that a pill couldn't touch—and then as my periods got farther apart, I'd have three to four weeks of total sleeplessness. Which drove me to HRT (hormone replacement therapy), fast.

While I'm on the subject of HRT, how (you may well ask), if estrogen makes the stress system more reactive, can estrogen supplements make sleep better, as many women and some studies suggest that they do? Findings are equivocal: some studies say that they help sleep, some that they don't, and a recent survey of the literature concludes that there's evidence both ways. When, in 2002, the Women's Health Initiative study came out with the bad news about HRT—linking it to increases in breast cancer, stroke, heart disease, and dementia—many women stopped taking it, and many experienced insomnia. Most of my friends stopped it then, and all but one complained that their sleep got worse. Most of them rode it out and eventually got back to their usual sleep. The few I know whose sleep continued to be disturbed went back onto the hormones, usually at a lower dose. Anecdotal reports in the popular press suggest that as many as 50 percent of women who stopped hormonal supplements at that time started taking it again, at a lower dose, citing insomnia as the cause.

When I tried cutting down estrogen, it felt like an electric current applied to my heart, *ker-pow, wham, jolt,* leaving me wired for the rest of the night. Twice this happened, and back I went on full-dose estrogen. My sleep is at the best of times so dicey, so barely there, that I'll do anything to hold on to what I have. I have since managed to taper to half a dose, slowly, over the course of more than a year; and I'm staying there, though I don't like the risk. But neither do I like what's happening to my memory, and there's evidence that estrogen has a beneficial effect on memory, that it may help buffer the hippocampus from the effects of cortisol. My hippocampus needs all the help it can get.

One reason estrogen might help sleep is because of the way it interacts with certain neurotransmittal systems. It enhances the action of GABA, the major braking system of the brain. It enhances the action of serotonin, decreasing serotonin uptake and making more serotonin available, the way the selective serotonin reuptake inhibitor antidepressants do. Or it may be that hormone supplements simply keep hormone levels more constant, thereby eliminating the fluctuations that cause the trouble. Or it may be that estrogen lowers temperature. What I'd like to know is, does it help mainly those women whose insomnia is hormonally sensitive?

Progesterone is also complicated: on the one hand, it raises temperature; on the other hand, it has a sedative effect so strong that some researchers suggest it be taken before sleep. When I've taken it at night, it seems to make my sleep worse; when I take it in the morning, I feel no effect either way. But there was a month when I cut it out, and my sleep was just awful, so I think it may help, though not in a simple way. The natural micronized progesterone that I take, Prometrium, is chemically identical to the progesterone the body produces, and the form of estrogen I take, Estrace, is supposedly also bioidentical. (I had a bad reaction to Premarin, which is urine from pregnant mares, and I don't like what they do to mares to obtain it.) I tell myself this makes it better, but who knows?

Whether or not a woman chooses to take HRT depends on a complex set of risk-benefit calculations that only she can make. Time will tell if I've made an unwise bargain.

Aging

It's difficult to sort out the effects of menopause on sleep from the effects of age, since sleep quality gets worse across the lifespan for men as well as women. "The harassed middle aged," as A. Alvarez writes, "are in love with sleep in the same way as the young are in love with love. Chastity is the torment of youth, insomnia of age, and at neither stage of life does it ever seem possible to get enough of what you want." *I'm not the sleeper I used to be* is a lament I hear from many people my age. *I used to sleep through alarm clocks, fire drills, earthquakes. Now I can barely sleep through the night,* says a friend.

Insomnia is said to be as high as 40 to 60 percent among the elderly. Many causes are cited: the aches and pains and illnesses that come with age, the medications people take for them, the higher incidence of sleep-disordered breathing and depression. You don't have to look far for reasons to be depressed and anxious in the final decades of life: loss of friends and family to death and illness; loss of income and social standing; futures that hold increasing frailty and death. But sleep becomes lighter, shallower, more fragmented even in people without psychological or physiological problems. "Age-related changes in sleep are apparently independent of any medical or psychiatric disorders," concludes a 1990 survey of the research; "even carefully screened elderly adults who report no symptoms and have no discernible disease have changes in the sleep-wake pattern." Slow wave sleep, the deepest kind, drops off to as little as five minutes by the time we're sixty. Older people make up for the sleep they lose at night by sleeping when they can, and sleep becomes less consolidated, more distributed around the clock, as it is with infants.

Age brings a weakening of the pressure to sleep and a disturbance of the timing of sleep. If you deprive younger subjects of deep sleep, they'll make it up the next night with "rebound" sleep, but older subjects don't rebound like this, a sign that the sleep pressure is diminished. In young sleepers, the temperature nadir occurs in the latter part of the sleep period, but in elders, the nadir occurs earlier, and so also does the rise in temperature, and we wake up earlier and more often. Body temperature in the elderly tends to be generally higher during sleep, and temperature highs and lows are less extreme, resulting in a blunted circadian rhythm. There is a decrease in the nocturnal secretion of melatonin and growth hormone, a 50 percent dampening of the sleep-inducing hormone prolactin, and a general elevation of stress hormones. The neurophysiological reasons for these changes are not well understood. It may be relevant that there's a loss of neurons in both the sleep switch (the ventrolateral preoptic nucleus) and the circadian clock (the suprachiasmic nucleus).

The sleep of insomniacs has many features of a sleep system in decline. Insomniacs also have less slow wave sleep, diminished sleep pressure, higher body temperature, a flattening-out of body temperature rhythms with highs and lows that are less extreme, higher levels of cortisol and norepinephrine, and an inability to sleep in a consolidated block. The sleep of insomniacs is also, as Swiss researcher Jean-Michel Gaillard observes, "unpredictable and highly variable." Normal sleepers progress regularly, predictably, through the sleep stages, spending thirty to forty minutes in stages 3 and 4 (deep sleep), a short period in REM, and returning to deep sleep for another thirty to forty minutes, with REM lasting only a few minutes in the earlier part of the night and becoming longer in the later part. They move through four to six *cycles* of ninety minutes each (a cycle is the passage from light to deep sleep through REM and back to light), spending 20 to 30 percent of sleep time in deep sleep and about that much time in REM, progressing through deep and shallow sleep several times a night, surfacing for a few moments but not remembering. (This pattern is called the *architecture* of sleep.) Normal sleepers tend to have sleep patterns so consistent from night to night that researchers who've worked with them can predict what's coming next. But "insomniacs exhibit significantly greater night to night variability," says Ismet Karacan.

Insomniacs not only get through fewer sleep stages; we rarely, one night to the next, progress through them in the same way. I don't think I've ever got through the five to six stages I see Bob get through regularly. I may wake up after three hours, or two, or one and a half, or three and a half, or four, or sometimes five. I may make it through two cycles, or one—and when I wake up, I come fully awake. To reiterate that insomniac quoted in a sleep study in 1976, "I never know when I'm going to have a really horrible night or just my usual lousy one." The unpredictability alone is sufficient to drive you nuts.

Gaillard saw the "differences between normals and insomniacs" as being "in some way similar to differences due to age in normal subjects." *Precocious senescence* was his term for insomnia. Precocious is something I'd like to have been in musical talent, but not in senescence. So what happens, I'm wondering, if you've been precocious in senescence, when you enter actual senescence? As I hear my friends beginning to complain about the kind of sleep I've had for decades—shallow, broken, nonrestorative, with frequent awakenings—I don't know whether to feel smug at being ahead of my time or to dread that my sleep may deteriorate further, as theirs has. But maybe it won't. University of Washington sleep researcher Mike Vitiello says that "after 60, things don't change significantly. Most of the sleep changes occur before 60, so it's not a continuous steady decline into decrepitude."

Scientists have long puzzled at the different rates at which people age. In the final decades of our lives, the differences between human beings are greater than in our early years, especially in terms of mental acuity, with some elderly performing as well as younger subjects on cognitive tasks and others doing very poorly. They now think that it may be the cumulative exposure to stress, "the wear and tear resulting from overactivity of stress-responsive systems," that makes the difference. "Chronic stress can accelerate the aging process," say Sapolsky and colleagues.

Sleep deprivation is a stressor, and as such, it adds to the wear and tear. "Decreased sleep quality," say Van Cauter and her colleagues, "accelerates senescence." Our joints and muscles tell us this is so, and so do our mirrors. A thirty-something insomniac wrote me, *I feel like I'm sixty, and some days I look it, but my mother is sixty-three, and she has more zip than I do. What am I going to feel like when I'm her age, if I live to be her age?* I look at my friends who sleep well, and I see that they are the ones who are aging well: they look great, their energy is good, not wired the way mine gets, not the kind that goes on buzzing in their sleep.

In a survey of over nine thousand elderly persons living independently, 57 percent reported having insomnia most of the time, and those who had the worst insomnia had the worst health and the most depression. Do they have the worst insomnia because they have bad health and depression, or do they have bad health and depression because they have insomnia? The deterioration of sleep in the aged, say Laughton Miles and William Dement, may at least partially account for those decrements associated with age, frailty, cardiovascular disease, cognitive impairment, memory loss, depression, aches, and pains.

"We can no more be cured of aging than of birth," write Sapolsky and his colleagues, but we can try "to slow and soften the sharpest edges of the biological unraveling that constitutes aging." A big part of this is protecting ourselves against the ravages of stress, and a big part of that is guarding our sleep. I think about those bred-to-be-insomniac fruit flies that fall down a lot, die young, and can't learn.

The effects on memory concern me the most. We all know that a bad night's sleep can interfere with certain kinds of recall, the ability to access things we thought we knew. Says Josh, the student taking synthetic cortisol for his kidney transplant, *My vocabulary has just gone, I can be stalled for fifty seconds, looking for a word.* With all that cortisol coursing through his system, this might not be a problem that goes away with a good night's sleep. Elevated cortisol levels damage the hippocampus, which is, as we saw, the part of the brain that damps the cortisol release back down—and which is also the part that is crucial to the formation of new memories.

In people who've had Cushing's for one to four years, a condition in which tumors cause the adrenals to "secrete tons of glucocorticoids," a magnetic resonance imaging study found "that their hippocampi had shrunk." "It's been known for decades that they get memory problems[;] . . . it's known as *Cushingoid dementia,*" says Sapolsky. Some people with posttraumatic stress disorders, including Vietnam vets and survivors of childhood sexual abuse, have "major . . . atrophy of their hippocampus. The more severe the combat exposure . . . the worse the atrophy." In people with long-term major depression, a magnetic resonance imaging study turned up "selective atrophy of the hippocampus." In the elderly, the size of the hippocampus has been found to correlate with cognitive function.

McEwen and Sapolsky found that the effects of Cushing's reversed when the glucocorticoid exposure was stopped; this also happened with patients who'd been taking steroids, who suffered similar cognitive impairments. But they point out that most of these studies look at exposure for only a few years, not over the course of many years. One study that looked at former depressives and posttraumatic stress victims years to decades later suggested that "whatever is happening is not readily reversible," as Sapolsky says.

Too much cortisol not only shrinks hippocampal neurons, it interferes with the creation of new neurons, the process called *neurogenesis.* It was long believed that brain cells could not regenerate themselves, but research in the past twenty years has demonstrated that new neurons are produced throughout adulthood in several regions of the brain, including the hippocampus. However, this process is arrested in the presence of high levels of cortisol. Studies now find that sleep deprivation also arrests it, reducing the proliferation of cells in the hippocampi of rats. On a brighter note, it's been found that exercise and learning new things may facilitate the development of new hippocampal neurons (and so may estrogen). A study I especially like found that mice who ran on their exercise wheels whenever they wanted to generated "significantly more newborn cells in their hippocampus" than mice who were forced to exercise. Nice. I never for a minute believed that anyone ever learned well under coercion. The moral of this study is, find an exercise wheel you like—and more important, get a life you like, one that's in accord with your predispositions rather than at war with them.

Insomniacs are said to have bad memories. We say we do—and the few studies I find say we do, too. *My memory's shot to hell, long gone, faded away; some days I just feel like I'm in a fog.* I hear this lament again and again. *I feel like I'll disappear into a fog altogether. One of these days I'll forget my own name.* In Gabriel García Márquez's *One Hundred Years of Solitude,* the inhabitants of a village afflicted by a "plague of insomnia" lose first their childhood memories, then the names and functions of everyday objects; finally, they lose all sense of who they are and sink into oblivion. I can well imagine. Entire subjects have disappeared from my brain, entire languages, whole areas of knowledge. When I hear people talking about something they learned in college, something they read a year ago, I'm amazed. With me, nothing sticks; conversations I have had with people, the people themselves, vanish without a trace. And yet the baby my mother describes in her letters had an extraordinary memory, or so it seemed to her. Where did that memory go?

There's a possibility so bleak I can barely bring myself to describe it: a fall from a horse when I was fourteen. I remember riding that morning; the next thing I knew, it was afternoon and I was lying on the ground, people standing around waiting for me to come to. The horse had arrived back at the barn without me; the stable hands came out looking and found me up the hill, crumpled in a heap. How long I was out or how it happened, I don't remember. I never told my parents. I put it out of my mind so completely that I actually forgot about it—until I started reading about the connection between head injury and insomnia. There's not a lot of research on this, but from what I can piece together, sleep disturbances occur in 30 to 70 percent of people who've had head injury. Studies find a decrease in both REM and slow wave sleep, an increase in the number of awakenings, and the persistence of sleep complaints "even a long time after trauma." I didn't notice any headaches or trouble with my vision after my accident, though I have had bad headaches and poor vision as long as I can remember. Fourteen was the age when I became aware of my sleep problems, but it was also when I became aware of lots of other things—in fact, I have little memory of much before.

I don't know how to think about this, but I suppose it's possible that that conk on the head jolted some crucial neurons loose, taking memory with it, and taking sleep.

There are many routes that might lead to this place: neurological impairment, inborn or acquired, stress systems that are especially vulnerable to stress, stress systems ratcheted up by repeated or prolonged exposure to stress, dysregulated hormones that feed into a cycle perpetuated by stress. It's what researchers mean by *multifactorial*. Only this doesn't begin to describe it.

CHAPTER 7

Rock, Hard Place

The Drugs

They're bad for you, but so's sleep loss bad for you. You're between a rock and a hard place. I go with the pills. That way at least I get some sleep.

I hate them. I use them. I need them. I wish there were something better.

I asked my psychiatrist about one of the new sleeping pills that's coming on the market. He's so disgusted with the pharmaceutical industry's perpetual next-big-thing he didn't even want to talk about it.

It is difficult to get a fix on drugs, since this society is nutty on the subject, pill-popping, on the one hand, and hysterical about drug abuse, on the other hand. An insomniac trying to decide what medication to use or whether to use a medication at all encounters a tangle of contradictory attitudes, from the hidebound to the hyped up, and may well find such contradictions in himself or herself. Direct-to-consumer drug advertising, made legal in 1997, barrages us with the message that there's a pill for every ill, and for ills we might not know we have. We turn to the Web to find out what insomniacs say, and we hear wildly conflicting accounts. Since no two people react to a drug exactly the same way, responses are all over the place:

It saved my life.
It was ruining my life.
I don't know what I would have done without it.

I wish I'd never heard of it.
It was a wonder, I was sleeping again.
It was a horror, I felt like I'd never sleep again.

We turn to doctors, where we find further versions of hysteria and hype. *I swear, they think I come in just looking for drugs, like I'm a coke-head or methhead.* Hypnotics, as sleep meds are called, are Schedule IV drugs, so designated by the Controlled Substances Act, which categorizes substances according to their medical uses and potential for abuse and dependence. Schedule IV drugs are not as bad as Schedule I, II, or III, but they are nevertheless *controlled* substances, under the jurisdiction of the Justice Department and the Drug Enforcement Administration. FDA guidelines suggest limiting their use to seven to ten days, to a maximum of a month, yet many insomniacs take these drugs for much longer. The law turns longtime users into potential "abusers" and puts us in an adversarial relation with the doctors we turn to for help.

Web postings bristle with rage at doctors who make us feel like criminals when we ask for something to help us sleep. *They take this oath that says "do no harm." But when they have something that works and they refuse to give it to you, I call that doing harm!* Most of us have been through the kind of runaround a friend tells me about:

> *I went to my doctor, asking for a benzodiazepine because that's the only thing that really works for me. He said no, no, they're addictive. He then proceeded to tell me that whenever he has a problem sleeping, he just writes his worries down on a piece of paper, and tears the paper up—"like so," and he held up a piece of paper and ripped it in two. Like, that's all there is to it. I just stood there, stunned.*
>
> *So I said, look here, I really am under quite a bit of pressure right now and there are a lot of people depending on me. Are you really afraid I'm going to become an addict?*

This man is a neuroscientist at a major university, but in the eyes of this doctor, he's a kid with his hand in the cookie jar. Then too there's the humiliation of having pills doled out one by one: *I begged my GP to give me some Restoril. He gave me four pills to "reset" my sleep pattern and get me on track—four pills, is he kidding? That might get me through the week.* A further problem with this pill-by-pill policy is stated by a friend: *So, the big one comes, the city's in rubble, and there you are with three Ambien left.* If you live in the San Francisco Bay Area, you think such thoughts. I have thyroid supplements stockpiled, but when disaster strikes, I guess I make do with whatever Ambien I happen to have left in the bottle.

But there is also rage at doctors who, as William Styron says, "promiscuously prescribe." In his account of his breakdown in *Darkness Visible,* Styron describes an "insouciant doctor" who told him he could take Ativan "as casually as aspirin." He got badly strung out on Ativan, then on Halcion. I hear this sort of criticism from many people: *He had his pen out, I swear to God I hadn't been there five minutes, and he was writing a prescription. That's all they do anymore.* And another: *I told him I'd upped the Restoril from 15 to 30 and I'm now up to 45 mg, and he said it was okay, it wasn't addictive, I could take it for the rest of my life. I tried to explain that it made me a zombie, but he didn't seem to hear.*

Doctors are in a kind of no-win situation: they get blamed for underprescribing, they get blamed for overprescribing, and they're not actually well trained in pharmacology; it's not a big part of their medical school education. So they rely on drug companies for information, on sales reps and advertising, on drug-sponsored Continuing Medical Education events like those I attend at the sleep conferences. It's easier to digest the sound-bite-size chunks dished out by the drug companies than to dig out information for oneself.

Drug companies spend about thirteen thousand dollars a year per doctor—$100 million a day—to get them to prescribe their drugs. An army of representatives, eighty-eight thousand strong, one for every four to five doctors, hangs around the halls of the hospitals and visits their offices, wielding "weapons of mass seduction: food, flattery, friendship—and lots of free samples." "The pressures to prescribe are enormous," says one doctor. "You constantly have people at your door." The hospital parking lots are so overrun with them that a Lilly rep on her way out may rear-end a Pfizer rep on her way in. The gifts go far beyond the pens, flashlights, key chains I raked in at the conference exhibits and include briefcases, stethoscopes, tickets to sporting events and musicals, all-expense-paid vacations in Aspen, Hawaii, the Bahamas. Most of the drug company reps are babes, television-pretty, miniskirted, long dark stockings and stiletto heels. You can spot them a mile away at the conferences, chatting up the guys, batting their eyelashes, peddling their wares.

Physicians believe that they're beyond being influenced by all this (actually, they believe that they *themselves* are beyond influence, but that *other* doctors may not be). And yet there are hundreds of studies that show that when physicians have frequent contact with sales reps, when they accept honoraria, research support, dinners, massages, vacations, when they attend Continuing Medical Education events, it makes a difference in what drugs they prescribe. Drug companies wouldn't spend this kind of money if it didn't. "We physicians think . . . we are shrewd and they can't put things over on us but, in fact, we are putty in the hands of these people," says Joe Gerstein, physician and associate professor at Harvard. "Doctors have been taught only too well by the pharmaceutical industry," says Marcia Angell, former editor of the *New England Journal of Medicine* and author of *The Truth about the Drug Companies*, and what they've learned is a "drug-intensive style of medicine." Besides, as an insomniac wrote me, *Drugs are what's quickest and easiest in these days of Mangled Care—just write a prescription and send us on our way.*

So there's all this hoopla, on the one hand, and all this heavy-duty restriction, on the other hand, and you wonder if anybody, anywhere, is giving a thought to what works best for the insomniac. We blithely assume that the drugs we're prescribed are those best suited to our needs and problems, but it looks to me like this is the last thing on anybody's mind. So many other forces determine which drugs get pushed on us and which get withheld—and which drugs even get developed—that the individual insomniac gets lost in the shuffle. Which throws the responsibility back on us, the consumers, the users, the insomniacs, to find our way through this maze.

The way I took was long, painful, and somewhat dangerous. I tell it as a kind of cautionary tale, in hopes that it may help others do better.

Benzodiazepines

I was given my first Ativan in 1980. A doctor at my HMO prescribed it to "break the pattern of insomnia," as he said. He gave it casually, with the best of intentions, and with no warnings.

The first of the benzos, Librium, had been introduced in the United States in 1960. Valium followed, in 1963. Both drugs were advertised as giving "natural sleep" and were prescribed liberally, indiscriminately, for whatever ailed you, whether it was insomnia, menopause, marital upsets, muscle spasm, aches and pains, or boredom. "Whatever the diagnosis—Librium," proclaimed the center-spread advertisement in a leading medical journal. "Give me Librium or give me death" was a comic slogan of the 1960s. Valium, like Librium, soon became a household word. By 1972, it was the most frequently prescribed drug in the United States, and Librium was third. "Anybody got a Valium?" cried Mary Hartman on *Mary Hartman, Mary Hartman,* a popular late-night comic soap opera of the 1970s—and everyone in the scene reached into his or her pocket or purse. The little yellow pill was dubbed "Mother's little helper" by the Rolling Stones, on account of the vast numbers of housewives who took it—a two-to-one ratio of women to men, with most of the advertising aimed at women. By the early 1970s, it was being taken by one in ten Americans. "Valiumania," the *New York Times* called it.

Dalmane (florazepam) was launched several years after Valium, and it too became a best-seller. It was the first benzodiazepine introduced specifically as a hypnotic, that is, a sleeping pill; Librium and Valium were both tranquilizers. Ativan (lorazepam), also a tranquilizer, followed in 1972, and Restoril (temazepam), a hypnotic, came in 1977. Klonopin (clonazepam) was introduced a few years later. The shorter-acting Xanax (alprazolam) was introduced in the early 1980s, followed by Halcion (triazolam) in the late 1980s. Each drug was promoted as safer and more wondrous than the one before.

The benzodiazepines were welcomed as safe and nonaddictive alternatives to the *barbiturates* (phenobarbital, Nembutal, Seconal), the type of drug used for sleep earlier in the century. Safer, they certainly are: their effective dose is farther from the lethal dose, so they're harder to overdose with. The barbiturates had been implicated in as many as 10 percent of suicides, among them Marilyn Monroe's and Judy Garland's, and they were seriously addictive. Yet they, too, had been advertised as absolutely safe and without toxic effects. It took nearly fifty years, from 1903 to 1950, to establish that they were dangerous. It would take twenty years to establish that the benzos were, too.

When the benzodiazepines first came on the market, it was not known how they worked. It was only in the late 1970s that it came to be understood that they bind to the receptor sites of the neurotransmitter GABA (gamma-aminobutyric acid), the main inhibitory or braking system of the brain, specifically, to the GABAa receptor. They increase receptor receptivity to GABA, thereby accentuating its activity, which causes a decrease in activity of the neurotransmitters—norepinephrine, serotonin, acetylcholine, dopamine—and a general slowdown of brain activity. Each of the benzos targets a different subtype of the GABAa receptor, which is why each drug has a slightly different action: some have more *anxiolitic,* or antianxiety, effects, and others have more hypnotic, or sedative, effects. But they all have "a general quietening influence on the brain." The problem is that the neurotransmitters whose activity is being suppressed are also necessary for other functions—attention, memory, coordination, muscle tone, hormonal secretions, heart rate, blood pressure control. Benzos decrease muscle tension and anxiety, but they diminish alertness as well, slowing reaction time, impairing memory, and sort of generally bludgeoning the central nervous system.

By the late 1960s, studies were turning up evidence that they were not as benign as had been believed. Dr. Ian Oswald, of the Department of Psychiatry at Royal Edinburgh Hospital, looking at the EEGs of people on benzodiazepines, found that they "do not induce natural sleep," and that when the drug is discontinued, a "backlash effect" makes the insomnia worse than before the drug was started—what we call *rebound*. Oswald found that "a number of measurable neurophysiological functions took over five weeks to return to normal." In the United States, Anthony Kales was also finding problems of withdrawal and was turning up evidence that the effects these drugs had on sleep actually lasted no more than a few days. But the dependence risks continued to be downplayed, and by the mid-1970s, as many as 20 percent of adults in the United States and other Western nations were taking benzos on a regular basis. Hospitals routinely prescribed them for inpatients, which helped with ward routines but sent many patients home with a habit. By the mid-1980s, estimates were that between two hundred thousand and five hundred thousand people (depending on the criteria used) were dependent on benzos.

It was the users, the consumers, who blew the whistle on the problem, by telling their stories. In 1979, Barbara Gordon, a TV celebrity, wrote of her withdrawal from Valium as a journey "to hell and back"; her book, *I'm Dancing as Fast as I Can*, became a best-seller and was made into a film in 1982. When Gordon told her psychiatrist, "I'm growing too dependent on pills," he interrupted, "But I've told you many times, Miss Gordon, they are not addictive. They can't hurt you." In 1982, the London Broadcasting Company did a series of ten programs about drug abuse and received hundreds of responses, most of them from women addicted to Valium and Ativan. The phone lines jammed and letters poured in, to the amazement of everyone, since these drugs were "known" not to be addictive. A survey reported in *Woman's Own* in 1984, to which over seven thousand replied "in frightening detail," found that "most had been taking tranquillisers for over four years, most had tried to quit, and most had failed." The problem was particularly acute in England, where the recommended dose was twice that in the United States: in England, four to six milligrams of Ativan was regularly prescribed for mild anxiety, and six milligrams was recommended for "moderate" anxiety. (Six milligrams of Ativan is the equivalent of sixty milligrams of Valium; two milligrams was the most I took, and it put me under the rug.) "These painfully ignorant doctors have created the biggest drug addiction problem this country has ever known"; they have made "a nation of junkies," said Dr. Vernon Coleman, a British general practitioner who saw the dangers early on and described them in his newsletter, *Life without Tranquillisers.*

"Evidence of benzodiazepine dependence was there all the time," wrote Charles Medawar, who founded in England, in 1971, the watchdog group Social Audit, an offshoot of Ralph Nader's public interest network. But "patients tended to be patronized. . . . Their experiences were for many years overlooked, and their views scorned[,] . . . disregarded, their opinions barely canvassed—though they had the raw data the whole time." Doctors had been told benzos were not addictive, and, believing the claims of the drug companies over the reports of their patients, they failed to see the evidence that they were. They assumed that when people continued to take them year in and year out, it was because they really worked. The intense insomnia and anxiety patients reported when they tried to stop were interpreted as evidence that they still needed the medication, and perhaps needed more of it. Dr. David Healy, a courageous and outspoken psychopharmacologist from the University of Wales College of Medicine, wrote, "Where they might have expected care and concern, many patients attempting to discontinue treatment have had the frustrating experience of being told authoritatively by their GPs that the difficulties they are having are the emergence of the original problem and that they need to continue with treatment, perhaps for the rest of their lives."

When a doctor was faced with incontrovertible evidence that a patient was really hooked, the patient was said to have an *addictive personality,* to be *dependence-prone.* The drugs were known not to be addictive, so only addicts or *latent addicts* could become addicted: "The abuse arises, not from some inherent property of the drugs, but rather from psychopathology in the user," according to a 1970 account, an explanation perpetuated by no less an authority than Freud, who maintained that it was the personality of the user and not the nature of the drug that was the decisive element in addiction. (Freud continued to believe, throughout his life, that addiction to cocaine "was not, as was commonly believed, the direct result of imbibing a noxious drug, but some peculiarity in the patient.") "True addiction is probably exceedingly unusual," testified the president of Hoffman La Roche, maker of Valium, Librium,

and Dalmane, to the U.S. Senate in 1979, "and when it occurs, is probably confined to those individuals with abuse-prone personalities who ingest very large amounts." A version of that claim is made today, about
the users of current medications: "Dependence liability relates to patient," I hear at the 2005 NIH Insomnia Conference. "In drug users and
alcoholics, there is abuse liability." *The doctors won't accept that it's the
drugs doing it,* says a U.K. insomniac. *They always say it's you.*

Yet here were benzo users who were becoming addicted even when
they stayed within the recommended dose, as attentive physicians
(mainly British) were coming to understand. "We thought only addictive
personalities could become dependent. . . . We got that wrong. What we
didn't know, but know now, is that even people taking therapeutic doses
can become dependent," says Malcolm Lader, professor of clinical psychopharmacology, Institute of Psychiatry, London. Here were users
becoming addicted who had no history of drug abuse.

Like me.

The Ativan Experience

The semester I started taking Ativan, the spring of 1980, I was on a leave
without pay. I had taken this leave to finish a book, it was costing me a
year's salary, and the time was being trashed by sleep loss. Day after day,
I was too wrecked to work. My doctor thought that the drug would
"reset my sleep pattern," as he said, so he gave me Ativan. (Sometime in
the course of my decades with it, Ativan went generic and became available as lorazepam, but I got used to thinking of it as Ativan, so Ativan
I'll call it.) In 1980, enthusiasm for the benzos was still high. "The Ativan Experience," promised a 1978 ad. It did not say what that experience was going to be.

Ativan has a shorter *half-life* (time it takes for half the drug's concentration in the blood to disappear) than the older benzos—Valium takes
20 to 100 hours, Dalmane takes 40 to 250, Restoril takes 8 to 22, and
Ativan, 10 to 20 hours. Though not technically a hypnotic—that is, approved by the FDA for the treatment of insomnia—it was still, as of
2002, the most recent year for which I have information, the eleventh-
most frequently prescribed medication for sleep.

Ativan, at first, was pure bliss. "The Angel Ativan," as poet Lynn
Strongin calls it. It was glorious to sleep through the night and be awake
during the day, unlike the twilight zone I mostly inhabit, half awake

nights and half asleep days. But when I went back to teaching the next semester, I couldn't deal with the rebound insomnia I got when I tried to stop, so I kept taking it for the entire term. And the next term, and the next—and this went on for eighteen years. I was going to a lot of conferences those days, traveling and giving papers, and Ativan enabled me to forget, for long periods of time, that I even had a sleep problem. Ativan enables users to forget lots of things, as I was to discover. It was moderately troubling that I had to increase the dose to get the same effect. I'd bite off little pieces, but then those pieces became bigger pieces: one and a quarter, one and a third, one and a half. By the end of the term, I was up to two milligrams a night and moving in a fog.

At some point during those years, I began to notice a lot of aches and pains. I began moving like an old person. My hips and knees ached so badly that I wondered, some days, if I was going to make it up the four flights of stairs to my office. I chalked it up to age, but my friends didn't seem to be aging this fast. One night I got up on a chair to swat a mosquito and toppled over backward. I was astounded—my balance had always been so reliable. I was lucky my head hit the rug and not the bedpost, which it missed by inches. I now know that motor and memory are what's most impaired by the benzos. I now think I was getting those aches and pains because Ativan was wiping out my deep sleep, which is where important restorative processes are thought to occur. Benzos also reduce REM. If you believe, as most researchers do, that REM and deep sleep do essential things, this is worrying.

Some people never experience restful sleep with a benzodiazepine: *It was dreamless [sleep] and I would wake up feeling exhausted.* Many feel *flattened out, damped down, zomboid, emotionally blunted, depressed, anesthetized, like I'm sleepwalking* (these are terms I hear): *I feel as if my own self was at some stage—removed. I gradually went missing.* It was years before I felt this bad with Ativan. Critics say that the benzos lose their effect after a few weeks; some say they lose it after a few days, and that what you're getting after this is a placebo effect. I think I continued to feel the effects; I know, so does everyone—but when I'd wake up after two to four hours, I could count on drifting back to sleep, which I can't do on my own, and I don't think I was just imagining this. I think that my usual hyperarousal was generally *unhyped*, along with my alertness. I could plotz down in my aunt's big recliner and nod off to sleep.

Every summer and school break, I'd stop it cold—not the recommended method, but school breaks are short and I was in a hurry. In fact, it's "a dangerous and unacceptable method of detoxification," as I later read. It felt like somebody had scooped out my brain and left a throbbing mass of protoplasm in its place. It was days before I could read again. The light felt like stab wounds, my eyes streamed tears, my right eyelid twitched. The rebound insomnia made me feel like I'd never sleep again, and I'd think, this time I've gone and done it, destroyed my capacity for sleep, fragile at best, now totally blitzed. It's like all the white nights of insomnia you've managed to put off come marching out to get you, along with all the nightmares you might (or might not) have had. I don't usually mind my dreams; even the bad ones are usually interesting—but being pinned under earthquake rubble or facing a firing squad, I could do without. What happens when you stop the drug is that the excitatory mechanisms it's inhibited are let loose, with a vengeance, and you get this rebound overactivity. The mechanisms that the benzos have damped down—and these include nearly every excitatory mechanism in the nervous system—are put "in a hyperexcitable state," explains Dr. Heather Ashton, a British psychopharmacologist who ran a benzo withdrawal clinic for twelve years (and helped a number of insomniacs who wrote me). Your GABA receptors have to learn how to work on their own again.

One Christmas when I cold-turkeyed it, I thought I was having a heart attack. It was like a vise closing around my heart, a fist squeezing it hard. I was lucky I didn't have a seizure—some people do. When I stood up, I felt like I was going to throw up or pass out, so I lay in bed the whole day. I know now that my symptoms were typical of benzo withdrawal: dizziness, extreme thirst, loss of appetite, light sensitivity, impaired concentration and memory. Symptoms I didn't experience, but which some people do, are tingling, crawling, burning sensations in the skin, breathlessness, panic. The withdrawal syndrome from any drug, explains Ashton, is a mirror, or opposite image, of the effects the drug has had. The dreams that the benzos have suppressed come back in the form of vivid dreams and nightmares; muscle relaxation is replaced by twitches, spasms, tension, rapid heartbeat; tranquility, by insomnia, anxiety, nervousness. The only way this rebound principle does *not* work is, alas, with memory loss: the drug impairs memory, and the withdrawal makes it worse.

By the end of a summer, I'd be back to my usual broken sleep, my dreams would be back to normal, and I could hold a phone number in my head almost long enough to write it down. I'd tell myself, I will *never* do this again, but then the semester would start up, and I would do it again. At some point, I had to admit that I was only going through the withdrawal to get the drug out of my system so it would have an effect when I went back on it. I did not know then that "recovery after long-term benzodiazepine use is not unlike the gradual recuperation of the body after a major surgical operation." I did not know that it's harder to withdraw from benzos than it is from barbiturates, a process that "typically passes in no more than 30 days." Some say it's harder than coming off heroin: "with heroin[,] usually the withdrawal is over within a week or so. With benzodiazepines . . . very unpleasant symptoms [may persist] for month after month." Some say symptoms go on for years.

I got into a pattern of going to my mother's for Christmases and long breaks, where it didn't matter that I was a basket case. I'd sit at the kitchen table with my mother and aunt, then in their eighties, flipping through magazines and chatting. My friends thought it odd, these long disappearances. I talked to no one about what I was going through. I wouldn't have known how to talk about it. Then one Christmas, I went to Mother's, intending to spend the break coming off the pills, hanging out with her and my aunt, only this time it was their turn to be indisposed. My mother went into decline and died in May; my aunt died six weeks before her, in March. During that period, when I was their primary caretaker, and then, later, reeling from their loss, I did not stop taking Ativan for two and a half years, and I stayed at 1.5 to 2 milligrams the whole time. Coming off it that time was beyond awful, but at least I knew enough by then to taper it off gradually. It took six months, an entire sabbatical, before I was back to my usual sleep.

A doctor once told me I was lucky to find a drug I tolerated as well as Ativan, that I got so much mileage out of. *Mileage?* I guess you could call it that. Ativan allowed me to carry on a career and to get through the worst nightmare of my life, my mother's and aunt's deaths. But *lucky* is an odd word to describe that roller coaster of withdrawal and addiction I was on for two decades, that sinking sense I always had that I was going to have to pay for this sleep and pay dearly, and the fear, never far from me then or now, of what this was doing to my brain and body. When I look back on that time, I'm amazed I survived it.

Ativan Issues

Ativan turns out to have problems other benzos do not. Researchers had assumed that the shorter the half-life, the faster the drug clears the body, and the less problematic the drug would be, in terms of hangover and problems of withdrawal. But it doesn't work that way. In fact, it turns out that the shorter the half-life, the more *acute* the withdrawal: effects are felt immediately after the drug is stopped and are felt more acutely. When my friend Roberta was first given a medication, she was given the older, longer-acting Dalmane, and this became her mainstay; she never went through the horrors of withdrawal I did. (She still takes it occasionally, though not every night. She doesn't have to—it's so long-acting.) In fact, now when doctors withdraw people from Ativan, they sometimes first switch them to Valium or Dalmane, which allows a more gradual reduction of dose. Yet it's not just its half-life that makes Ativan the worst, since Restoril has a similar half-life and is not so problematic. "When somebody comes into my office and says that they've been trying to stop their lorazepam, my heart sinks, because I know I shall have twice as much of a problem as getting them off, say, Valium," says Malcolm Lader; "the symptoms are more severe, they're more persistent, more bizarre, and people are much more distressed by them."

There is some debate about what to call the condition I was in, during those years I took Ativan—whether to describe it as *addiction, habituation,* or *medical dependence.* Many people prefer the term *dependence* to *addiction*, since addiction has associations with hard-core drugs. (The word *drugs,* for that matter, has associations with hard-core drugs: some people prefer to call them medications. I use both words, more or less interchangeably, because I think of them both ways: they serve useful purposes, as medications do, and they can badly mess you up, as hard-core drugs can do.) Dependent I was, no question of that, and it was not "just psychological." If I stopped the drug for one night, I felt a fist around my heart: that drug was part of my body, brain, and nerves. Addicted? *Addiction* is usually associated with pleasure seeking and a craving for the drug, and I crave chocolate and popcorn more than I ever craved Ativan; insofar as I derived pleasure from it, it was the pleasure of sleep. But addiction is also associated with exceeding the prescribed dose, with "drug-seeking behavior"—and exceed it I did. A kindly old physician wrote me a prescription for one milligram per night, assuring me that "that much Ativan never hurt anybody." I never told him that there were times I took twice that. I never told him about my trips to Mexico.

Whether you call it addiction, habituation, or dependence, I was hooked, and it was hell coming off it. Not everyone becomes addicted, however, even to Ativan. Ilene was given this drug to help her *forget* chemotherapy (it's prescribed for such things on account of its "well-known amnesic action"); she took two milligrams for a few months, and had no trouble stopping. Do I have a more "dependent personality" than Ilene has? Maybe so. If a thing is addictive, I become addicted—I've battled my way free of cigarettes, coffee, chocolate, and there were times in my life when I drank more than was good for me. But why did Ilene never feel that fist around her heart? The physiology of addiction is not well understood. One theory is that the faster you move the drug out of your system, the more likely you are to feel the withdrawal— and I do seem to have a hair-trigger reaction to drugs and to most other things: a few sips of champagne, and I'm up; a few sips of coffee, I'm alert. But drugs have never been my thing. Even in the 1960s, when everyone I knew was smoking dope and dropping acid, I was never drawn to drugs, except for the diet pills I snitched from my father's sample cabinet—which I loved.

I hear many cautionary tales like mine, and worse. I hear, *If I had known when I started what it would be like to stop taking this drug [Ativan], I'd never have started.* I hear, *Anyone who uses these drugs should be told they can ruin your life.* But I also hear stories of people who take benzos year after year and seem to do okay. A Berkeley psychiatrist told me, "These drugs are supposed to be so bad for you, but I meet in my profession lots of people who take them for years and years and do fine—and no, they don't have to increase the dose." An insomniac told me, *I've kept my dose of Restoril to thirty milligrams for years now, and I sleep. My doctor doesn't have a problem with this and neither do I.* Peter Hauri points out, "In our sleep clinics we see all the failures. We don't see the thousands of people who take the standard dose of Dalmane, . . . are satisfied with the pills, and live to be a ripe old age." These testimonies suggest that some people get away with long-term use. I did not. And on the basis of my experience, I'd be cautious about taking a benzodiazepine to "break a pattern" of insomnia.

I now take Ativan occasionally, when I'm traveling or at a conference, and sometimes during the school year, but I tolerate it less well than I used to. I feel more next-day lassitude, and even with one milligram, I stumble over Shakespeare when I read aloud in class—the tongue doesn't do what the brain tells it to do. (This happens with Ambien, too.) The older you get, the more sensitive you become to the effects of the benzodiazepines, especially the cognitive effects. The liver and kidneys become less effective at eliminating medications, so they hang around your system longer; concentrations build up and side effects become worse. Sleep researchers who have studied the effects of the benzos on the elderly report more falls, fractures, and greater cognitive and memory impairment. And yet a 2004 study found that "more than 40 percent of all benzodiazepines are prescribed to people over sixty-five." And another 2004 study, a survey of 192 long-term users of benzos over sixty-five, found that "the majority of patients reported no warnings from professionals about adverse effects," and that "half had tried to stop at some time but most attempts had been short-lived."

Over sixty-five? By sixty-five, I want this drug out of my life. Ativan is not a friend I want to grow old with.

You'd think that sleep medications would be carefully scrutinized in the elderly, since so many older people take them. But no. Most clinical trials *exclude* people over sixty-five because they're complicated to study; and drug companies don't usually even specify lower doses for the elderly. "We test drugs in young people for three months; we give them to old people for 15 years," says Dr. Peter Lamy of the University of Maryland School of Pharmacy. And most doctors are clueless. A recent study of physicians who treat Medicare patients found that 70 percent of the doctors who took an examination on prescribing for older adults failed the test—and these were the interested doctors, the ones who agreed to take the test; most of the doctors contacted did not reply.

And women? It is known that sleep meds affect us differently, yet we're still excluded from most studies. It is known that Restoril "has a 73% longer half-life in older women than in younger women," and that women seem to respond "more poorly to tricyclics compared with men and . . . better to SSRIs." Considering that so much advertising is aimed at us and that we're the primary consumers, it would be nice to know more. In 1993, the FDA issued guidelines urging drug companies to look for sex differences in the ways drugs are processed; but guidelines are only guidelines.

Today it is generally acknowledged that the benzodiazepines are addictive. There are Websites for benzodiazepine dependency and withdrawal. But there is still tremendous denial. An insomniac wrote me, *When I went off Klonopin, I stopped sleeping entirely. The doctor said, oh, no, it couldn't be the drug.* Another told me, *I try telling my doctor, every time I try to go off this drug [Klonopin], I stop sleeping entirely. He says it's just the insomnia coming back and I should probably not stop. I tell him my insomnia hadn't been that bad when I started taking it in the first place.*

As a long-term user, I'd like to know something about long-term effects. These drugs have been used extensively for fifty years, but their effects over time have barely been looked at. Daniel Kripke, who made a lasting impression on me with his Grim-Reaper slide to illustrate "the dark side of sleeping pills," at the first sleep conference I attended, says that chronic use may "damage the sleep system" the same way long-term use of alcohol does (which also binds to GABA receptors), even "after long abstinence." (Some alcoholics never return to normal sleep.) I think I did return, "after long abstinence," to what's "normal" sleep for me; I may sleep a little worse now, but then I'm decades older, too. My aches and pains now seem in a more normal range for a person my age.

But I have many questions. I have a sense that the benzos and non-benzos and even Benadryl affect my vision the next day. When I come in out of bright sunlight, after doing something strenuous like swimming, I get a weird wavy effect off to the edge of my vision. It only happens after I've taken a sleep med. It's hard to describe, something like the shadow a ceiling fan might cast against a fluorescent light; it strobes with my pulse. My vision is worsening alarmingly. I have a retinal wrinkle that puckers the visual field of my right eye so there are no straight lines on that side of the world. There's also a "pseudo hole" in that retina that I've been told, grotesquely, to "keep an eye on"; and I do actually see it— on days after I've taken a sleep med—like a small, opaque contact lens that's wandered off course, making a greenish dead spot; sometimes it zigzags across my line of vision. "Blurred vision and other complications related to the eyes" are listed among the withdrawal effects from benzos, but that's the only clue I find. *What* "other complications," I'd like to know. Or maybe I wouldn't.

Since the benzos suppress deep sleep, they may affect the hormones released during deep sleep, and what that does over time is anybody's guess. More than one study links them (and certain antidepressants) with cancer. They also produce *anterograde amnesia,* meaning that you can't remember things that happen after you consume them: *you can't form new memories,* which is why they're useful for chemotherapy. This effect wears off as the drug wears off, so we're told. But in 1988, a legal action began in the United Kingdom on behalf of several hundred people seeking compensation for dependence on Ativan, their main claim being that long-term use had left them cognitively impaired. By 1992, over twelve thousand claimants had joined this action. Valium and several other benzodiazepines were involved, but the number of claims against Ativan exceeded all the rest put together. The case dragged on, the drug companies fighting it every step of the way, until finally it reached the point where legal costs threatened to exceed the amounts claimed, so it never came to court.

I have no idea if these drugs have permanently dumbed me down; I can't remember what I was like before. I never experienced any amnesic episodes, or none that I remember, but of the thousands of hours of books on tape I listened to in those years, I remember almost nothing. With an insomniac, of course, you can never tell if a memory problem is due to drugs or just plain lack of sleep. Ditto for coordination: benzo use increases the risk of falls; insomnia left untreated may lead to falls. Rock, hard place.

A 1994 study of twenty-one long-term benzo users followed these patients up after six months' abstinence and found that, on a simple battery of routine tests of cognitive function, there was "significant impairment in patients in verbal learning and memory, psychomotor, visuo-motor and visuo-conceptual abilities, compared with controls." "The impairment does not necessarily diminish with time," says a 1993 study, with a coolness that chills my blood. Ashton says that "cognitive impairment due to benzodiazepines does not always recover completely, although it improves after withdrawal." She refers to a study done ten months after withdrawal, which found that "cognitive impairment, though slowly improving, persisted for at least this time." She adds that "on the available evidence there is no reason to think that any such changes would be permanent," but that "long-term benzodiazepine use may add to age-related cognitive decline."

It's one of my greatest terrors, memory loss, and the subject of my nightmares. I have something urgent to do, I'm responsible for something, only I can't remember what it is or how to do it. I was involved in a jewel heist the other night, I knew the combination to the safe, only I couldn't remember what it was; I was punching in numbers desperately, wildly, but they were the wrong numbers, time was running out, I knew I'd be caught.

I think of my Aunt Sady, living out her days in a Brooklyn apartment, increasing her dosage of sleeping pills year after year (barbiturates, those would have been, or maybe Librium or Valium; I never asked). She became vaguer and vaguer until she was totally lost. She was diagnosed with Alzheimer's, but was it really Alzheimer's? I'll never know.

Xanax and Halcion

"I watched closely, amazed and appalled, as Xanax burst onto the scene as the new 'safer' Valium," writes Jay Cohen, author of *Overdose*. "Upjohn launched a torrent of advertising that emphasized Xanax's superiority over

Valium," and "it quickly became a best-seller." In 2000, it was first on the list of the ten most commonly prescribed psychiatric medications in the United States (Ativan was fifth, Ambien was seventh, Valium ninth). In 2002, it was the tenth-most frequently prescribed hypnotic.

The first published study on the dependence risk of Xanax concluded that the risk was low. But Cohen says that he "saw far more dependency, more quickly, and of greater severity with Xanax than ever with Valium." Its short half-life—six to twelve hours—can produce withdrawal reactions even while patients are still taking the drug. Accounts of withdrawal from Xanax, even from people who have been taking no more than the prescribed dose, make my experience coming off Ativan sound like a walk in the park. In her book on chronic headaches, Paula Kamen describes anxiety attacks so extreme that she had to move back in with her parents to get through them; and they went on for months. (This is, ironically, the drug that's prescribed for anxiety attacks.) Withdrawal may be accompanied by paranoid and other psychotic reactions. Medawar draws attention to "the small print warning of the Xanax label: 'Some patients may prove resistant to all discontinuation regimens,' i.e., once on, never off."

"Xanax is the worst," said a psychiatrist friend who's had long experience prescribing drugs. "It has the most rapidly developing tolerance; it's the most difficult to stop." And yet I know people who've found it a mainstay for many years, though they take it only occasionally, not every night.

Halcion was approved in the United States in 1982, and it came on the scene with all the usual hoopla, hailed as the ideal sleeping pill, as safer and more effective than all previous medications, leaving no next-day hangover. By 1989, it was "Upjohn's second biggest moneymaker" (second only to Xanax), according to a *Newsweek* cover story. But in that same year, negative publicity began appearing in such prominent places as the *MacNeil/Lehrer NewsHour* and *20/20*. It was patients, again, who blew the whistle. In 1988, San Francisco writer Cindy Ehrlich published a powerful piece in *California* magazine, recounting how, after a few weeks on Halcion, even at a low dose, she was "babbling nonstop" to her therapist, telling her thoughts "about suicide, nuclear war, alien invasion," and how her therapist kept throwing more drugs into the mix, adding Xanax, an antipsychotic, an antidepressant. She and her therapist "sat staring at each other for six months, wondering why I was going off my rocker, and neither of us thought it might be a drug reaction." Ehrlich later discovered that the irritability, confusion, agitation she was experiencing were described as side effects of Halcion in the *Physicians' Desk Reference,* the leading drug reference among physicians, though they were implied to be rare. She also discovered that they'd been in the medical literature since 1979, when a Dutch psychiatrist, in a letter in *The Lancet,* described exactly her constellation of symptoms.

Halcion achieved real notoriety in 1990, when best-selling author William Styron, in *Darkness Visible,* linked it to his breakdown. Styron was, as he says, "consuming large doses" at the time of his breakdown. He acknowledges that his own "carelessness was at fault in ingesting such an overdose": "I was headed for the abyss, but I believe that without Halcion I might not have been brought so low." In fact, people are driven to overdose because the half-life of Halcion is so short (two hours) that the user is practically withdrawn each day, experiencing what Edinburgh researcher Ian Oswald describes as "daytime rebound anxiety." Three years later, Styron said that he was "stunned by the volume of the mail" he received, amazed that 15 to 20 percent of those who wrote to him described "their own Halcion-induced horrors, homicidal fantasies, near-suicides and other psychic convulsions."

"This is a very dangerous drug," says Anthony Kales. It is dangerous not only to the user but to others. In 1990, the FDA "tallied the numbers of hostile acts reported in association with 329 prescription drugs. Halcion ranked number 1, followed by Xanax." A man in San Diego started setting fires; a woman in Virginia shot her husband; a man in Michigan stabbed his wife. None of these people had histories of mental illness or violence. In 1991, Kales established that half a milligram of Halcion consistently produced next-day memory impairment, far more so than Restoril; he and others joined Oswald in suggesting that it be taken off the market. (Upjohn slapped a suit on Oswald for a million pounds—and Upjohn won.) Halcion was banned in Holland for over a decade; it was banned in Britain, Norway, Finland, Bermuda, and Jamaica. It went on to become the best-selling benzodiazepine in the United States and the world. It was not, however, on the list of the top sixteen drugs prescribed in 2002.

I never went near either of these drugs. Better the devil I knew, I figured, and stuck with Ativan. But a 1997 review of Halcion concluded that it is actually no worse than the other benzodiazepines in terms of amnesia, depression, psychosis, aggression, bizarre behavior, and anxiety.

The Age of Ambien

When Ilene told me she'd been prescribed Ativan to help her *forget* the experience of chemotherapy, and that it had wiped out not only the bad stuff but portions of the good stuff (returning to Hawaii several years later, she remembered that she'd driven up the volcano only after she was halfway up it again), I decided it was time to find something else. When school started that fall, I began taking Ambien.

Ambien (zolpidem) appeared on the scene in 1993, perfectly timed to step into the gap left by the failure of Halcion. By the end of the century, it had achieved blockbuster status, over a billion in sales, and it kept going up, to over $2 billion in 2005: "11 billion nights and climbing," boasts an ad. Ambien, like the other so-called nonbenzodiazepines—Sonata (zaleplon), Lunesta (eszopiclone), and indiplon—was developed to be faster and shorter-acting. It is wonderfully fast-acting, but it's also so short-lived, with its half-life of two to four hours, that it's out of my system before the night is over; I wake up, heart pounding, receptors all perked up demanding more. When I first started taking it, I managed to take it only during the week, which I could never do with Ativan, but soon I was taking it weekends, too. It has a nice long skinny shape that allows you to bite it off in little pieces, but then those little pieces became larger pieces, until I was up to ten to fifteen milligrams a night, exceeding the recommended dose (five to ten milligrams) and the recommended limit of ten to twenty-eight days.

The nonbenzodiazepines are chemically different from the benzodiazepines. They bind to the same GABAa receptors, but they affect fewer receptor subtypes; they bind more selectively and, being "cleaner" drugs, do not (usually) have the withdrawal effects that the benzos do; and they produce less tolerance and dependence. Ambien is said to interfere less with normal sleep architecture and to allow deep sleep, but I read contradictory things about this. When FDA approval of the drug was announced in 1993, the announcement said that "changes in the sleep EEG with zolpidem . . . are almost identical to those caused by the benzodiazepine hypnotics." Spectral analysis of the EEG, a refined computer analysis, shows that Ambien's effects on the EEG are comparable to the benzos', increasing stage 2 sleep at the expense of deep sleep. Several of the doctors and researchers I talked to flat out reject the inflated claims made for Ambien over the benzos: "Not a dime's worth of difference between them," said a Berkeley psychiatrist who did not mince his words: "Doctors shouldn't fall for their own bullshit. We don't really know how these drugs work."

I felt, as I felt with Ativan, that I was not getting the restorative effects of deep sleep—my aches and pains were bad as ever—and I hear many of the same complaints about Ambien that I heard about the benzos: *I never feel like I get real sleep from Ambien. I feel not myself, out of sorts, off balance, depressed, spacey, like there's a thick glass pane between me and the world.*

The nonbenzos are said not to affect memory, but amnesic effects were described in the literature from the start. A student tells me, *I often don't recall what I've read the night before when I take an Ambien. I can't tell you how many nights I've wasted studying—it just doesn't stay with me.* I read, *The memory loss that you are experiencing at night will gradually start occurring during the day if you take it for too long.* Ambien is claimed not to be addictive, and it was not, for me—but it is, for some people. *I am absolutely addicted to this medicine,* writes a twenty-one-year-old person who's been taking it for five years. *It is addictive, no matter what doctors may tell you. I had a horrible time coming off it.* And now these effects are being described in the literature.

But what was truly alarming to me were the personality changes. Paranoia. I began to lose confidence in the classroom. I'd do things to sabotage myself, start the class off with a question I hadn't a clue how to answer, let the discussion wander off into corners and out on tangents, make a lot of unwise moves. I began to feel insecure, like I was losing whatever it is that enables me to hold a class. Students can smell fear.

I've heard many stories about the bizarre effects Ambien has on personality and behavior. A woman I know found her husband on the closet floor, pulling the clothes down around him; another time she found him rearranging all the living room furniture. *When I was on Ambien, it caused me a weird psychotic breakdown,* wrote the San Francisco insomniac quoted in the last chapter. *Normally, I'm very stable. But after a week of taking Ambien, I lost it. I was in a crowded church. I started to feel the world close in on me. I had to get out.* The Web is full of such accounts, along with reports of people waking up to find their beds littered with candy bar wrappers and crumbs, with no recollection of these binges. Early in 2006, stories began appearing in the media: a woman ate a whole tub of margarine, another gained a hundred pounds before realizing that Ambien was the problem. Sleep researchers knew about the sleep-eating, but I don't think anyone was prepared for the reports that started coming out, also in early 2006, about people sleep-driving while under the influence and having no next-day recall. Ambien has been implicated in so many accidents that it's made the "the top 10 list of drugs found in impaired drivers" in ten laboratories that test drivers' blood samples. A New York lawyer has filed a class-action suit against the makers of Ambien, citing reports of people driving under the influence of the drug, or "eating raw eggs and even a buttered cigarette, and sleep-shoplifting DVDs."

Early in 2007, the FDA called for stronger warnings on sleep aids. "These drugs do things we do not understand," as Kripke says.

Sonata came on the market with great fanfare, a few years after Ambien. *I asked the doc if he'd given me a sugar pill,* said one person I talked to, which I'm afraid sums up my experience with it—which is too bad, because it is (or it is claimed to be) a relatively benign drug. I do know people who have occasional or moderate insomnia, who are menopausal or perimenopausal, for whom Sonata works beautifully.

After my year on Ambien, I went back to Ativan. After that year, I went back to Ambien. Ambien works for me, now that I know how to use it—not every night, and only in the second half of the night, and keep the dose low. After the two to four hours of sleep I can usually get on my own, I nibble off three to five milligrams from that long skinny purple pill (all sleeping pills should be shaped like that, so we can calibrate doses). It gives me about an hour per milligram, up to a maximum of five hours—even if I take ten or fifteen milligrams, I never get more than five hours. The sleep is never as good as my own sleep, but the difference between the two to four hours I get on my own and the seven to eight hours I can get with a few milligrams of Ambien is the difference between walking and hobbling through my life. I try to do this no more than three, four, or at most five days a week. The problem is that five days becomes six days, and three milligrams becomes five. . . .

Taking a sleeping pill is like having a bear by the nose.

The Drug Most Taken: Trazodone

Ambien can advertise itself as "the #1 sleep agent" because it is the most frequently prescribed drug that has been FDA-approved for insomnia. But it is not actually the drug most often prescribed for insomnia: trazodone (Desyrel) is. Trazodone is not technically a "sleep agent" or hypnotic (which is why Ambien can claim it's "#1"). It is an older type of antidepressant, related to a category of drugs called *tricyclics,* which includes Elavil (amitriptyline) and Sinequan (doxepin), drugs that were not developed for sleep but which may have sedating side effects. (Trazodone is technically an "atypical tricyclic," though it's usually grouped with the tricyclics.) As the use of benzos fell off in the early 1980s, doctors began prescribing these more and more: in 2002, amitriptyline ranked third on the list of drugs most prescribed, and doxepin, fourteenth. Other antidepressants used for sleep are Serzone (nefazodone), which is closely related to trazodone but was taken off the U.S. market in 2004 for its liver toxicity, and Remeron (mirtazapine), which is notorious for causing weight gain but may be very effective with insomnia—it's fourth on the list of drugs most often prescribed. The older antidepressants suppress REM, more than the benzos do—if you don't like your dreams, you may be glad of this, but if you do like your dreams, you may not. These drugs are thought to target several systems—the serotonin, norepinephrine, GABA systems, among others; they're "dirty" drugs, in that they do not target selectively. But again, it is not really understood how they work. "First you figure out *what* the drug does, then, if you're lucky, you find out *how* it does it," as a researcher told me.

Every time I ask a doctor at my HMO for something to help me sleep, trazodone is the drug I'm offered. For years, I refused it, having had a dismal experience with Elavil in graduate school. But a few years ago, I decided to give it a try. The doc who recommended it seemed so sure it would help, and I liked him, so instead of dropping the prescription into my purse, where it would dissolve into the mulch of gum wrappers and shredded tissue at the bottom, I took it to the pharmacy and got the pills. I was amazed at the quantity they gave me, a great fat bottle of one hundred. Ambien, you milk out of them piece by piece (and pick up the tab yourself); Ativan, you go to Mexico for (or did, before the Internet); but trazodone is given out like candy. It costs next to nothing, since it's long been off patent, and there are no restrictions on it—it's not a controlled substance, so doctors feel easy prescribing it. You could take this drug forever, as far as anybody is concerned.

I then had to find a time to take it. It's not easy to experiment with sleep medications, since you're risking the whole next day. I couldn't chance it before a teaching day and it seemed a shame to take it on a night I felt I could get to sleep on my own, so it was months before I found the right time, a Saturday night when it looked like sleep wasn't going to come but there was nothing urgent to do the next day. I took fifty milligrams—nothing. I took another fifty milligrams—still nothing (the dose that had been suggested was one hundred to two hundred milligrams). Afraid to mix it with anything else, I toughed out the rest of the night—sure enough, it was one of those nights when sleep didn't come at all. All I got from that drug was the same excruciatingly parched mouth that I remember from Elavil.

But maybe, I thought, I just didn't take enough, or maybe I waited too long that night to take it. Finally, a few months later, I found a time when there was nothing pressing the next day. I'd just read a study that described a lifelong insomniac who had success with a dose of 200 milligrams. It was a Saturday night, I was feeling mellow, so I thought, well, maybe if I take 200 milligrams all at once, it will get me past my usual three-hour wake-up call. But I couldn't quite bring myself to swallow four of these fat white tablets, so I stopped at three (150 milligrams). I was reading, waiting for the drug to kick in, and at some point I found myself reading the same sentence over and over, head unpleasantly fuzzy, so I turned off the light—and then suddenly I felt this great surge of cardiac energy, my heart started pounding, and I thought, *Uh-oh.* I managed to drift off, but three hours later I was wide awake. I lay there listening to a book on tape, and eventually I got back to sleep, but it was that sort of sleep where you're aware of yourself sleeping. I came to at 7 A.M., parched, head aching. I got up and was staggering, really reeling, went back to bed, feeling dizzy and queasy, and lay there just incredibly tense; my limbs were unhappy no matter what I did with them. I would have gotten up, except I felt so awful, and I had a book on tape that made the dark more appealing than anything I could imagine doing with the day, so I listened to Richard Ford's *Independence Day,* and dropped back to sleep around 10 A.M. and slept till 1. Woke up feeling hungover, depressed, parched, and headachy, still sort of lurching. I found myself, in the middle of leaving a message on Ilene's phone machine, forgetting what I'd called to say.

"Well, did it make you sleep?" asked a friend who's used trazodone for years, and who had urged me to try.

"I don't know what you'd call it, but it wasn't an experience I'd care to repeat."

I have heard many success stories with trazodone—*I am a different person now. I feel as if I missed the entire first half of my life in a haze of exhaustion. . . . For me, trazodone is like insulin.* But I have also heard stories like mine: *Yikes, what a chemical lobotomy that was!* said a friend. *I've been taking 150 milligrams trazodone and I'm getting sleep,* wrote an insomniac, *but I have this tendency to stare out the window a lot. I don't feel like myself. My doc says it can't be the drug, but I never felt like this before, spacey all the time.* I hear complaints about racing hearts and weakened limbs and muscle twitching, and I hear withdrawal horror stories. *Don't believe anyone who tells you this drug is not addictive; it took me weeks of withdrawal hell to get back to the way I was sleeping before.* And I hear stories of doctors who turn a deaf ear to their patients' complaints: *He told me there was no such thing as withdrawal from trazodone, and if I had a problem when I stopped this drug, I should increase the dose.*

The speakers at the sleep conferences are critical of the older antidepressants used for sleep. They say that docs prescribe them so liberally because they're not scheduled drugs, that they're practicing "regulatory-based rather than evidence-based medicine"—which I well believe. They say that trazodone can aggravate cardiac arrhythmia (irregular heartbeat)—which I also believe, given the dramatic effect it had on my heart. They say that it can cause cognitive impairment, and I believe that too, given the way it fuzzed me out. They say that it was the thirteenth-most-common psychotropic drug associated with emergency room visits in 2000, and that it hasn't been sufficiently studied to warrant its prescription for sleep.

All this is pretty damning and pretty convincing, and yet plenty of people do well with this drug and keep it at a low dose through the years. Ambien has worked better for me than trazodone, by far, but I'm skeptical about the way the newer drugs are being pushed. The Ambien bandwagon has big bucks behind it. I know—I've been to its booth at the fair and come away with its prizes.

Russian Roulette: The SSRIs

"And then something just kind of changed in me. . . . I became all right, safe in my own skin. . . . One morning I woke up and I really did want to live, really looked forward to greeting the day." So writes Elizabeth Wurtzel in *Prozac Nation,* in 1994, one of several best-sellers inspired by this blockbuster drug (*Listening to Prozac* was published the year before). Prozac (fluoxetine) burst on the scene in 1988, and soon everybody was taking it, everybody was talking about it and hearing tales of lives miraculously transformed by it. "Chances are, someone you know is getting better because of it!" boasts a Prozac Website. By 1994, it was the second-best-selling drug in the United States. And more than a medication, it was a "media event," with cover stories on *Newsweek* and *New York Magazine.* More than an antidepressant, it was "bottled sunshine." It was a "lifestyle drug," "the personality pill," as *Time* magazine trumpeted: people were taking it to feel "better than normal," to become new, "improved" versions of themselves, smarter, more self-assured—and thinner. Claims were made for it that were as extravagant as, well, the claims that had been made for Librium and Valium.

The tricyclics were the mainstay of antidepressant treatment until the late 1980s, when the SSRIs overtook them. They are called *selective serotonin reuptake inhibitors* because they inhibit the reabsorption of serotonin, so that more of it remains available. After Prozac came Zoloft in 1991, then Paxil in 1993, to be followed by Celexa and Lexapro, and Effexor and Cymbalta, which affect norepinephrine as well. They are given for everything from obsessions, compulsions, phobias, panic disorders, and posttraumatic stress syndrome to shyness, kleptomania, eating disorders, PMS, migraines, and getting through the holidays. They are handed out as benzos used to be, after five to ten minutes' conversation. They are the most heavily marketed category of drugs in America, and by 2001, they were the best-selling: Zoloft was the sixth-most-frequently prescribed drug in the United States; Paxil was seventh; Prozac, ninth; Effexor, twenty-third; and Celexa, twenty-fourth. (Ambien trailed that year at twenty-seventh—though four years later, it was fourteenth.) Americans spent more than $9 billion on them, according to a 2003 report noting that this "exceeded the gross domestic product that year of each of two dozen African nations."

My students are given SSRIs when they break up with a boyfriend, get nervous about exams, want to improve their class performance, when the family dog dies. "It is estimated," says a 2005 study in the *New England Journal of Medicine,* "that 25 to 50 percent of U.S. college students who are seen in counseling and at student health centers are taking antidepressants." College counselors are now concerned about how many students come to college who are *already* taking them. "Antidepressant prescriptions to children increased three- to five-fold between 1988 and 1994," reports Dr. Julie Magno Zito, professor of pharmacy and medicine of the University of Maryland. "Preschoolers . . . are now the fastest-growing group of children receiving antidepressants," reports James Gorman in 2004. (Never mind that these drugs have hardly been tested in children, and when they have been tested, they have not been found to be effective.) The assurance with which doctors prescribe them is extraordinary, given how little is known about them and how short a time they've been tested, even on adults—six weeks. "Fundamentally," says Dr. Thomas Kramer, "we have no idea how these medications work." The official story is that they work by making more serotonin available, but if it was that simple, they'd kick in immediately, but they don't—they take weeks to get up to speed. They change the climate of the brain in ways that are not understood.

In 1997, thirteen-year-old Matt Miller, who had been given Zoloft for depression, hanged himself. His parents began looking for answers on the Web and found a lot of other parents with similar stories. "Common to all of them," reports Greg Critser in *Generation Rx,* "was the intense violence of the suicide or suicide attempt, the fact that the youths had not been on the antidepressant very long, and that no one had warned them that SSRIs could cause a condition known in the medical literature as *akathisia,* a state of internal restlessness and agitation so intense that taking one's life can appear to be the only way to relieve it." These parents could not get anyone to take them seriously until, in late 2003, the U.K. equivalent of the FDA advised against the use of SSRIs, except for Prozac, by anyone under eighteen. A year later, the FDA, after much deliberation, required antidepressants to carry a black box warning, the strongest warning possible, indicating significant danger of self-harm. David Healy, author of *The Anti-Depressant Era* and *Let Them Eat Prozac,* has looked at every study of SSRIs ever done and claims that the makers of these drugs knew of these dangers all along.

The SSRIs are regularly prescribed for insomnia, though insomnia is one of their well-known side effects. (Forty percent of Prozac users require sleep medication.) Insomnia is depression, goes the thinking; the SSRIs are good for depression—therefore they must be good for insomnia. And sometimes they are—there's a wide range of response to these drugs, wider than to the benzos, which may make them worth trying for sleep. But doctors should warn patients about the insomnia effect—and that it may not go away: *Zoloft made me crazy. I only took it three days but I couldn't sleep for weeks after that.* A woman I interviewed swears that her insomnia was triggered by Prozac: *I took Prozac for ten days and stopped sleeping. That was the beginning. The Prozac really triggered it. He should never have prescribed it—he knew I had a sleep problem.*

One-half the dose of Zoloft I'd been prescribed sent me over the moon: head fogged, I stumbled into bed, a little alarmed but consoling myself, well, at least I'll get some sleep—then came that surge of cardiac energy I'd felt with trazodone, only this lasted all the next day, until I got to the pool to swim it out. It wired me like those diet pills I used to take in college, except that it fried my brain. When I described this reaction to a psychiatrist at a sleep conference, she looked at me like I was, well, on drugs, and assured me this was a totally idiosyncratic response. (*They always make you feel like you're the only one who's having this reaction,* as more than one insomniac has observed.) And yet "agitation," a "restless agitation that ranges from jitteriness to a sensation described by some people as 'jumping out of their skin,'" is a well-known effect of the SSRIs. I've been told if you hang in there with the SSRIs long enough, they may lose their stimulating effects, but I wasn't hanging around to find out; anything that speeds me up like this is doing me no favors.

It's common practice to prescribe a benzo or a sedating antidepressant to counteract the stimulation: *Zoloft made my sleep much worse, so he said I should take a Restoril. Now my sleep is worse than ever. I'm dizzy and don't feel right.* Sleep specialists recommend such cocktails, one drug to pick you up, another to calm you down. But they're not for everyone: *I had a grand mal seizure once when taking Zoloft and Elavil—I quit that psychiatrist real fast.* They're not for me: if I chew off three milligrams of Ambien the same night I've taken an antihistamine, it puts me into a fog that lasts all day.

The SSRIs are claimed not to be addictive, but there are many studies and massive anecdotal evidence that they can cause significant withdrawal problems. Trawling through Charles Medawar's Website, the Antidepressant Web, I read of symptoms like the ones I experienced with Ativan: heart pounding, extreme insomnia, headache, dizziness, nausea, nightmares, sweating, irritability, lethargy. Addiction problems are most often reported in relation to Paxil (paroxetine, called Seroxat in the United Kingdom), the SSRI most often prescribed for insomnia. Paxil has been approved not only for depression but for panic disorder, obsessive-compulsive disorder, and social anxiety disorder (shyness), a problem most of us hadn't known was a medical disorder until SmithKline's public relations efforts convinced us it was. I've been offered this drug for insomnia, but on the basis of my night and day with Zoloft I won't go near another SSRI. Now I learn that "at least 25% [of those who take Paxil] and perhaps over twice that many, depending on what is being measured and who's counting," have withdrawal problems, and these problems can be fierce: *My brain has turned into liquid, my brain swooshes around in my skull. It feels as if static electricity is shooting through my brain; I can feel it travel down my arms into my hands. The world spins.* These feelings of electrical shock are so common as to have a name: *brain shivers.*

To Medawar and others who have been keeping track, it looks like "history has been repeating itself in a rather sinister way." For the past

150 years, "doctors have been prescribing an uninterrupted succession of drugs for mental distress, each time believing they were not addictive and that patients had only themselves to blame if addiction set in." Morphine was not thought to be addictive, nor was heroin, nor cocaine. The barbiturates were declared to be safe and effective, then the benzos, and now the SSRIs look like "a re-run" of that experience. Medawar describes "a pattern of error" in which "one drug after another, officially proclaimed as not addictive, has later proved to be just that." Says Medawar, "The clear message of history is to beware."

But rather than heeding the lessons of the past and becoming more cautious about new drugs, physicians are becoming more cavalier. They're prescribing more drugs than ever before—the number of prescriptions filled in the United States rose from 1.9 billion to well over 3 billion in the decade between 1992 and 2002—and they're prescribing newer drugs. "In the last seven years," writes Dr. Dan Shapiro, University of Arizona College of Medicine, "I have watched our residents prescribe the newest medications almost exclusively." Direct-to-consumer advertising, made legal in 1997 (only in the United States and New Zealand), is pushing this trend. By 2004, drug companies were spending $4.35 billion for ads on prime-time television, on billboards, on buses, and in magazines, flooding the market with hyperbolic claims that confuse patients and physicians alike and driving drug prices over the top. Now, in addition to the pressures to prescribe they get from drug companies, physicians have to deal with pressures from patients.

New drugs are dangerous drugs. "I tell my patients the drugs you see advertised on TV are the ones you don't want to use. Let other people use them first," says Dr. Brian Strom of the University of Pennsylvania School of Medicine. People assume that FDA approval guarantees that long-term studies have been done, that thousands of subjects have been studied over long periods of time, but in fact studies may last no longer than a few weeks and involve no more than a few hundred subjects—young, healthy male subjects, at that, which makes the drug look safer than it is. New drugs are becoming even more dangerous as they're being rushed to market faster, a trend that's also driven by industry pressure. Within a twenty-five-year period, 20 percent of new drugs were found to have adverse effects unknown or undisclosed at the time of approval, effects as serious as liver damage, damage to the heart and bone marrow, reports a 2002 study in the prestigious *Journal of the American Medical Association*. "It's a form of Russian roulette, really, to be using such drugs," says Dr. Sidney Wolfe, director of the Public Citizen Research

Group, one of the authors of this study. Cautious physicians say they won't prescribe a drug the first year it's out—"and if it's a family member, wait five years," as my father used to say. The watchdog group Public Citizen suggests seven years.

Excellent advice, if you can follow it, but in the real world, people are desperate, desperate for sleep, for relief from depression, from pain. So this is advice that most insomniacs (including me) do not heed.

What will the SSRIs do over time? Time will tell, or rather, the people who take the drugs over time will tell. We the users are the guinea pigs. The Internet gets the word out faster, spreads the news about the bad effects of drugs, by putting us in touch with one another. The manufacturer of Paxil kept insisting that the drug was not addictive, all the while the Internet was "groaning with evidence" that there were tens of thousands affected by a problem that officially did not exist—and in June 2003, Glaxo-SmithKline revised its estimate of risk of withdrawal symptoms from one in five hundred to one in four. But even with the Internet, it takes time for the bad news to be heard by the committees that issue the warnings and do the recalls, and meanwhile the drug is out there in the world.

Health care professionals generally agree that the SSRIs do more good than harm. I've known depressed people for whom they've been truly miraculous, so transformative that taking a sleeping pill seems a small price to pay. Occasionally these drugs are even wonderful for sleep. If you're getting some good from an SSRI or from any other drug I find problematic, listen to your body and to your doctor (assuming you have one you can trust), and not to me. Stay tuned to your body, if you can. It's not easy to monitor our own conditions when we're taking a drug that alters our conditions and there's so much else going on in our lives, but it's important to try.

In the future, scientists will be able to tell us how our genetic make-ups affect our responses to drugs. It's now known that the subtlest genetic variation can make all the difference in the way we respond to a drug. A mutation that makes women (but not men) redheaded, for example, also makes them more responsive to opiates. *Pharmacogenomics*, which studies how our individual genetic codes affect our responses to drugs, may someday spare us a lot of painful experimentation: we'll go to a doctor, have our blood taken and our DNA assessed, and with this information, the doctor will tell us which drug works best. "The age of personalized medicine is coming," a biologist friend assures me. "They'll test you for any one of the thirty or forty or so genes associated with insomnia—genes relating to reuptake factors, whole body regulators, and circadian and hormone regulators—they'll design drugs to affect those pathways, and, voila, you'll sleep!" But for the time being, we need to stay tuned to our bodies—as I did not, in my Ativan years.

The Next Big Thing?

When Ambien achieved blockbuster status at the end of the 1990s, the drug companies woke up and smelled the opportunities. Insomnia, says David Southwell, chief financial officer of Sepracor, maker of Lunesta, is "like depression before Prozac." "There is such a huge, untapped market of insomniacs out there who aren't seeking treatment, or who are getting suboptimal treatment." The marketing analyst group Spectra Intelligence reports that the global market for sleep-wake disorders is, as of December 2005, $4.3 billion and likely to increase to $11 billion by 2012. It's a plum of a market, since there are so many of us, and we get worse with age—and that big bulge in the population, the baby boomers, is getting on in years.

But "it's always very risky to try a new route," says Emmanuel Mignot, and risk is not something the big drug companies are inclined to take. To hear their hype, you'd think they were champions of innovation, but they have not in recent decades been highly innovative. They're more inclined to take the easier path, of modifying a chemical compound here or there, and leaving the basic research to federally funded researchers. The discovery of the most important drugs in the past few decades began with basic scientific work at the NIH or at academic research laboratories supported by government money. The drug companies piggyback on publicly funded work, stepping in to do the developing and marketing once it looks like the drug will be a go (and the consumers get to pay twice—first, with our tax dollars, and then when we buy the drug).

Most of the drugs that have come on the market in the past few decades have been "me-toos," modified versions of older drugs, slight variations that do not provide "significant clinical improvement" over existing drugs but have been altered enough to qualify for a new patent. Copycat drugs are known quantities, and as such, they are reliably profitable, which is why the industry makes so many of them. The drugs are not innovative, but the ad campaigns are over the top: they have to be,

because people have to be persuaded that there's a reason to take one
"me-too" over another, as Angell says.

Angell estimates that the industry spends close to $54 billion on pro-
motion, what with its direct-to-consumer advertising, sales representatives, gifts, perks, bribes, buckets of free samples, "educational" events,
and more drug company lobbyists than there are members of Congress
(twenty-one of them actually were, in 2000, former members of Congress). Fifty-four billion dollars is nearly twice the $28 billion the U.S.
government spends on all biomedical research. The cost, of course, gets
passed on to the consumer: in 1990, a brand-name prescription cost
around twenty-seven dollars, and a decade later, the average cost was
sixty-five dollars, making the pharmaceutical industry the most profitable in the nation, with rates of profit more than three times the average of other corporations.

Now the industry is moving in on the insomnia market, positioning
itself to penetrate this "under-penetrated market," as one biotech analyst
calls it. Drug makers spent $298 million advertising sleep meds during the
first eleven months of 2005, more than *four times* what they spent on this
type of advertising in all 2004. With several new drugs in the ring and more
in the wings, drug companies are launching "an advertising effort that industry watchers say could rival the saturation campaign for erectile dysfunction drugs." This may turn out to be, as a market analyst predicts,
"one of the epic marketing battles in the history of pharmaceuticals."

Anyone watching prime-time television in the fall of 2005 would have
seen the Lunesta moth flit across the screen, iridescent green against a
deep-blue background: "Lunesta, for a fresh start." Chances are, they'd
have seen it many times. Lunesta (eszopiclone) came on the market early
in 2005, with a flurry of advertising that promised "rapid sleep onset, . . .
improved sleep maintenance, . . . no evidence of tolerance," and "no
next-day residual effects in most patients." Every medical or sleep journal I see these days, every magazine I pick up in the physician's or den-
tist's office, has glossy ads that boast its effectiveness "night after night
after night." Sepracor, a small company based in Marlborough, Massachusetts, tested their drug for six months, which no other company had
dared to do, and it paid off, big time: users did not develop tolerance or
show adverse effects. Lunesta became the first sleeping pill not limited to
twenty-eight days' use, the "first and only hypnotic agent approved for
long-term use." With the FDA's lifting of the limit, "a taboo in the use
of sleeping pills had been broken," announced the *New York Times*.

"Within two months of its launch, Lunesta prescriptions hit 50,000 per week," reported an analyst. As of March 2007, Sepracor had spent $500 million on advertising (much of its television campaign was tied to the new season of *Desperate Housewives,* watched mainly by women), and Lunesta's performance "massively exceeded analysts' expectations." "In the twelve years I've been in practice," said a San Francisco sleep doctor, "this was the only time I've had a line of people out the door waiting to try a medicine." Now "people come in all the time and tell me they want to try that new sleeping pill with the butterfly on it," said Dr. Daniel Carlat, of Tufts University School of Medicine.

But Lunesta is not a new drug. Eszopiclone is a me-too, nearly identical to *zopiclone,* which has long been available as Zimovane in Europe and Imovane in Canada. Zopiclone bears much the same baggage as the other non-benzos—dependence, withdrawal symptoms, suggestions of cognitive impairment; in fact, it was denied approval by the U.S. FDA. A 1990 *Lancet* editorial described it as "another carriage on the tranquilliser train." While acknowledging that it "has fewer acute adverse effects than many existing compounds," the editorial dismissed manufacturer's claims that it's "not associated with the development of tolerance in long-term use . . . and that rebound insomnia is rare and minimal" as "inadequate to the point of being irresponsible."

Defenders of Lunesta claim that eszopiclone's tweak of the zopiclone molecule will address these problems. But the Drug Enforcement Administration's announcement of eszopiclone's scheduling, early in 2005, acknowledged that "in clinical trials, eszopiclone shows an adverse event profile comparable to that of other hypnotics," effects such as "amnesia, difficulty concentrating, memory impairment," and described its abuse potential as "similar to those of the benzodiazepines and the nonbenzodiazepine hypnotics." The main difference between Lunesta and existing treatments, wrote the editors of *The Medical Letter on Drugs and Therapeutics,* an independent source of information written for pharmacists and physicians, "may be that the manufacturer of Lunesta sponsored a 6-month trial and submitted the results to the FDA, while the other two manufacturers did not." In early 2007, when Ambien came under stricter FDA warnings for its associations with "complex sleep-related behaviors," Lunesta did, too. There have been, besides, carcinogenicity issues associated with both eszopiclone and zopiclone that did not turn up in connection with the other non-benzodiazepines; there were FDA discussions of the possibility of a cancer risk. The FDA *Pink Sheet Daily,* which covers pharmaceutical news, reports that "cancer risk" was at the "center of FDA approvability debate." (On the FDA label of Lunesta, some tumor growth in animals is described.)

I found Lunesta a bust, which didn't surprise me, since I figured if it was all that great, word would have reached us about Zimovane or Imovane long ago. It didn't get me past my three-hour wake-up call or make it easier to get back to sleep once I was awake, and it didn't act as quickly as Ambien. Also, it left a bitter taste that affected the way foods tasted all the next day, an unpleasant reminder of how long these drugs hang around in the system, and how they affect parts of our bodies unrelated to sleep. (About 30 percent of users experience this taste, I was told by a Lunesta representative). I doubt I could take this or any other drug "night after night" without developing tolerance or some other undesirable effect. Lunesta may have remained effective for the six months it was tested, and six months is longer than most drugs are tested, but this is a blip on the screen of a chronic insomniac. But I know people who swear by this drug, who say it's kept on working for several months, with no adverse effects. But I also know people who complain of a long hangover—not surprisingly, since Lunesta has less receptor specificity and a longer half-life than either Ambien or Sonata. I sense a general disappointment among insomniacs on the Web.

But time will tell, time and the patients. I do think there's a place on the market for the me-toos, contrary to what critics say; sometimes a tweaked molecule makes a difference, since everybody's response to drugs is so different. Lunesta is probably worth a try—if you can afford it. It's even more expensive than Ambien, and most insurance does not cover it.

From the maker of Ambien, Sanofi-Aventis (a recent merger of two French companies, Sanofi-Synthelabo and Aventis, and now the third-largest drug company in the world), comes a new, improved version of, well—Ambien. Ambien CR (continuous release) has a first layer that dissolves quickly, to release half of it, and a second layer that dissolves more slowly to release the other half. Not exactly a breakthrough. You sort of wonder why they didn't think of it before—and they probably did, but the timing assured that, when Ambien went off patent, the company would have a whole new patent. A lot of us have been eagerly awaiting the Ambien generic, which will bring the price down from three dollars a pill and may encourage our HMOs to be more generous with it. But now, if we want a longer-acting Ambien, we're still in for that crushing price.

Indiplon is another nonbenzo that's being developed in two forms, longer and shorter acting. Pfizer was working on this drug in conjunction with Neurocrine Biosciences, a small biotech company in San Diego, gearing up for a major advertising blitz, when, unexpectedly, in mid-2006 the FDA turned the drug down; then Pfizer dumped it. No break-throughs here, though great claims are made for it—rapid sleep onset, excellent safety profile, minimal side effects. Maybe it really will be wonderful—assuming it gets FDA approval—as fast-acting as Ambien, only longer lasting, with its half-life of five to six hours. Probably it will be like the rest of them, better for some people but not for others. Another me-too that's in the pipeline is Silenor, in phase III clinical trials as of fall 2006, which sounds like warmed-over doxepin. But then doxepin helps some people, so maybe this will, too—at a greatly increased price.

Many people are disgusted that, with all this hoopla, there isn't more to choose from. "If they put a third of all the effort they put into promoting into discovering new products, we might be getting somewhere," says sleep researcher Irwin Feinberg. Most of the hypnotics on the market (as I write in early 2007) target the GABA neurotransmitter system, the same system targeted by Librium half a century ago, though the sleep-wake system involves many mechanisms besides GABA, as we've seen.

There is one exception. A few months after it approved Lunesta, the FDA approved Rozerem (the generic name is ramelteon), produced by the Japanese drug giant Takeda. This is a melatonin receptor *agonist* (that is, it intensifies the action of the melatonin). It has, like Lunesta, been approved for long-term use, but—unlike Lunesta or any other sleep med— it is not a controlled substance: it's the first-ever FDA-approved hypnotic that's *nonscheduled,* because it does not work on the GABA system. But the effects aren't all that spectacular: in the studies submitted by Takeda to the FDA, ramelteon increased total sleep time, on average, by only eleven to fourteen minutes. There was concern among FDA scientists that it might raise levels of prolactin, which sounds nice to me, since I suspect it was prolactin that gave me blissful sleep when I was pregnant, but which may be a concern to premenopausal women and younger men, since it can interfere with the proper functioning of the ovaries and testes. I hear that it's eight to seventeen times more powerful than melatonin, though it's not a more concentrated dose of melatonin: it is chemically different from melatonin. Since melatonin never did a thing for me—and since this drug is better at getting you to sleep, which isn't my problem, than keeping you asleep, which *is* my problem—I'm not eager to rush right out and try it. But if you've had success with melatonin, as many people have, you might check it out.

I ask researchers about new developments whenever I get the chance, but my questions are usually met with awkward silences or brush-off answers. Drug companies guard their secrets like the crown jewels (they're worth as much). You have to go by what's in the public domain, which consists mainly of press releases put out by the company and industry-sponsored studies, and these make the drug sound like the promised land.

One of the developments that researchers had high hopes about has just fallen on its face. Gaboxadol was being developed by the European drug company H. Lundbeck in conjunction with Merck. It worked on the GABA system but, unlike the benzos and nonbenzos, seemed to increase both deep sleep and REM. It was said to increase sleep pressure, to mimic "the effects of a physiological increase in sleep need." Harvard sleep researcher Clifford Saper speculated that it might "activate [the sleep switch] rather than working on its target," thereby creating a sleep that's more natural and restorative, perhaps even strengthening memory. It sounded too good to be true, and it was. In late March 2007, Merck canceled the project: the drug turned out not to be so effective, and "unusual side effects—including hallucinations and disorientation—showed up in the studies."

Mignot never thought that Gaboxadol would "activate the sleep switch." He says that a more productive approach would be to turn off the wake switch by damping down the effects of the wake-up neurotransmitter hypocretin. A drug of this sort is being developed by at least two companies. Swiss biotech company Actelion is announcing success with animal and human studies; "I think it may be the beginning of something quite exciting," says Thomas Scammell, professor of neurology at Harvard Medical School. Actelion is hoping to have a drug developed by 2012.

Mignot refers to a "tide that's coming." The scene, he says, is "clearly changing," as many companies are at work on targets other than GABA, and some are studying GABA receptor subunits other than those currently being targeted. Some companies are looking at drugs that might damp down the stress system, though results have so far been disappointing. Yet another approach is a synthetic version of pregnanolone, a neuroactive steroid that also functions at the GABA site, going by the catchy name of CCD-3693. At least one company is at work on melatonin agonists. There are eight serotonin antagonists in development (antagonists damp down, agonists hype up), three by Sanofi-Aventis, maker of Ambien. One of these, eplivanserin, is in phase III development and expected to be the first of this kind of drug to market. Industry watchers are betting on this category, which is not likely to be classified as a controlled substance.

We'll see. Let's hope we'll have, within the next decade, a wider variety of drugs to choose from, and perhaps something that will more precisely target our specific problems.

A Drug We Almost Didn't Get, and Don't Quite Have . . .

There is a new drug on the scene, or somewhat on the scene, that looks like it may give more natural sleep than the others, with fewer bad effects. But it's extremely difficult to get a fix on this one, or to get a fix *of* it, either, since gammahydroxybutyric acid, GHB, is the notorious "date rape drug" of the 1990s. Approved by the FDA in 2002 in the form of sodium oxybate, or Xyrem, for the cataplexy associated with narcolepsy, and approved in 2005 for "excessive daytime sleepiness," this is the most highly restricted and controversial of substances used for sleep.

GHB has been around a long time. It was first synthesized in 1960 by the world-renowned French researcher Henri Laborit, who was looking for a way of getting GABA to the brain and found a molecule that moves easily across the blood-brain barrier. Like GABA, GHB occurs naturally in the brain and body. It is closely related to GABA, and it is thought to work on the GABA system, though on GABAb rather than GABAa, as the benzodiazepines and nonbenzodiazepines do, or possibly "on its own receptor," Mignot speculates. Unlike the benzodiazepine and benzodiazepine-like drugs, GHB actually increases REM and deep sleep, promoting the release of growth hormone and the restful hormone prolactin. It has been studied in animals and humans, attracting the attention not only of top sleep researchers like Eve Van Cauter but of people who are interested in life-extending substances.

The GHB story is a longer and stranger story than I can tell here. The short version of it is, I think, that several forces came together—thrill-seeking kids who got messed up by home brews and dangerous drug mixtures, a media in search of sensational stories, politicians and law enforcers who wanted to look tough on drugs—and these converged to make a brouhaha that demonized the drug, nearly succeeding in getting it banned and stirring up clouds of controversy that have not settled to this day.

Until 1990, GHB was readily available in health food stores, where it was bought mainly by bodybuilders; the growth hormone it releases makes it useful for "buffing up." But in November 1990, the FDA announced that it was "an illegally marketed drug" and forcibly removed it from health food stores. It seems that some overzealous bodybuilders had been taking excessive amounts of it and got messed up. Conspiracy theorists claim that the FDA was deliberately removing from circulation a substance that would have put major drug companies out of business. I don't know about that, but I do know that making it illegal made it truly dangerous, since people continued to use it, only they got it from illegal sources. GHB does, alas, have recreational uses—bad news for those of us who are only looking for a night's sleep. It is (said to be) relaxing and disinhibiting, promoting euphoria and mellowing people out, much like alcohol—so I hear (sleep is all it does for me). GHB became popular at "raves," all-night dance parties attended by hundreds of kids, where throbbing electronic sounds, strobe lights, drugs, and alcohol kept the juices flowing.

Suddenly the media were full of scare stories, and we were hearing about GHB the party drug, the nightclub sex drug, the killer aphrodisiac, the date rape drug. Pieces appeared on CNN, 20/20, ABC News, and in Newsweek, Seventeen, the Los Angeles Times, the New York Post, associating it with overdose, murder, rape, and warning of an "epidemic of abuse" of "a date-rape drug that, when slipped into a woman's drink, can render her helpless." "Liquid X [Ecstasy]—A Club Drug Called GHB May Be a Fatal Aphrodisiac," pronounced a Time magazine headline.

But there's a lot in the media coverage that doesn't stand up to scrutiny. "The dose of GHB required to knock someone out isn't much lower than the one that kills," says the Time magazine article that labeled GHB the "fatal aphrodisiac"; yet the scientific literature describes a wider margin of safety than this. Nobody actually knows how many deaths resulted from GHB on its own, since "well over half of all patients who present with GHB intoxication have abused other drugs as well," reports a 2005 review in the New England Journal of Medicine. When it was taken with substances like alcohol, Ecstasy, methamphetamine, cocaine, Rohypnol (a benzodiazepine known as roofies)—as it usually was—it became dangerous indeed. Nor is it known how often it was actually used in date rape, since—says the 2005 review—"most of the published evidence of GHB in this role is anecdotal." But the story had all the right elements—sensationalism, sentimentalism, a cautionary moral—and the media were off and running with it. And, like any story repeated often enough, it assumed the status of truth.

A decade or so earlier, in 1983, Dr. Martin Scharf, head of the Tri-State Sleep Disorders Center in Cincinnati, had received permission from the FDA to treat narcoleptics with GHB and began doing clinical trials at his own expense. Why, you may ask, would narcoleptics, who have difficulty staying awake, want to take something to make them sleep? Well, the reason they can't stay awake is that they're exhausted: their sleep is as fragmented as their consciousness. Scharf found that GHB, which gives deep sleep, was spectacularly effective with cataplexy. Bob Cloud, former director of the Narcolepsy Network, describes what cataplexy feels like: "Imagine a puppet on strings and suddenly the strings, which are your muscle tone, are immediately let go and so you fall to the ground, and your head comes down and whips against . . . the sidewalk or table corner or whatever." Some people also experience dreams, terrifying hallucinations, while being conscious. (With cataplexy, REM invades consciousness—which accounts for the dreams, and the paralysis as well.) Cloud had "numerous daily episodes of complete body collapse, such that I couldn't leave my office or home without risk of harm to myself or others." When he began taking GHB, his cataplexy disappeared almost overnight. "It saved my law practice. It saved me from disability."

Scharf studied the drug for seventeen years. "It wasn't 'the date rape drug' when I started working with it," he told me; "it gave people their life back. I had a wonderful experience in terms of helping people, but it was bankrupting me because I did this all without a grant." Since GHB is not patentable, he said, "nobody wanted to spend the money to do the research." No patents, no profits, no drug, is the way it usually works, but Scharf was in a position to pursue his interest: "I could do it because I owned my own sleep center. So it was the right thing to do, and nobody else was in a position to do it. But in 1995, when I was really struggling, I phoned the FDA and asked them to find a company to develop this drug. They said, Well, there's this new company, Orphan Drugs, let's try that. I offered Orphan all my data, free, and they went for it."

The FDA had approached several companies to develop GHB, and the only company it could find was Orphan Medical, a small firm of sixty people, founded in 1994, dedicated to the development of "orphan drugs." Orphan drugs are called "orphans" because nobody wants to sponsor them. They are for rare diseases, diseases that affect fewer than two hundred thousand people, which is not enough to make development profitable. It took patient lobbying and the leadership of Abbey Meyers, founder of the National Organization for Rare Disorders, to get these diseases the attention they deserved. Meyers organized patient advocates and lobbied for legislation that would motivate the drug industry to develop drugs for them, and the Orphan Drug Act was signed into law by President Reagan in January 1983, mandating that the FDA find companies to develop drugs for rare diseases and work with these companies to promote drug development. The new law provided financial incentives, tax credits, exemption from certain fees, and the right to market the drug exclusively for seven years; these were necessary not only because the patient populations were small but also because many of the compounds used in treatment of rare diseases were unpatentable and therefore unprofitable.

Based on the results of Scharf's clinical trials and on Orphan's commitment to perform further trials, Orphan was given the go-ahead to develop GHB. "Marty Scharf is why we have this drug at all," Mignot told me. The story makes you wonder how many other unpatentable substances are out there that might help us, that never found their Marty Scharf.

Meanwhile, in 2000, President Clinton signed the Hillory J. Farias and Samantha Reid Date-Rape Drug Prohibition Act into law. The new law made GHB a controlled substance and very nearly made it a Schedule I drug, which would have put it on the same list as LSD, heroin, methamphetamine, marijuana, and cocaine, drugs that have the highest potential for abuse and "no medical use." That would have put an end to it, in terms of research or use. But patient advocates from the Narcolepsy Network testified before the FDA, along with scientists like Mignot and Jed Black of Stanford's Center for Narcolepsy. Black called it "a great drug. . . . We haven't had a case where there hasn't been an improvement." So GHB was designated a Schedule III agent for use with narcolepsy, but a Schedule I agent in terms of possession or distribution, making these a felony. In the fall of that year, Orphan submitted a New Drug Application, and a few years later Xyrem, GHB in the form of sodium oxybate, was approved.

Xyrem was approved without off-label restrictions, which would have restricted its use to narcolepsy and forbidden doctors to prescribe it for any other purpose. This is important: it leaves the door open for insomniacs. But physicians are still not prescribing it even for narcolepsy. Most narcoleptics continue to be treated the old way, with a stimulant to keep them awake during the day and an antidepressant to counteract the cataplexy (antidepressants are prescribed because they suppress REM, but they cause daytime sleepiness, which no narcoleptic needs more of). Physicians are reluctant to prescribe Xyrem because GHB had such bad press, and because it's so tightly controlled. The "risk management plan," devised by Orphan in its eagerness to get the drug approved, is an elaborate surveillance system designed to prevent "diversion." The doctor faxes a special prescription form, provided by an Orphan sales rep, to a special pharmacy. The pharmacy then conducts a check on the physician to make sure she or he has a license to prescribe Schedule III meds, and it checks with the state medical board to make sure there are no actions pending against the physician. The pharmacy also runs a check on the patient, making sure that there is such a patient and that a prescription has been written for him or her. The drug is then FedExed from a single national pharmacy, which is built like a fortress and guarded as carefully, with "locked, steel-reinforced concrete holding areas for the medication, and 24-hour security and surveillance." The patient is sent only a month's supply at a time and has to be there to sign for every delivery or designate someone who will sign. If that person is not available to sign, the deliverer makes only one redelivery attempt, and if that's missed, back it goes, so the package doesn't hang around a warehouse or on a delivery truck. Patients and physicians are sent videos and brochures describing the distribution process and the strict criminal penalties for illicit use.

So it's a strange situation: GHB, which appears to have, as Mignot says, "a favorable side effect/efficacy profile," is very difficult to get hold of. And don't even think about trying for it by other than legal means—you could end up dead, and in jail to boot. And in case you have any ideas about bringing it across borders, the FDA has issued an "import alert" that puts Xyrem on the list of the "Ten Most Dangerous Drugs."

Insomniacs and GHB

Of all the things I read or heard about GHB, what struck me the most was something said by Jed Black at an FDA hearing: "It is unexpected that a medication that objectively markedly improves sleep quality also improves measures of daytime alertness [as Xyrem does], as this finding has never been observed with traditional hypnotics or sleep aids." Unexpected? You mean, all those years, all those drugs I've taken to sleep, do not improve daytime alertness?

Yes, I think this may be the case.

The first time I tried Xyrem, I woke up feeling foggy, and I thought, Oh, no, another disappointment, another drug that does one thing for young, healthy males and something else for sixty-something females. But then, after an hour or so, came this amazing clarity. I felt so alert I hardly recognized the condition: I had a day writing unlike any I could remember, when the words, the ideas, the images just came pouring out, and the energy lasted well into the night (too well, in fact—it didn't turn off). I had a mind not stumbling and sluggish and forgetful of what I was thinking the second before, but clear, searching, focused. I think the initial grogginess may have come from having slept so deeply: my body was in a state of shock from so unusual an experience. I now take it once, twice, at most three times a week. Not every day is like that first day, but many days are. There are other things I like about it: it always works, unlike the benzos and nonbenzos, which occasionally don't grab hold, which leaves me facing the day both sleep-deprived and drugged. And it seems sometimes to leave me less hungry.

But this drug is tricky. You have to experiment to find the dose that works for you. I don't dare take it when I need to swing into action the next morning, catch a plane, for example, because I'm not sure how long I'll need to come fully out of it; and I'm not sure it's great for coordination. It usually lasts three to four hours (two sleep cycles), so that to get a full night's sleep you may have to take it twice. One dose is all I can tolerate—only after I've had a few hours' sleep of my own—though others do fine with two. Some complain that two bouts of three hours each isn't enough sleep for them, though others say that four hours of sleep with Xyrem is better than seven to eight with other sleep meds, since the sleep is so deep. It *is* a delicious sleep, and it sometimes brings deep dreams.

It's different from anything I've ever taken. I feel its effects throughout my body in a way I've never felt any other sedative (it's been used as an anesthetic in Europe), which made me uneasy at first, but now I don't notice. Sometimes when I come to after three hours, I can drift back to sleep again, though often I can't: I wake up with a tension, a restlessness in my limbs. I think this may be because it suppresses dopamine, so when it wears off, you get a dopamine rush and a rebound energy (which some people experience as agitation).

I look on the Web, and I see that there are many insomniacs who know about this drug and have tried to get it, mostly without success. I hear of people at the end of their rope, having tried everything else, strung out on the benzos and the nonbenzos, going from doctor to doctor and finding that doctors are "scared to death" of it. (The best bet for finding a doctor who will prescribe it, according to Talkaboutsleep.com, is to

find an alternative doctor or a physician used to dealing with fibromyalgia, since Xyrem works wonders with the pain of fibromyalgia: people
with fibromyalgia and chronic fatigue syndrome have had their lives
transformed by it.) Then comes the issue of paying for it, when insurance
won't cover it. The cost is off the scale: the average annual wholesale
price for the nine grams taken by narcoleptics nightly is $9,924 a year.
(I got lucky—I found an enlightened doc at my HMO.)

Xyrem is a drug doctors have very little experience with, so even those
who are willing to prescribe it are unlikely to know much about it. On
the Web, you find the wide range of responses you find to any sleep
medication—some people love it, some have a bad reaction, many have
mixed feelings. Some complain of the morning spaciness I first felt; some
say they felt that spaciness at first but it went away (as I think it has with
me); some wake up clear and energized from day one. A few speak of
muscle cramps. (I had these at first, but I upped my calcium and magnesium and they went away, as maybe they would have anyway, since this
drug has effects that disappear with use.) I gather that I'm not the only
one who feels cold and looks pale and puffy around the eyes the day after
I've taken this drug (the puffiness could be water retention from the salt;
if you need to restrict sodium in your diet, this is probably not the drug
for you—sodium oxybate packs a hefty dose of sodium). Some speak of
weight loss (which would not be a problem for me). Some say it gives
them a stuffy nose (it unstuffs mine).

Some feel that it's "too potent and weird" to be good for long-term
use. It *is* potent: "it's a hammer," as Mignot says. Me, I love that wave
that takes me under. But I can see how some people might find it
frightening—and if I were responsible for the welfare of a child or an
older person, I wouldn't take this drug; I wouldn't trust myself to respond to an emergency. It is dangerous when taken with alcohol, sedatives, tranquilizers, opiates (but so are other drugs); nor should it be used
with antihistamines or painkillers, nor by anyone with epilepsy. I come
across a few complaints about depression, a red flag for me, since there
have been times I think it's left me low. Its effects are less predictable than
those of Ambien, which remains my mainstay.

I'm learning my way with this drug, getting a sense of what it does for
me and to me. I wish more were known about it. I do find it reassuring
that there are narcoleptics who've been taking it for decades. Bob Cloud
testified in the 2001 FDA hearing that, during the nineteen years he's
taken it, "I have never changed the dose. I have never experienced tolerance. I have never noted side effects. Simply stated, the drug is as safe and

effective as it was on day one." When I asked him, in 2006, if he'd still say the same thing, he said, "Yes." But I wish there were more research. "It was miserable doing research on it," Martin Scharf told me, "People are scared to death of it. I took an enormous beating from the FDA, being reprimanded for violating procedures which didn't even exist at the time I was working on it. It was a very bitter experience. Where I expected a pat on the back, I received a poke in the eye. But we kept with it."

What especially interests me about GHB, and what interests the researchers who work on it, is the deep sleep it gives. Deep sleep is, as we saw, the kind of sleep we lose with age. This is where the restorative processes that keep minds and bodies toned are thought to take place. Loss of sleep is the bane of growing old, augmenting other losses that come with age: loss of vigor, health, work, loved ones. Most medications on the market today are a parody of what we need, dumbing us down and increasing the risk of falls. I don't know about falls with this drug; I can't swear that it doesn't affect my coordination (or maybe it's just that I get so mentally focused that I forget to look where I'm going); and I know nothing about what it does to memory. But those clear, energetic days I have after taking three grams of Xyrem the second half of the night make me think it can't be all bad.

But please do not take what I say as an "endorsement" of this drug or of any other I've described as helping me or anybody else. This drug is not for everyone; no drug is. You need to find your way with these medications, research them thoroughly, come to your own conclusions. And GHB does have abuse potential, no question. This is not a simple issue, nor is it always rationally decided, though I will state it simply here, quoting a physician friend who himself takes Xyrem for a sleep disorder: "Because a few people abuse a substance, does that mean it should be withheld from those in need?" He faces this question on a daily basis with the pain medications he prescribes. "Say 2 to 10 percent are going to abuse a medication—what about the other 90 percent who are tremendously helped by it?"

What's an Insomniac to Do?

There is, as we've seen, a lot of hype in the air. For the first time in history, a mass audience is being barraged with ads for drugs to help us sleep. Says Jerry Avorn, author of *Powerful Medicine,* "The sinister purpose of the ads is to convince people they have ailments they didn't know they had—like a medical condition called 'insomnia' that needs a chemical treatment."

The results have been dramatic. Sanofi-Aventis "pumped $55 million into U.S. print and TV ads for Ambien in 2002," and annual sales of the drug "jumped to $1.5 billion, nearly twice the level in 2000." For the $350 million Sanofi-Aventis put into advertising Ambien and Ambien CR in 2005 and 2006, it acquired 27.6 million of all 44 million prescriptions for sleep medications those years. The use of sleep meds in the United States doubled between 2002 and 2004, according to a study by Medco Health Solutions, a pharmaceutical benefits agency—and among children and very young adults, it rose 85 percent. This exponential increase is driven by direct-to-consumer advertising—because it's not happening in the European Union.

The effect of this onslaught has been to normalize the use of sleep meds, making it seem like the most "natural" thing in the world. "The ads and the drug company websites suggest that these drugs are safe and imply that they may even be necessary," since lack of sleep is bad for health, writes Bonnie Morris in "Sleep Anxiety Leads Many to the Medicine Cabinet" in the *New York Times* in 2005. "And to look good, of course, you have to get rest."

But these are not look-good, feel-good drugs. They should not be taken casually. Reports of the sleep-eating, sleepwalking, and sleep-driving associated with Ambien that poured out of the media in early 2007 are a sobering reminder that these drugs are not toys. I do think the media exaggerate the dangers, as the media have been known to do. Considering how many of us have taken Ambien through the years, and considering that many (most?) of the more dramatic incidents occurred when the person had been drinking, or when she or he had taken the drug and then had not gone right to bed, I don't see too much cause for alarm. It was clear to me when I was taking fifteen milligrams of Ambien every night that it was affecting my personality in ways that were not good; but I've since learned how to use it, and it serves me well. I'm actually sort of dismayed to see this drug that's a lifeline for me suddenly demonized.

No sleep medication is problem-free, as those of us who take them know, or should know. None gives deep, natural sleep through the night and keeps on working, without adverse effects, night after night after night; none is a magic bullet that repairs or supplies what's deficient in our systems, the way insulin "fixes" diabetes. Since it's not yet *known* what's wrong with our sleep systems, what glitch or deficiency makes such fragile sleep, much more will have to be learned before researchers can develop a substance (or substances) that fixes the problem; and for that to happen, more basic research is needed, much more than sleep and insomnia are now getting.

The best drug is no drug, as far as I'm concerned. My best days, in terms of mood and mental clarity, are days that follow seven to eight hours of my own, undrugged sleep. Since my body has never been exactly generous with that kind of sleep—it happens maybe a dozen times a year—I often, I usually, take something for sleep. Rock, hard place: lack of sleep is bad for mood, health, and memory; sleep meds are bad for memory, health, and sometimes mood. I go with the meds because they make it possible for me to have a life, to be out and about in the world, teaching classes, writing books. Whether the kind and quality of life I buy with the meds is ultimately worth the risk, whether it will cut my life short, whether doing without sleep would have cut it shorter, I don't know. We each of us have to make these risk-benefit calculations for ourselves.

The question then becomes, how to minimize the damage?

I have found that alternating drugs and trying to confine my use of them to the second half of the night is a way of keeping them effective and getting some sleep of my own, which is the best kind of sleep. After the two, three, or four hours I get on my own, I take Ambien or Xyrem to finish out the night (Ambien more than Xyrem). But I also like to have a six-to-seven-hour drug on hand, Ambien CR or Restoril. The benzodiazepines are still, sad to say, the only thing that gets me through a whole night (many of the insomniacs and many of the doctors and psychiatrists I've talked to come back to the benzodiazepines because they find this to be the case); though the next-day hangover I've been getting with them lately is definitely worse.

Doctors understand the principle of rotation—they rotate meds themselves, to keep from getting habituated. But imagine coming to a doctor and saying, I'd like some Restoril, 7.5 milligrams, and some Ativan, 1 milligram, and a whole bunch of Ambien, 5 milligrams, and oh yes, a few bottles of Xyrem. Good luck convincing anybody that you want more drugs in order to take *fewer* drugs.

For chronic insomniacs who've been made to feel criminal when they ask for sleep meds, who've been denied meds by doctors afraid to prescribe them, the recent climate of liberality has been a boon. But I fear now that the media scare stories will unleash that drug hysteria that's never far from the surface in this country, the polar opposite of promiscuous pill popping—extremes that seem somehow weirdly related, flip sides of the same irrationality. We are a nation of extremes: with half our population obese and the other half starving itself to fit a grotesque, health-damaging image of thinness, we're not good at happy mediums. I fear we may now be in for a backlash with sleep medications: the last time I asked, my HMO turned down my request for Ambien. So here I am again, scrambling around looking for drug sources, which is time-consuming, costly, and demeaning. (And no, I won't risk the Web.) Surely there is some sane middle ground between the hysteria and the hype.

Surely doctors can find some means of differentiating one patient from another, can find ways of working with those of us who need sleep meds, taking us through careful trial and error, informing themselves and us of the risks and benefits of each. "When it comes to their own values and preferences, our patients are the experts, not us," writes Jerry Avorn in *Powerful Medicines*. "In balancing the hazards and benefits of a given prescription, we [physicians] must learn about their perspective as much as they need to hear about ours." And we could use some follow-up, some monitoring. This may be too much to ask, in this age when much prescribing is done to get us *out* of the office, not back in. But it would be nice. We need doctors to prescribe according to our best interests, insofar as they can determine what those are, and not according to which drug is being pushed hardest or which drug has the most scare stories and restrictions around it.

"Finding what works is an art more than a science," as a psychiatrist friend tells me, "and sometimes it's just blind luck—you stumble around and hope you'll stumble onto something that works." It would be nice to have the art, the science, and the help of the professionals in this; but in fact, most of us never have. Many people feel they've been better served by Internet forums and support groups than by doctors. "As someone who has taken cocktails or psychiatric medications as prescribed by medical providers for more than 19 years," writes a woman to the editor of the *New York Times*, "I can attest that the professionals do not always know everything there is to know about medications, nor do drug label warnings always provide an adequate understanding of how drugs actually work. . . . Internet forums and online research, on the other hand, enhance my ability to advocate for myself."

If it's beyond the capabilities of doctors and psychiatrists to figure out what's best for us, it's hard to ask patients to take this on—but we, finally, are the ones who must take it on. We need to get on the Web and spend whatever time is necessary to research the available meds, informing ourselves of their risks and benefits, and informing our physicians, if need be. We may have to educate our physicians (which does not mean rushing in with the latest ad; ads are intended to sell us the drug, not educate us about it, contrary to what the drug companies would have us believe). Check out the package insert before taking a drug—if the pharmacist doesn't give it to you, ask for it, and if she or he has thrown it away, find it on the Web. Know what dose you're taking, make sure it's the lowest dose possible. (I'm always shocked to hear, "Uh, you know, it's the purple pill," when I ask someone what dose she or he is taking; and physicians are often equally oblivious, starting us out on a higher dose than we need, or prescribing "nightly" when "as needed" is what's needed.) "Read, ask, think," writes Jay Cohen, in *Overdose*. "Use all reasonable resources, including books, medical journals and the websites of respected institutions and experts, as well as websites of patients who present credible information." Make sure you know what you're putting in your body.

And doctors, please hear us when we tell you what we know; take our word as much as you credit the claims of the drug companies. For our word has got to be the last word. The final verdict on drugs must be with the users, the consumers, we who bear the marks of these substances upon our bodies and our brains.

CHAPTER 8

Change Your Attitude, Change Your Ways

Behavioral Modification

It took me four months, but now I'm sleeping better than I did before. I feel like I'm back in control of my life.

I was sleeping better before I started this program. It's not like it says in the book, instant success. I've been at it for two and a half months. I've never been tired like this before.

Above all, keep regular hours. Ben Franklin's dictum, "early to bed, early to rise," has been confirmed by numerous sleep researchers. Get a life, Ben.

Deborah Bishop and David Levy, *Hello Midnight*

This was the hardest chapter of them all, the part of the story that took the most soul-searching, where I'm most uneasy about generalizing from myself. It gives me no pleasure to point to the limitations of an approach that has helped many people and has much to recommend it. I know how hard the behavioral modification researchers work. I've followed them around the conference circuit; I see their commitment, their dedication to a difficult cause, their efforts to help us sleep without drugs in a drug-driven culture: this is not the corner of the sleep world where there's money to be made. I respect them, and I respect the insomniacs who've made behavioral modification work for them.

But it's not for me.

The idea behind behavioral modification is that insomnia has been precipitated by a stressful event or events, and has then settled in, like a bad habit. Like Pavlov's dogs, conditioned to salivate at the sound of

218

a bell they've learned to associate with food, insomniacs have developed wake-up associations with sleep and bed. "When the stressors fade away," writes Charles Morin, leading proponent of behavioral modification and author of *Relief from Insomnia,* some people "may have developed negative reactions to stimuli normally conducive to sleep (e.g., bed, bedtime, bedroom). What used to be a place and time for relaxation and sleep is now associated with frustration, anxiety, and sleeplessness. . . . Over time, a conditioning process leads to a vicious cycle of insomnia." This is the view enshrined in the DSM-IV, which states that "most cases" of primary or psychophysiological insomnia "have a fairly sudden onset at a time of psychological, social, or medical stress." The insomnia may then persist "long after the original causative factors resolve, due to the development of heightened arousal and negative conditioning."

Behavioral modification is a group of therapies aimed at reconditioning us. *Stimulus control therapy* aims at getting us to associate the bed with sleep. Go to bed only when sleepy, use the bed only for sleep and sex, avoid naps and so-called *sleep-incompatible behaviors,* such as reading, watching TV, eating, talking in the bedroom. *Sleep restriction therapy* requires that you restrict time in bed to the time you spend asleep. If you think that you get five hours' sleep, you should go to bed at your usual time and set the alarm for five hours later. When you wake up before the alarm, make yourself get out of bed—some say after ten minutes, some say twenty, some give a "quarter of an hour rule." Then go to another room and watch TV or read. When you begin to feel sleepy, go back to bed, but if you don't fall asleep in ten to twenty minutes, repeat the process, getting out of bed and going to another room again. However little sleep you've had, get up to that alarm without fail, seven days a week. The idea is that, by restricting time in bed to the time you actually sleep, you create what Morin calls "mild sleep deprivation," which results in more consolidated and more efficient sleep. When you find yourself sleeping 90 percent of the time you spend in bed (i.e., attaining 90 percent *sleep efficiency*), and sustain this for five consecutive days, you may extend your time in bed by fifteen minutes. But if your sleep efficiency drops below 85 percent, reduce your time in bed to match your average sleep length for the past five days, but do not reduce it to less than five hours.

All this, of course, requires careful monitoring, which you do by keeping a sleep diary, noting, whenever you make a change, precisely what effect that change has.

Behavioral modification proponents believe that we bring our sleep problems on ourselves by worrying too much about our sleep and having mistaken notions about how much sleep we need; *cognitive restructuring* aims at changing our attitudes and assumptions. Cognitive restructuring, together with stimulus control therapy and sleep restriction, is called *cognitive behavioral therapy* (CBT). *Sleep hygiene* is also important: sleep in a dark, quiet place; cut out caffeine, alcohol, big meals, and stimulating activity late in the day; and don't exercise too close to bedtime. Relaxation therapies are also advised. These include deep breathing, *progressive muscle relaxation,* where you concentrate on tensing and relaxing first one muscle group, then another, until your whole body is relaxed, and *imagery training,* where you visualize pleasant or neutral images. Biofeedback, meditation, and yoga are sometimes recommended.

It's given me my life back. The Web forum Sleepnet.com tells many such stories. People post on this forum for months, even years, and you can follow their stories, hear about their efforts to restrict and regularize their sleep, watch them struggling their way through to better sleep (or not). This forum functions like a support group, with people urging one another on, advising, cajoling, scolding, consoling, providing encouragement. (It's perhaps no coincidence that it is associated with Stanford, since the Stanford Sleep Disorders Clinic has had success with support groups.) People who post here recommend readings that have helped them: Gregg Jacobs's *Say Good Night to Insomnia,* Peter Hauri and Shirley Linde's *No More Sleepless Nights,* Charles Morin's *Relief from Insomnia,* and John Wiedman's *Desperately Seeking Snoozin',* which many insomniacs find inspirational because it's written by someone they identify with, a "recovering" insomniac, as he calls himself, a man who has reformed his sleep by rigorously, religiously, adhering to what he and others call "the program."

And yet, as Charles Morin acknowledges, "not many people are using CBT, it looks like." Why not? asks Edward Stepanski in a 2002 survey— "Given that behavioral treatments have been available for many years, why have they not gained greater acceptance?" Stepanski concludes that it's because they're "time intensive" for the practitioner and "demanding for the patient." "Demanding" is an understatement.

I've been doing this three weeks and I don't think I've had more than an hour [of sleep], at most two, the whole time. It's not getting better—it's getting worse.

I'm in my fifth week of sleep restriction, restricting myself to 5 hours, bed at 1, up at 6, but I'm still not sleeping more than 4 hours. Should I make myself get out of bed an hour earlier? How do you deal with being tired all the time?

I gave myself 6 hours, and after a week, I was sleeping almost 6 hours, then raised it to 6 and a half and it all went to pieces. So I started back at 5 hours, increased it slowly and it went to pieces again. It's been 6 months and I'm still not back up to 6 hours. I spend my days just trying to stay awake.

As I read the postings on Sleepnet.com, I am in awe of the efforts people make, their persistence and determination to "keep a positive attitude" through long periods of sleep deprivation. They're a hardier lot than I am; they are also, I suspect, much younger. But I talked to one woman who'd been doing sleep restriction for two and a half months— who *was* my age. *It worked at first,* she said, *got me up to six hours' sleep—a miracle!* But then when she tried to get up to more than six hours, she fell back to less. When she cut back the time she allowed herself in bed to five and a half hours, it was still, after two and a half weeks, not working (this was when we talked). She told me she was considering cutting back time in bed to five hours. My heart sank at this—she sounded so exhausted, and her life seemed so focused on sleep, as it has to be when you're going through this monitoring and keeping track. I told her how impressed I was by her dedication.

Well, what else am I supposed to do? she shot back. *It's the only alternative to drugs.* Which is why people persist with it.

How much are people helped by these methods? Gains are, as researchers admit, "modest." Though Morin and others have found that patients' satisfaction is "significantly enhanced" and benefits are sustained "for at least six months after treatment," "sleep duration is increased by a modest 30 minutes," with a usual ceiling of six hours, according to a 1999 review of fifty studies. "The time it takes to get to sleep and time spent awake after sleep onset, the two main target symptoms of treatment, often fall below or near the 30-minute cut-off criterion used to define insomnia," he says. "Treatment is not effective 100% of the time, and it never makes them good sleepers. There's some improvement, but . . ."

How many people, what proportion of insomniacs, are actually helped by behavioral modification methods? Morin guesses that 70 to 80 percent are helped, based on his surveys of studies—70 to 80 percent of *the subjects of these studies,* that is. How representative are these subjects? Subjects are carefully screened so as to eliminate anyone who uses drugs or has psychological or physical problems. Few of the studies keep track of the people who drop out, and none tell you about the people who wouldn't dream of going near such a study.

And what *kind* of insomniac is helped by the methods? That's the interesting question to me, the one nobody's asking.

My Take

My own experiences with behavioral modification have not been encouraging.

I count among these experiences my time in the 9 to 5 world, working in publishing. I was not rigorously adhering to "the program," but I was waking to a 6:30 alarm for nearly a year. Actually, I wasn't waking to an alarm; I was awake when the alarm went off, and had been awake since my usual two- to four-hour wake-up call. I could not get up and go to another room—my roommate was asleep in the only other room. Probably I lay there fidgeting, I don't remember; it was a long time ago. What I do remember is that I went through that year in a haze. I was able to do it because I was twenty-three, excited to be in New York, working at my first real job. I was surrounded by amiable co-workers who took a lot of coffee breaks, and the work wasn't nearly as demanding as graduate school had been: all I had to do was show up and do a bit of writing and chatting. Even so, I got sacked, not because I did the job poorly, but because I rarely showed up on time.

My point is that a year on this schedule didn't make a dent in my sleep pattern, though I never, in those days, took a nap or a pill. I've never understood why, if regularization and restriction are all they're cracked up to be, so many people who work 9-to-5 jobs, whose schedules impose regularity and restriction and don't allow napping, are still plagued by insomnia. In fact, strict schedules often make insomnia worse: *The problem got really bad for me when I got an 8 to 5. . . . It didn't get easier as the months went by.*

So, a few summers ago, I set aside a time to give "the program" a real try. I went to bed at my usual hour, 3 A.M., set the alarm for 8, and when I woke after a few hours, I made myself get out of bed if I wasn't back to sleep in fifteen minutes—which I never was. There are not a lot of other rooms to go to in my house—my study is out of bounds, since it reeks of work, so that leaves the living room, which is cold, uncosy, and close to the street. I'd sit there and read the paper or watch a video, waiting to get sleepy. But I don't get sleepy once I'm up and out of bed, and the sky would grow light and the traffic would start up and the birds would begin their racket, and there was no point to going back to bed—even if I did start to get drowsy, the idea of the alarm about to go off made sleep unthinkable. So I went for most of that time on two, three, or four hours a night, with an occasional five or six. But I wasn't in my twenties, and I didn't have an exhilarating walk down Park Avenue to an office full of congenial co-workers and the excitement of a new job. "Stay active and be around people," say the books, and it's excellent advice, if you can do it. But everybody I know works during the day, so, short of walking down to the corner grocery and striking up a conversation with the produce man, there wasn't a lot I could do. I was home alone, with the grueling task of writing this book.

Gregg Jacobs, author of *Say Good Night to Insomnia,* assures us that "it is only performance of monotonous or sedentary tasks such as driving, or the ability to produce creative solutions to problems, that seems to deteriorate after one sleepless night." Well, writing is all about "producing creative solutions," so there went that. As research shows, creativity, flexibility of response, ease of association—"divergent thinking," as it's called—are among the first casualties of sleep loss. I did manage to get myself to the library to read some journals and do some xeroxing. I spent a lot of time in hot baths, since everything hurt. I read a lot of memoirs, saw a lot of videos. I got through most of the piles of newspapers and magazines stacked in the hall. I cleaned out a closet. I swam occasionally, but for days at a time I was too wiped out even to do that: I'd get that throaty feeling like I was coming down with something (and I did get two colds that summer). My weight was creeping up. I was too wrung out to schedule evening events, so I was spending a lot of time alone. It was depressing.

Sometimes I'd get up to five and a half hours' sleep, and I'd stay at that for a few nights running. There were a few times when I got up to six hours for two or three nights in a row, and I'd feel like I was getting the hang of it, but by then I had such a backlog of exhaustion that I was still too dazed to work. I'd always drop back down again to three or four hours, my default position, and then creep up to five for a few days. *Sleep management,* as I recall, is a euphemism for torture. "Doctors are stunningly casual," writes Paula Kamen, about recommending things "that have effects that can tear apart one's world and grind everything to a sudden, unexpected halt." Kamen is talking about medications here, but this can be said of sleep restriction as well. *I'd like to see them do it,* as more than one insomniac has commented. Proponents claim that behavioral modification, unlike drugs, has "no adverse side effects," but, as Wallace Mendelson points out, "if you got this kind of next-day sleepiness from a drug, that would be seen as an adverse drug effect, but if patients stumble around from stimulus control, it's okay." I'm inclined to agree with whoever posted this comment on Talkaboutsleep.com: *One day people will look back on sleep restriction with a kind of horror at the barbaric medicine practiced in the early 21st century.*

Did I give it enough time? *How do I know how much time is enough?* is a lament I hear from people who've quit after two, three, four, or five months. Experts say you need "several" months, whatever that means. I guess you never know—maybe if you'd hung in there a week longer, you'd have made it work. It seemed a very long time to me, most of the summer; then, come September, I was back in front of the classroom, and that was that. Did I adhere strictly enough? There were times I'd get really ragged and I'd reach for an Ambien, turn off the alarm, and go to sleep. And occasionally, I'd take a nap. Rigid adherents of the program say no naps, no pills, but Hauri and others say it's okay to take a pill now and then, and even a nap, as long as it's early enough in the day. Bob and I went away for a few weekends that summer, and I backslid. So I guess I'll never know if I gave it "enough time."

I could see that I might get up to as much as five or six consolidated hours of sleep, and might stay there for stretches of time—if I followed the rules strictly and forever. But studies suggest there's this six-hour ceiling. Behavioral modification proponents tell us that's okay, we just need to curb our expectations about how much sleep we need: "This ceiling effect suggests that it may be unrealistic for older adults to expect more than 6 hours of sleep and that the uninterrupted nature of sleep is clinically more important than its total duration," says Morin. But then they wonder why their subjects' moods and daytime functioning aren't much improved. Could it be because they're not getting enough sleep? (A psychiatrist friend comments, "As is often the case with psychotherapy studies, the outcome is *statistically significant,* but not a *significant benefit* to the patient. The two meanings of *significant* are confounded.") Six hours is sometimes all I need, but as a steady diet, with an occasional dip into less, it's subsistence sleep. But I think that's the way sleep restriction works: you stay slightly sleep-deprived so you'll fall asleep and stay asleep, but if you make up your sleep debt, your hyperarousal hypes back up.

Sleep researchers warn us about the dire consequences of skimping on sleep—but then they advise insomniacs to accept this six-hour ceiling. Why do I feel there's a double standard at work here? One set of rules for people, another for people who can't sleep.

The program is very unforgiving:

> *I was doing great, but I went to a party Saturday night, and now I'm back to where I was before. I have to start over. No more parties for me.*

> *I'll feel like I've beaten it, but just a few nights off schedule and I'm sleeping as bad as I ever did, and it takes a month of strict restriction before I'm back on track.*

It is very demanding: *I have to start unwinding hours before I go to bed: if I do anything in the evening, it's impossible to sleep.* And the worse your insomnia, the more rigorous you must be, say the books.

Curb my expectations? Okay, I'm over sixty, I don't expect to be turning cartwheels, but neither do I want to feel less good than I know I can. If I made this a permanent way of life, I'd be waking to an alarm not only weekends but summers and school breaks and vacations. I'd have to do this forever, to keep myself in the state of "mild sleep deprivation" necessary to keep my sleep consolidated. I'd be in that slightly dopey state I hate, fighting sleep, eating too much, longing for caffeine—even on days I don't have to be. Never again that delicious sense of having fully slept, slept in, slept it off, made up for the days of dragging through—though it usually takes medication to get me there, it's a luscious feeling, and it mends my soul.

The program is too strict for me, its yields are too sparse. I could not see it as a permanent way of life. As one man said, looking back on his experience of two years, *It produced some change but not enough to be worth the agony. I still wasn't getting enough sleep to feel really good.*

But this is anecdote, and this is me. What does the research say?

The Research

Most of the fifty studies surveyed in the 1999 review headed by Morin looked at sleep onset insomnia, that is, how long it takes a person to get to sleep. Fewer than ten looked at sleep maintenance problems, at staying asleep and returning to sleep, though that is the kind most people—certainly elderly people—actually have. Some of the studies reviewed found that older adults were less responsive to behavioral methods than younger people. So in order to address the question of "late-life insomnia," Morin and colleagues did what has become a landmark study, "Behavioral and Pharmacological Therapies for Late-Life Insomnia," published in the premiere U.S. medical journal, the *Journal of the American Medical Association*, in 1999.

The researchers found that cognitive behavioral therapy was more effective than drugs, and more effective even than drugs combined with CBT. They looked at 78 subjects, 20 of whom were treated with temazepam (Restoril), 18 of whom were treated with CBT (ninety-minute sessions for eight weeks), 20 with a combination, and the rest with placebo. The combination of drug treatment and behavioral therapy had the best results initially, but a follow-up interview twenty-four months later indicated that behavioral modification alone had the best results over time. Slightly over half of the CBT subjects achieved 85 percent sleep efficiency or more, which is the "typical cutoff score used to distinguish clinically impaired from normal sleep"; subjects were sleeping, a year and two later, an average of an hour longer, up from five hours twenty minutes to six hours twenty minutes. It was an elegant study, referred to in many subsequent studies, though the sample size (a total of 78 subjects, 18 of whom received CBT and another 20 who received a combination of CBT and drugs) was, as Morin admits, relatively small. Subjects were carefully screened and, as in all such studies, highly motivated.

"Insomnia in Aged Found Treatable," read a *New York Times* headline. A 2004 study headed by Gregg Jacobs that "replicated and extended" Morin's findings also got *New York Times* mention. This study also compared CBT with both pharmacological treatment and placebo and found that CBT produced the greatest changes in terms of time to fall asleep and sleep efficiency and "yielded the greatest number of normal sleepers after treatment." The researchers found that 57 percent of those who received CBT, that is, 8 out of 14, attained 85 percent sleep efficiency. Subjects went from around five hours' sleep to nearly six hours—that six-hour ceiling again—but mood and daytime functioning did not seem improved. The sample size was, again "relatively small"—14 of the 63 total received CBT. As Jacobs says, "Because this sample consisted mainly of individuals who responded to newspaper advertisements, the results may not be generalizable fully to patients with clinical insomnia or patients who are more refractory to treatment, such as drug-dependent patients."

This is a question that haunts this research: will what works with a small group of carefully screened, self-selected, highly motivated subjects actually work with "real world" insomniacs? Sample sizes are small in nearly all these studies: half of the fifty studies Morin reviewed in his 1999 survey looked at fewer than 30 subjects, and the rest did not look at many more. There are further problems. As Allison Harvey and Nicole Tang point out in their 2003 review of the literature (this literature is much reviewed), "None of the studies we reviewed reported the number of patients who refused treatment." Nor did most of the studies report the number that did not complete the treatment or the proportion that did not benefit. The researchers conclude that, for these reasons and others, many studies of cognitive behavioral therapy "fall short of the current standards" for study trials, as described by the Standards of Practice Committee of the American Academy of Sleep Medicine.

Also problematic is that most of these studies are based on sleep diaries, that is, on self-report, and when objective measures are taken they often contradict the subjective accounts. (This was why Morin's 1999 study was a landmark: subjective accounts were confirmed by polysomnography.) I'd be the last to side with objective measures when they come into conflict with subjective report, but I do find it interesting that the subjective account is so readily accepted in these studies. Elsewhere, when the subjective is not confirmed by polysomnography, it's taken as evidence that insomniacs "exaggerate" sleep disturbance.

So—sometimes insomniacs are believed, and sometimes they are not?

The discrepancy between subjective and "objective" points to another question that haunts this research: how much of the improvement that's being reported is actually a placebo effect? Most of the behavioral modification studies that had a control group using placebo found that placebo "significantly improved sleep," reports Stepanski in a 2000 review. *Placebo,* from the Latin, "I will please," is a treatment or therapy that has no therapeutic value but is administered as if it did. Doctors in military field hospitals in World War II began taking the placebo effect seriously when they found that an injection of saline might numb pain as well as morphine. The placebo then became a cornerstone of clinical trials: one group of patients receives the therapy being tested and a "control" group receives the placebo.

Peter Hauri's work on biofeedback illustrates the placebo effect in a striking way. In one study, Hauri looked at two types of biofeedback and found that one type was more effective with patients who had muscular tension and another was more effective with patients who did not. In a follow-up study, Hauri found that even those who received the "inappropriate" biofeedback treatment reported that their sleep had improved, though "objective" measurements—sleep lab evaluations—"painted a very different picture," saying that it had not. Some principle may be at work, he speculates, "such as the rekindling of new hope or the relatively intensive interaction involving sleep researcher, biofeedback technician, and patient," that makes the patient feel there is improvement.

Merely being in a study seems to help some patients. The encouragement and optimism of the practitioner, the relationship that develops between patient and practitioner, the attention the patient gets, all make a difference. The placebo effect tends to be especially high, as high as 30 to 40 percent, in conditions where the subjective state is key, such as depression, anxiety, pain—and insomnia. Some people say this is why alternative approaches have such high success rates, because alternative therapists tend to be great believers in their methods, more so than many practitioners of conventional medicine, who often merely dispense the latest drug a drug company rep has dropped off. I can vouch for the commitment and enthusiasm of the behavioral modification proponents I've seen at the conferences, and for the energy, charm, and charisma of people like Charles Morin, Colin Espie, Tracy Kuo, Rachel Manber, Jack Edinger, Michael Perlis, Michael Irwin. Does it matter if the effects are "real" or placebo? I don't think it does, not with insomnia, where the subjective experience is everything: if you think your sleep is restorative, then it is.

But it seems that some large claims are being made on the basis of not much evidence, not many subjects studied, and not all that much improvement.

In fact most of the behavioral methods are ranked as not having a "high degree of clinical certainty," according to standards of efficacy established by the American Academy of Sleep Medicine, which ranks methods according to how many studies and what quality of studies have been done. Stimulus control therapy, which aims to retrain the insomniac to associate bed and bedplace with sleep, is the only strategy ranked as *standard*, that is, as having "a high degree of clinical certainty." Progressive muscle relaxation and biofeedback are ranked as *guidelines*, that is, as having "a moderate degree of clinical certainty," "probably efficacious." Sleep restriction and cognitive behavioral therapy, which combines various of the other therapies, are ranked as *options*, that is, their efficacy has "not been established"; evidence is "either inconclusive or conflicting." For sleep hygiene education and imagery training, there is also "insufficient evidence" to recommend them either as single therapies or in combination with others.

I was surprised by these ratings. I was surprised that *paradoxical intention*, which asks the patient to engage in the most feared behavior—which, for an insomniac, is staying awake—had a higher degree of clinical certainty than sleep restriction or CBT or sleep hygiene. The theory is that insomniacs have "performance anxiety" associated with sleep and fall asleep most easily when they're not trying to, but I can tell you how this would work with me: tell me I have to stay awake, and I'll say, "Phew, what a relief! What would you like to talk about? Or would you like to watch a DVD?" (Ask Bob. Or read my mother's letters, which are full of my infant ploys to stay awake; I was a sleep escape artist even then.)

I was surprised that sleep hygiene, much of which is just good common sense, came in so low in the AASM ranking. But on second thought, maybe I'm not so surprised, since I've never actually found that following the rules makes my sleep better, though breaking them can certainly make it worse. Research confirms this sense: "few studies have demonstrated superior efficacy [of sleep hygiene or sleep restriction] over reliable placebo intervention." I was surprised that the combination therapy, CBT, came in lower than stimulus response alone. CBT has been shown to be very effective with obsessive-compulsive disorder and panic disorders, but its success with insomnia seems less impressive. As Harvey and Tang summarize in their 2003 review, "A significant group of patients [19 to 26 percent] do not respond . . . and many patients who do respond do not improve enough to be classed as good sleepers following treatment."

The situation is confusing because the AASM states as its official position that "sleep hygiene [and] behavioral therapies . . . are . . . highly effective." And yet according to the AASM's own standards of efficacy, these methods are not ranked as highly effective. I'm not sure what to make of this contradiction. Has it been decided that we *ought* to believe these methods work, because if we believe, we'll work harder at them, and then they'll have a better chance of actually working? Or is it that the sleep research community is so eager to look like it has something besides drugs to offer insomniacs that it chooses to ignore the uncertain grounds on which its claims are made?

Insomnia is "readily treatable," "easily treatable," I hear at the meetings, again and again. Millions of insomniacs disagree.

What Kinds of People Does It Work For?

Since, as Morin says, there is "significant variability" in the way people respond to behavioral modification methods, "we need to explain why some improve and others do not." Very true: yet I find hardly any research that actually tries. I find endless reviews of the studies that have been done, overviews, surveys, meta-analyses; I've never seen a body of research that's so thoroughly reviewed (a sign of the honesty of its researchers—or their insecurity?). But "only one study has directly examined whether treatment response was mediated by initial insomnia severity," says Morin. (I *think* that statement means, "whether those whose insomnia is more severe respond worse or better to treatment." Do they really have to talk like that?) A 1997 study observed that, of fifteen subjects, those who responded rapidly to behavioral modification methods had increased arousal at bedtime, whereas those who responded slowly were likely to be spending more time in bed; but this was a one-page abstract, and the suggestion was not followed up. A study of paradoxical intention speculated that this method might work better for those "who can readily identify with experiencing 'effort to sleep,'" which makes sense, but I don't think this idea was tested.

What you'd guess is that those insomniacs respond best whose insomnia is actually caused by the problems that the methods are designed to address. If you really are trying too hard to sleep, maybe being told to stay awake will put that right. If you really are spending vast amounts of time in bed, it would help to know that you should go to bed only when you're sleepy, and that when you can't sleep, you should do something else. If you really do have exaggerated notions about how much sleep you need, it would help to know you can live on less than eight hours. If your insomnia really is caused by drinking too much caffeine or alcohol, then cutting these down or out might be transformative— though this is a "pretty low-hanging fruit," as a physician friend comments. (They're *all* low-hanging fruits, if you ask me. I'm struck by the contrast between the way the professionals talk about insomniacs—as if we're six years old and none of this ever occurred to us—and the sense I get talking to insomniacs, that they're a sleep-wise, savvy bunch of people who know things like this and much besides.)

Do insomniacs really have worse habits, do they engage in more so-called sleep-incompatible behaviors, than normal sleepers? Do they have unrealistic expectations about how much sleep they need? Do they have worse associations with the bed than other people? The studies that have looked at these questions (there are only a few) suggest—no.

"Good sleepers have been shown to have the same prevalence of bad sleep habits as do poor sleepers," summarizes Stepanski in a 2000 survey of the research. Two studies headed by Stephen Haynes set out to investigate whether insomniacs "engage in a significantly greater number of sleep-incompatible behaviors in their bed and bedroom," whether they spend more time in these behaviors, whether they have more irregular habits than noninsomniacs. The researchers found that they did not, and when they did, there was no significant relationship between these behaviors and their problems sleeping. In fact, a 1986 study headed by Ruth Davies instructed insomniacs to engage in "sleep-incompatible behaviors," telling them to stay in bed when they couldn't sleep and spend thirty minutes in wakeful activities such as reading, watching TV, listening to the radio. The study found that their sleep complaints were reduced nearly as much as they were with insomniacs who got out of bed and went to another room. This group neither regularized nor restricted their sleep, and yet their sleep was significantly improved after four weeks, and remained better a year later. The crucial thing was to stop the wheels spinning, change the channel (as we'll see).

A 1995 study by Canadian researcher Catherine Fichten and her colleagues divided 634 older, noninstitutionalized residents into good sleepers, poor sleepers, and poor sleepers who weren't troubled by sleep loss, and found that all three groups had similar sleep hygiene, spent similar amounts of time in bed and napping, had similarly erratic bedtimes, irregular lifestyle, and so on. The researchers found that "sleep practices (e.g., naps, bedtimes) are not implicated in chronic poor sleep," and that *"many commonly held assumptions about sleep disruptions in older individuals are myth rather than reality"* (my emphasis). Nor was psychological distress the cause of the insomnia, according to this study. Nor did the data "support the hypothesis that older poor sleepers have unreasonable expectations": good and poor sleepers alike wanted approximately seven hours, which was the amount the good sleepers actually got. Fichten maintains that "lifestyle changes" do alleviate people's sleep difficulties, but this does not mean that maladaptive lifestyle practices are the cause of their insomnia, any more than the success of aspirin at alleviating headaches means that lack of aspirin causes headache. That is, even when the methods work, their success tells us nothing about the etiology of insomnia; it brings us no closer to an understanding of the cause.

Many cases of insomnia can, of course, be explained in terms of conditioning. A stressful event or events—an illness, divorce, a sick child, the death of a loved one—disrupts a person's sleep, and then insomnia settles in like a bad habit. Here's a friend's account: *I was always a light sleeper, but my divorce pushed me over the edge. I went through a bad time, and I've never slept since.* Here's another account: *My insomnia came on rather suddenly. One of my kids got sick one summer—just the flu, but it lasted a few weeks. I was very anxious about it and didn't sleep. That was twenty-five years ago. I have suffered severe insomnia ever since.* And another: *I started a real bad bout when I had my first child. Whenever he would wake up and I had to take care of him, I could never go back to sleep. . . . With each subsequent child (I had three) I had the resultant insomnia.* Some women say they never sleep so well again after they've had children: *I slept with one ear open the whole time they were growing up. They became good sleepers after a few years, but I never did again.*

I'd bet that reconditioning methods would work best with those whose insomnia has been conditioned—but I've found no research that looks at this.

Do "most cases" of insomnia actually fit this model, as the DSM-IV claims? A 1997 study of 348 patients found that "31% could not recall a specific event associated with the onset of their insomnia." Hauri, as we saw earlier, found childhood-onset insomniacs who could not remember a stressful event that had brought on the problem, and whose insomnia remained consistent through stressful and nonstressful periods.

"Quite frankly, there isn't much evidence" that most insomnia is actually due to conditioning, admits Kenneth Lichstein, a speaker at the 2005 NIH insomnia conference. There is strong evidence, Lichstein says, that insomniacs have "negative thinking, selective attending to negative thoughts, self-fueling exacerbation. . . . The irritants in their lives aren't different [from other people's], but what is different is their perception of the irritants." I'll come back to "negative thinking" later in the book, but here recall those findings cited in the conference chapter, that people respond differently to sleep loss, "by an order of magnitude," and suggest that chronic insomniacs might be finding the irritants of their lives more irritable because they're worn down by chronic sleep loss.

One way you might find out whether people are negatively conditioned toward the bedplace is to look at the way they sleep away from home. If they sleep better away from home, whether on vacation or at a sleep clinic, you might surmise that they have wake-up associations with the place they sleep. But the studies that have looked at this have been "equivocal." (I can see why. When I ask myself, do I sleep better away from home, mostly I don't, sometimes I do—and mainly it depends on where I am and what I'm doing there.)

How about differentiating between insomniacs who have trouble falling asleep and insomniacs who have difficulty staying asleep, between so-called sleep-onset and sleep-maintenance insomnia? If people have difficulty falling asleep, it would seem more likely that they have negative associations with the bed; if the problem is staying asleep or returning to sleep, it might be more complicated. Glasgow researcher Colin Espie suggests, "To find out if there's evidence for conditioning, we should be differentiating the group that takes a long time to get to sleep from the group that takes less time." He (and others) even suggest that onset and maintenance insomnia may be different conditions and require different interventions. But the sad truth is, nobody knows. And nobody seems to be trying to find out.

What Comes Naturally

It may be that the behavioral modification proponents are having such a hard time whipping us into shape because sleeping in a consolidated block is not "what comes naturally." A series of fascinating studies done in the 1990s by NIH researcher Thomas Wehr suggests that this may be the case. So does a recent history of the night, *At Day's Close: Night in Times Past,* by A. Roger Ekirch, whose extensive research points to the possibility that the shape of sleep today, the eight-hour consolidated block, is an artifact of electric lighting and the industrial revolution.

Wehr placed fifteen subjects in fourteen hours of darkness—the length of a midwinter's night at the latitude of Washington, D.C.—in order to approximate the circumstances of preindustrial northern Europeans. For four weeks, subjects spent the hours between 6 P.M. and 8 A.M. in dark, windowless rooms, where they were allowed no artificial lighting or music and were instructed to relax and sleep. At first, they slept eleven hours a night, but once they'd paid off their sleep debt, which took a few weeks, they settled into a pattern of about nine hours a night. What was interesting was the way their sleep broke into two or more segments: they slept four to five hours, then lay awake in quiet rest for a few hours, then slept another four to five hours before they woke with the sun. The first segment was primarily deep sleep, ending with a bit of REM; the second consisted largely of REM; and in between they lay quietly resting, in a state between sleep and waking that was neither sleep nor active wakefulness, but "quiet rest with an endocrinology all its own." And they felt terrific, better than ever, in terms of mood and energy.

Wehr describes the long period between the two segments of sleep as "approaching an altered state of consciousness not unlike meditation," "a state not terribly familiar to modern sleepers." Temperature stayed lower longer, and there were higher levels of melatonin over a longer period of time. Levels of *prolactin*, a lovely hormone that keeps birds still when they brood their eggs and is essential to milk production in pregnant women, also stayed higher longer, remaining elevated not only during the hours of sleep, when it is normally elevated, but during the wakeful period between sleeps, which may be why this period was so tranquil. Prolactin has been shown to be stimulated by meditation. "Perhaps," speculates Wehr, "what those who meditate today are seeking is a state that our ancestors would have considered their birthright, a nightly occurrence."

When Wehr's subjects woke from their first sleep, it was usually from an intense REM period, accompanied by vivid dreams. The long period between the two sleeps allowed them time to contemplate their dreams, providing what Wehr describes as "an extended period of quiet wakefulness in which the effects of the dreams might reverberate in conscious awareness." Wehr speculates that this may be why people who lived in traditional societies attributed more importance to dreams than we do: the stretch of time between sleeps may have "provided a channel of communication between dreams and waking life that has gradually been closed off as humans have compressed and consolidated their sleep."

Wehr notes that his subjects were reverting to a sleep pattern typical of animals, whose sleep "occurs in multiple bouts throughout the night (or day)." Human beings are generally considered "an exception to this rule, because their sleep is usually consolidated." But if the older pattern is so close to the surface that modern Americans revert to it in a few weeks, it may be that our biological rhythms are more closely keyed to it than to the eight-hour block. Our sleep, Wehr hypothesizes, may have become consolidated because our long, sixteen-hour exposure to light "compresses and consolidates . . . sleep in an unnatural way." The consolidation of sleep into a solid eight-hour block, then, "may be an artifact of modern lighting."

Ekirch's history of night, *At Day's Close*, lends support to these speculations. Ekirch, a historian at Virginia Polytechnic Institute, finds evidence of segmented sleep in the Europe and America of two hundred to five hundred years ago. Combing through diaries, letters, legal dispositions, medical documents, and imaginative literature of the sixteenth, seventeenth, eighteenth, and nineteenth centuries in Europe and America, he found thousands of references to "first sleep," "first nap," "dead sleep," and "second sleep" or "morning sleep." City dwellers and tillers of the field, people from upper and lower social classes, used these terms as if they were completely commonplace and familiar and "required no elaboration." "There is every reason to believe," Ekirch concludes, "that segmented sleep . . . had long been the natural pattern of our slumber before the modern age, with a provenance as old as humankind."

During the period between sleeps, a lot went on. "Families rose from their beds to urinate, smoke tobacco, and even visit close neighbors. Remaining abed, many persons also made love, prayed, and reflected on the dreams that typically preceded waking from their 'first sleep.'" It was a pleasant period, according to many accounts. "People used this shrouded interval of solitude to immerse themselves in contemplation—to ponder events of the preceding day and to prepare for the arrival of dawn." It was a time for intimacy: as a sixteenth-century French physician advised, "After the first sleep," people "have more enjoyment" and "do it better."

Sleep seems to have become consolidated first in the urban regions and among the upper classes, where households and neighborhoods could afford lighting. As more homes and streets were lit, as more activity began to take place at night, the darkness receded and exposure to light lengthened. But references to "first sleep" persist even into the first half of the twentieth century. Wehr thought he was simulating patterns of "prehistoric" sleep in his studies, but the shape of sleep he discovered turns out to be as recent as that of our great-grandparents, perhaps even our grandparents. The consolidation of sleep into the pattern it has today is an astonishingly recent event in the history of the world.

There is evidence from many sources that sleep in times past was more fluid and less rigidly demarcated in terms of time and place than it is today. In paintings of the Flemish school, agricultural workers were depicted asleep in broad daylight, by the side of the field, or in the road. Through the seventeenth century, writes Lawrence Wright, in *Warm and Snug: The History of the Bed,* sleep took place without "much care for privacy or coyness"; warmth and safety were valued above privacy. "Until the 18th century," Wright recounts, "sleeping remained a communal activity, and it was common for several people, not just two, to share a bed." "In travellers' tales of inns and lodgings we find rooms and even beds being shared, and sometimes shared with strangers." (I try to remember this whenever I find myself cramped in with a lot of snoring strangers on an endless night flight.)

It was not only the exposure to longer light that made the shift in sleep patterns, but the transformation of life from an agrarian to an industrialized rhythm—and the two movements facilitated one another, since electricity was a product of the Industrial Revolution and in turn fed back into it. The new nineteenth-century factory system "demanded a transformation of human nature," writes British historian E. P. Thompson in *The Making of the English Working Class,* a transformation of workers' relation to time—and to sleep—that did not come easily, since early industrialized workers resisted clock time and discipline. "They were not enthusiastic about being rung to work at sunup and rung home at sundown (or later)," writes Ralph Keyes in *Timelock;* they were "still tuned more to the clocks of their bodies than to the mechanized kind." The agricultural way of life had been demanding, but it was governed by the natural rhythms of light and dark and the seasons; it allowed more room for variation and rest than factory work did. The virtues of hard work had to be drummed into workers, for the work was grueling, the shifts were long (fourteen to sixteen hours), and the profits were enjoyed not by them but by the owners of the factories. Getting them to accept the new discipline required threats, rewards, fines, and the inculcation of a new "work ethic." "Time-managers" policed the workplace with stopwatches and warned against lying abed. Sunday sermons preached hellfire and damnation to the lazy and dissolute and denounced "the slumbers of sin."

The new world hopped to the new beat more readily than the old, born as it was in Puritanism and steeped in the spirit of Ben Franklin, with his tireless promotion of industry and productivity ("time is money") and denigration of sleep: "Plough deep, while sluggards sleep, and you shall have corn to sell and to keep." Thomas Edison, maniacally energetic, boisterously self-promoting, and fixated on productivity and self-improvement, epitomized the entrepreneurial spirit of the Industrial Revolution. He is quoted as saying, "There is really no reason why men should go to bed at all. . . . Sleep is an absurdity, a bad habit." It's appropriate that he gave us the lightbulb, which did so much to beat sleep into retreat.

Sleep, by the end of the nineteenth century, had become synonymous with sin, sloth, a waste of time. So was born the sleep machismo that's been our curse ever since. And sure enough, sleep, by the end of the nineteenth century, was becoming problematic. Not that our ancestors enjoyed blissfully bucolic sleep: their sleep was often "restless," "troubled," "broken," "frightened"—these are terms Ekirch often found—disturbed by the proximity of other people, animals, hunger, fleas, cold, pain. But as life speeded up, marching to a faster tempo and a more mechanized beat, physicians began writing books and pamphlets deploring the problem of insomnia, attributing it to the faster pace and greater complexity of modern life. The first reports of a medication used for promoting sleep (bromide) were in the middle of the nineteenth century. Opium addiction became rampant, particularly among factory workers and upper-class women. Opium was available at the grocers; laudanum, a mixture of opium dissolved in alcohol, was the main ingredient of tonics widely used through the early part of the twentieth century.

There are not many cross-cultural studies of sleep, but anthropologists Carol Worthman and Melissa Melby, gathering together what is known about sleep in traditional cultures—the rain forest dwellers of Gebusi, New Guinea; the !Kung hunter-gatherers in Africa; the Swat Pathan herders in Pakistan; the Ache foragers in Paraguay; Balinese farmers in Indonesia—conclude that sleep in such societies is more fluid and polyphasic than in our own, retaining features it had in our past. Sleep in traditional societies occurs in social spaces, entire families huddled together in a small hut or around a fire. Communal sleep is safer: the presence of other people, the munching and bleating of animals, the fire kept going all night for warmth and protection, are reassuring rather than disturbing. Among the !Kung, "no one, including children, is told to go to bed"; "people stay up as long as something interesting is happening . . . then they go to sleep when they feel like it." In Bali, children learn to sleep in the midst of activity, "in almost any position" (as Margaret Mead observed), and retain this ability throughout life.

Women sleep with their infants and often with their children. There is a lot of physical contact, with the limbs of two and sometimes three sleepers intertwined. There are arguments that cosleeping, which is frowned upon in most Western societies (except for Sweden), is good for the infant, that having the mother's comforting presence and bodily contact reduces stress levels, helps regulate breathing, heart rate, and other physiological functions. "By sleeping next to its mother, the infant receives protection, warmth, emotional reassurance, and breast milk," as "nature intended," writes anthropologist James McKenna, who finds that infants who have been raised like this "become better adjusted adults." McKenna sees enforced separation as the source of many sleep disorders.

People in traditional societies slip more easily in and out of sleep than we do. The boundaries between sleep and wakefulness are less marked, the times and places of sleep are less fixed. In some societies, sleep conforms

to the biphasic pattern we know from siesta cultures, with most of the
sleep occurring at night and a nap in the afternoon, but more often the
pattern is polyphasic. "Africa, Asia, these are the polyphasic societies,
the world of opportunistic sleepers who sleep when the chance allows,"
writes Aminatta Forner. "People sleep like babies, intermittently through
the day." She recalls "the Thai taxi driver napping on his own back seat.
The office worker in Delhi lying on a park bench with an open newspaper across his face. In West Africa I sat for twenty minutes opposite a
snoozing clerk stretched across his desk. In time he roused himself and
guiltlessly attended to my business." Sleep in such societies "is tolerated.
Sleep is shameless," she says. It's not the "shameful" thing it's made out
to be in northern Europe and North America, where expressions like
"caught napping," "asleep on the job," and "asleep at the switch" reflect
the belief that an adult who sleeps during the day, especially in public
view, "must be unemployed, sick, drunk, or idle."

A psychologist friend speculates, "A hundred years ago, it was probably easier to be an accepted member of the family and community even
if you had odd sleep habits, or couldn't sit still, or couldn't read, or
abused morphine, or acted weird sometimes or whatever. But as modern industrialized society demands ever greater productivity, literacy,
impulse control, intelligence, and so on, from each person, male or female, child or adult, young or old, scientists will gradually develop an
endless lists of 'disorders,' ADHD, personality disorders, learning disabilities. Maybe sleep disorders are part of this group?"

Sleep as a Social Construction

What this brief look at other cultures and other times suggests is that
sleep may be differently "tuned" or organized under different sociocul-
tural conditions, as Worthman and Melby say. Western sleep is solitary,
bounded, consolidated, with transitions between sleep and wakefulness
that are few and brief, whereas non-Western sleep is communal, involving frequent transitions and a greater variety of in-between stages.

The malleability of sleep is apparent in the changes currently taking
place in Mediterranean and Latin American societies, where biphasic
sleep, until recently the norm, is being phased out, in the interests of efficiency. "In China recently, the widespread custom of *hsiuhsi,* or the afternoon nap, has taken a bashing from Western-style work schedules.
'Our businessmen are being told by people in your country that sleeping

in the afternoon is a sign of laziness,' a traveller recently heard. 'We are not lazy and do not wish to appear that way, so most business people have given up *hsiuhsi*.'"

Will these societies now sprout a whole crop of new and different types of sleep disorders? I hope some sleep researcher is asking that question.

But not everyone's sleep is equally malleable—variability again. Not all of Wehr's subjects reverted to segmented sleep: twelve did, but three retained their consolidated sleep. Studies of shift workers indicate that there are shifters and nonshifters, that some people's circadian cycles, as measured by melatonin release, shift easily and others' do not. Some people barely notice changes in the light, others are highly sensitive to such changes. Some are so sensitive that they become depressed in the winter, in a syndrome known as seasonal affective disorder. One of Wehr's subjects "became profoundly depressed and suicidal when he was exposed to short days and long nights and recovered when he was reexposed to long days and short nights." Some strains of hamsters are less responsive than others to a shortening of light exposure, as Wehr points out. Different strains of hamsters, different strains of us.

It may be that behavioral modification doesn't help more people to better sleep because it's pulling against patterns that are deeply engrained. It may be that, in trying to sleep in a solid eight-hour block, we're bent on a course of defying nature. Perhaps some of us are just "nonshifters" who refuse to be dragged from our archaic pasts into a postindustrialized age.

E.P. Thompson sees the preindustrial rhythm as more in tune with our natural clocks: "That this rhythm still characterizes students, the self-employed, farmers, and others" suggests that most people would probably work this way if they had control of their schedules. Left to our own devices, how would each of us sleep? How many odd and idiosyncratic sleep patterns would we find in ourselves? In my ideal world, we'd have the freedom to find out. I have a friend who slips in and out of sleep like a forager. He works a few hours, naps, then gets up and works some more, dropping in and out of sleep at any and all hours of the day or night. Luckily he's self-employed, highly productive, and has a wife who sleeps well enough to be unperturbed by his comings and goings. The term for him, I know now, is *free running*, a term he likes.

Sleep researchers assume that the sleep they measure in labs is universal across cultures, but they may be looking at the sleep of a select group of young, healthy, well-fed Westerners and a pattern that's a few generations old and mistaking it for a biological norm. The shape of sleep we take for granted may be specific to our culture, and to only a small part of it, at that, since sleep studies generally exclude women, the elderly, the poor. Throughout history and in traditional societies today, the fluidity of boundaries between sleep and wakefulness and the rest periods between sleeps have given access to a range of states and experiences we are losing; and it's not only our dreams we are losing, but a whole range of stages between sleep and wakefulness that would have been more accessible to people accustomed to slipping in and out of sleep, and that might, if we had a keener sense of them, enrich our understanding of sleep (as we'll see in the next chapter).

"We're going to have to reconceptualize what it means to sleep normally," concludes Wehr. "When modern humans find that their sleep is fragmented and interrupted by periods of wakefulness during the night, they regard it as being disordered," but it may be "that a natural pattern of human sleep is breaking through into an artificial world in which it seems unfamiliar and unwelcome." It may be that sleep disorders are so common because we're pitting ourselves against what comes naturally. Our sleep is fragmented when we're babies, and again when we're old; it seems that, as we age, "it gets harder to override it." If a third of the population complains of insomnia and a tenth sleeps as badly as I do— as National Sleep Foundation surveys suggest—you really have to wonder about that norm.

Sleep, as we see again and again, is more complex than our conceptions of it. If sleep is an "undiscovered country" (to twist Hamlet's lines on death) from which the traveler *does* return, the tales we return with often reveal more about ourselves than about the places we have been. Again and again, we see a tendency to impose a grid on this vast unknown, to clamp down a cookie-cutter pattern that reduces it to a size and shape that can be "managed," while sleep remains larger and more mysterious than our terms and categorizations for it. A way of enlarging our conceptions might be to open the conversation to other cultures and to the voices of others in our own culture—other than young, healthy, well-fed males.

A Take-Charge Kind of Thing

Managing sleep is what behavioral modification is all about. It feels like the behaviorists are performing the same sort of policing function with us that time managers performed with nineteenth-century factory workers, attempting to keep us in line, whip us into shape, so we'll be more efficient. A consolidated block of sleep *is* more efficient, as history shows. The countries that sleep efficiently conquered the world.

"It's so very American, the way they talk," a European sleep researcher muttered to me during a conference session. "The self-management approach takes the view that you need to be in charge of your own destiny," writes Morin, who, though not American, has got the Yankee spirit. It's the take-charge, take-control determination familiar from the many self-help and recovery programs that thrive in this country. It's the spirit of Norman Vincent Peale's *Power of Positive Thinking* (a book published in 1952 that sold millions of copies and is still in print), a message that says you are in control of your life, you are responsible for your successes and failures, you can do it if you try, it's all within your power: you are what you think you are; imagine yourself different and you will be different. The recovery movements combine this positive thinking with the sort of "kick butt, get a grip, just do it" talk that's in the air—that's *on* the air, every afternoon, in the advice Dr. Phil dishes out to audiences nationwide. This get-tough spirit comes down to us from our Puritan forefathers, who were famous for self-improvement books that urged a scrupulous accounting of every move and thought—not unlike the sleep diaries behaviorists insist that we keep, where we track every single thing about our sleep, monitoring our every move and its every effect. "Last night you didn't sleep well. Did you eat too much? Did you sleep too much the night before? Every day you must look at what occurred the night before and at what happened yesterday to affect your sleep. Scold yourself if you cheated." So says John Wiedman in *Desperately Seeking Snoozin'*. "I almost look at myself like a recovering alcoholic in that if I fall back into old habits, I will end up back where I started before my 'cure.' . . . I now know that I have to be careful, or I can 'fall off the wagon.' . . . I now consider myself a 'recovering insomniac,' I know that any time I cheat on the program, I have to pay the price."

I don't think this analogy between alcoholism and insomnia makes a lot of sense, but the language has wide appeal, as the popularity of Wiedman's book testifies.

People who post on Sleepnet.com echo these terms: *Last night I fell off the wagon and took a pill.* Some give pep talks to themselves and one another that are right out of *The Power of Positive Thinking: Imagine yourself sleeping well and you will. Tell yourself that you are good and you deserve to sleep. Insomnia is a bad attitude, a failure of will. Insomnia is self-doubt, self-loathing, a failure of self-esteem, a lapse into negativity.*

Love yourself, accept yourself, develop a positive attitude, and you will sleep. In recovery movements like Alcoholics Anonymous, you're urged to give yourself over to a higher authority, a belief in God; here the higher authority is not God but "the program." There is a strong strain of religiosity in some of these postings: *Just believe. You have to believe in the program for it to work. You have to follow it like Gospel. I have accepted this program, that it is going to work for me. I have faith that it works.*

And if it works, fine—anything that works is fine. It just doesn't work for me.

Insomnia "is nothing more than a bad habit," says Wiedman. With all due respect, sometimes it is and sometimes it isn't, and often there's not enough basis to say. There are many things insomnia might be. Behaviorists say that wherever it comes from and whatever causes it, you can cut into the cycle of negative conditioning and learn new habits. Maybe so. Maybe if you regularize your sleep, you can balance a hormonal or thermoregulatory problem. But maybe you can't. I hear many stories like this one: *I knew it was hormones, I knew it wasn't anything I was doing, but they kept telling me I just needed to get on a regular schedule. Finally I found a doctor who got me on hormone replacement therapy and a low dose of trazodone, and I got my life back.* There are some physiological problems that are not amenable to change by an alteration of habits.

The behaviorists say it's a "faulty causal attribution" to think this way. "For insomniacs, the erroneous belief that sleep is disrupted by something beyond their control, such as a chemical imbalance, leads to a sense of hopelessness and helplessness," writes Morin, and this "exacerbates the sleeping difficulty." But how can you be so sure a "causal attribution" is faulty when "little is known about the mechanisms [and] causes . . . of chronic insomnia," as stated in the 2005 NIH insomnia conference report? "How can you say what 'good' sleep hygiene would be, when you don't even know what good sleep is?" says my friend Ilene, drawing an analogy between insomnia and obesity, which she sees a lot of in her practice: "We thought we understood about weight loss; we were so sure: you lose weight by starving yourself. Now it turns out, the body goes into starvation mode when it's starved, so that when you go back to eating normally, you put on weight and gain back more. The relationship between food intake and weight gain is much more complicated than we thought. For all we know, there's something like this we don't know about sleep."

The flip side to the positive-think, take-charge talk is the self-blame generated when you can't make the program work or when you're not up to trying: if I were a stronger person, a better/more motivated/self-disciplined/clean-living person, I could make it work. *If I weren't such a fuck-off, I'd stick to this and make it work,* said a freelance computer programmer I talked to. This guy did not look like a fuck-off to me. He was a person who worked at home, whose work was close, fussy, demanding, who needed a way of relaxing evenings that involved friends, sociability, some drinking, and whose life was constrained by so many straightjackets that he couldn't bring himself to put on yet one more. The self-castigation I heard from him did not sound right.

What Kinds of People Does It Not Work For?

"Even though a particular intervention is efficacious," says Charles Morin—and I've heard him say this several times—"if it produces adverse side effects, is too time-consuming, or too costly, adherence is likely to be poor. Thus, regardless of how efficacious a given treatment is, if it is not acceptable to patients it may be of little clinical use."

Try following those rules in a college dormitory, as one of my students said, when I asked her if she had tried them. Try following those rules in a nursing home, said a doctor at one of the conferences. And would you really want to? Would a person who is old and infirm and in chronic pain be able to brutalize himself or herself by living on restricted sleep for however long it takes to find out if it's going to help? *How do you practice sleep hygiene in a trailer?* said a physician I interviewed, many of whose patients live in trailer camps. *How can you tell an overwhelmed single mother who lives in an inner-city hell to cut out stimulating activities in the evening and regularize her habits?* says a friend who's a social worker. These methods work best for the well-to-do, for those who can take time off from work or who don't need to work at all, and for people who have comfortable other rooms to move to. (It is perhaps no coincidence that Stanford, which has had success with this program, is located in one of the most affluent areas in the world.) *It won't cut it in corporate America,* as one insomniac said. "Telling someone whose life is disorganized—who has to fly all over the country for business, for example—to regulate their sleep patterns better is not helpful," said Dr. Merril Mitler, director of research at the Sleep Disorders Center at the Scripps Clinic and Research Foundation in La Jolla. It won't cut it for people who cannot tolerate a certain amount of sleepiness on the job, whose jobs are so demanding that they can't take time off, time out to

be comatose for however many weeks or months it takes to find out if
the program works for them. It won't cut it for those whose jobs impose
irregularity—shift workers or freelance workers whose assignments come
in irregular spurts. Bonnie, a freelance artist, was told by the doctors at
the sleep clinic she went to to "get a regular job":

> *Their whole thing is, find a line of work where you'll be in bed at 11 and
> up at 7. They said, if you're serious about getting sleep, you'll change your
> life.* NO, *I said, I've chosen to live the way I live* BECAUSE *my sleep is bad;
> this is the only way I could live.* . . . *They really made me feel terrible, like
> it was all my fault. But I mean, it has to work for who you are.*

I wish the studies that found a 70 to 80 percent success rate with CBT
had told us who these people are, what kinds of jobs they hold, what professions they work in, and what kinds of insomnia they have. If "subjects" were viewed as more than just head counts, as multidimensional
beings with thoughts and voices and lives they live, we might have this
kind of information. I'd bet that behavioral modification works best for
people whose jobs provide the kind of external stimulus that enables them
to get by with some sleepiness. Put me in a social situation full of interesting interaction, and I can make do on five hours' sleep. I can do conferences, committee meetings, errands, travel; I can hang out, schmooze,
and do simpler kinds of writing. But put me in a room alone, with no
props or distractions, and I look at the stacks of articles and materials I
need to get through for this book, and I feel I'm at the bottom of an
avalanche—though that same mountain, on days when I have my wits
and energy, looks like a challenge and kind of fun. Maybe if I did another
kind of work, I'd be less concerned about my sleep. *But I mean, it has to
work for who you are.*

When people tell us we're getting "enough sleep," I want to ask,
"Enough for what?" "Enough for who?" Enough for one day but not
another, for one kind of work but not another, for one kind of person
but not another (since sleep needs are so variable).

I suspect, too, that behavioral modification methods work better for
people who are, in their personalities and habits, more regular than I am.
My life and habits have never been regular. Rules and regulations make
me feel nervous, not secure. Some of the people I talk to, and some of the
people who post on Sleepnet.com, love the strictness of the program: *Just
do what it says and you'll be fine.* Others hate it: *My anxiety just goes
up when I know I have 20 minutes to get back to sleep. I really became*

afraid of not sleeping because my time in bed was so short. I was getting anxious about sleep in a way I hadn't been before. Another woman says, *They tell you, don't look at the clock, and I never had actually paid much attention to the clock, but when I was doing sleep restriction I was look-ing at it all the time, trying to figure out when I should get up.* I too was made anxious by the clock in a way I'm not usually (has it been fifteen minutes yet? Can I lie here another five?). Just knowing I had so little time to get back to sleep made it a sure thing I would not. The sleep jour-nal was also a problem: I found it crazy-making, all that keeping-track. The entire program was making me sleep-obsessed, which I realize sounds strange coming from someone who's written a long book on sleep, but there are more and less productive forms of obsession.

I follow a lot of rules in the course of a day, teaching, writing, mak-ing deadlines, meeting with students, meeting with colleagues. I jump through a lot of complicated hoops—be here, be there, be this, be that, now do it this way, now do it without the net, keep that smile on your face. I have a fair amount of self-discipline: I quit smoking after a decade and a half of heavy smoking, I gave up coffee, I weigh ten pounds more than I did in college, and I swim year-round, on cold, rainy nights in an outdoor pool. But I balk at bringing the rule book into the bedroom. Cut out "stimulating activities in the evening"? Evenings are when I relax, so-cialize, see friends. Take them away and you take away the only latitude in my life. So, yes, I eat out and drink wine with dinner and stay late at parties, I work later than I should, and sometimes it wrecks my sleep—and sometimes it does not.

I talk to other insomniacs who've come to conclusions like mine. *I was giving up too much. For those of us who aren't so desperate, it's just not worth it.* That may be the key: how desperate we are. *I was averaging maybe five to ten hours of sleep a week,* said a woman whose behavioral modification has brought her up to four or five hours of sleep a night, better than she's been for years. *That's* worth doing! If I'd stayed in that publishing job I got fired from for coming in late, six hours' sleep would have been a cornucopia, compared to the two to five hours I was limp-ing along on.

Frankly, I love sleep too much to voluntarily restrict it for the rest of my life. Sleep is a pleasure and a restoration and a friend. It soothes my aching bones and ailing psyche, knits the raveled sleeve of care. Some-times I'll lie in bed after I wake up, just lie there and think about my dreams, or sometimes I'll listen to a book on tape, because I know this is the only unregimented time I'll have all day—and sometimes I fall back to sleep, and even if I don't it can feel restorative, just lying there in the dark. To be always, for the rest of my life, waking to an alarm? If an alarm wakes me in the wrong part of a sleep cycle, it puts me into a grog and a funk that lasts the day: it does violence to both sleep and consciousness. I think I agree with whoever said there can be no hope for a society that wakes to an alarm.

It's not that the behavioral modification approach isn't right; it's just that it's not right for everybody. It is certainly worth a serious, wholehearted try, if you can find time in your life, time to take out of your life, and if you can see it as a viable way of living. It may work for you, and if it does, you'll have a sense of control you'll never have using drugs, which is, as I've said, like having a bear by the nose.

It may also be that you can cobble together some modified version of the program that works. Peter Hauri allows that some people do better watching TV and reading in bed, that some sleep better with naps, that some even do better with evening exercise. Joyce Wasleben, author of *A Woman's Guide to Sleep,* does not take a hard line on getting out of bed when you can't sleep, unless you're really agitated, because "too many women are driven today by 'should dos.'" Deepak Chopra advises, "Even if you are feeling quite restless, the best thing you can do is just rest easily in bed, eyes closed."

In the end, you and only you know what's right for you.

Professional Opinions

"Since the mid-eighties, the etiology of insomnia has been largely understood within a behavioral framework," wrote behavioral modification proponent Michael Perlis in 2001. He calls it a "compelling conceptualization." "Compelling" it may be, but you could also see it as a kind of "premature closure" that has brought us no closer to understanding the actual etiology of insomnia. The behavioral theory is a "top-down theory," says Eric Nofzinger, the Pittsburgh researcher who does neuroimaging of sleep; it assumes that "some unknown higher order cognitive process, such as rumination, . . . is driving the altered neurobiology in insomnia"; but we need first "to define the underlying brain mechanisms that regulate sleep/wake processes." As Michael Bonnet says, "We haven't understood the underlying neurobiological systems that make sleep happen. So meanwhile we're trying to talk people into behavioral changes, and that's okay in some instances, but doesn't really get to the root of it."

When I asked a Berkeley psychiatrist friend who runs insomnia support groups at a Veterans' Administration hospital if behavioral methods were effective, he said, "Yes." "Ironically," he added, "they seem to work best for the most seriously ill patients: the mere neurotics have less incentive to change." (This is an attractive, charismatic guy who I can well imagine having success with his groups.)

"Does the approach really address the problem? Does conditioning account for insomnia?" I asked him.

"It's the part we can change," he said. "It's what we know how to do. You don't look for the cause, you just drill this stuff in. You drum it in— this is when you should go to bed, this is when you should get up, this is what you can and cannot do in the hour before you go to bed. It's like physical conditioning: the worse your sleep is, the more careful you need to be—you need to be fastidious about monitoring your conditions."

"Isn't that a little like kicking the TV?" I said.

"Oh, it's not like it's understood. It's like everyone's sort of given up on the rest, because it's too difficult."

It may be that behavioral modification is all that can be done at this point. And even if it is not much more effective than placebo, placebo can be powerful. Yet insofar as its success is being used to suggest that the problem is under control, it seems to have allowed everyone to "sort of give up on the rest."

CHAPTER 9

Asleep at the Switch

The Clinics

Sleep like other Things is sold
And you must purchase your Repose with Gold.
Nicholas Boileau

On my third try, I make it in.

My first try was in the early 1980s, when I called the Stanford sleep clinic about getting into one of their studies. It ended with my beating a hasty retreat when I learned that they "didn't monitor for *that*"—*that* being the time of month in their female subjects. Since I've always had a strong sense of my insomnia as hormonally driven, this seemed a sorry waste of time.

My second try was about ten years later. I was coming off sleeping pills, on the downswing of the cycles of withdrawal and addiction I was hooked into for nearly two decades; I hadn't slept for nights. I thought, this can't go on. I dialed the number (Stanford, again) and got a recorded voice, one of those machines that shunts you through dozens of options, none of them what you want (not what a desperate person needs to hear), then tells you to stay on the line if you need help. Well, yes, I did need help, I needed at least to speak to a human being. Finally I got a girl whose voice, bored, disaffected, sounded like she'd rather be surfing, who couldn't quite get her mind around why I was calling—like, why would anyone call the Stanford sleep clinic with a question about how to get into the Stanford sleep clinic? Finally she got it: "Oh. Your doctor puts in a referral, and insurance decides whether to okay it." I guess that's what had her confused: it's all handled by other parties. Well, there was no doctor at my HMO who'd refer me out for anything as costly as this, so I asked her if I could self-refer and pay out of pocket, and what did it cost? She said she wasn't sure about the self-referral, but it cost thirty-five hundred dollars for a night (can I be remembering this right? It sounds so astronomical). I said thanks—and beat a hasty retreat off the phone.

That's twice.

My third attempt, a few years later, is not with Stanford but through my HMO. I've lucked into a doctor, a primary care provider, who is sympathetic, a young, bearded, teddy-bear type of fellow who radiates warmth and concern. His eyes do not glaze when I start talking about my insomnia: in fact, he's actually *interested*. When I tell him about my lifelong sleep problem, he tells me about *his:* he has "idiopathic hyper-somnia," meaning that he's sleepy all the time, for reasons unknown. He lives on caffeine and the wake-up drug Provigil: "My EEG shows no deep sleep, and nobody knows why. It's horrible, feeling tired all the time, fighting sleep."

"Yeah, I know." I ask him to help me find out what the EEG says about *my* sleep.

"I can put in a request for a study," he says, "but I don't think you'll have much luck with this HMO. Not that it's any worse than any other. But let me put it this way: it's easier for me to get a bone marrow trans-plant for a patient than to get a sleep disorder fully evaluated and treated, and it takes months less time. You wouldn't believe the runaround I've had trying to get treatment for my problem, only to be told, 'We're sorry you have this problem but that's the way it is.' You wouldn't believe how little sleep disorders are taken seriously."

I tell him yes, I would believe it. But I am a little shocked to hear that a physician can get no better help for himself than this. I tell him I'd re-ally appreciate it if he'd try.

He says, "Okay. But I don't think they'll go for it."

They do not go for it. He runs it through again, throwing all his weight behind it—and this time, it goes through. The first date we can find, what with their schedule and mine, is early November—four months after he'd put in the initial request.

I've been told to show up at 8:30 P.M. and to plan on being out by 7 A.M., which, given that my usual sleep schedule is more like 3 to 10 A.M., seems sort of ridiculous. It seems strange, too, that I'm to spend only one night, since insomniacs' sleep is so erratic, so variable from night to night. I've been told to bring my own pillow, sleepwear, toiletries, so I have them all packed and am about to leave the house, map in hand, steeling myself for the challenge of finding a part of Los Angeles I'd never heard of (this was when I lived in Southern California), when the phone rings. It's the sleep lab, telling me, "Your insurance turned down the request." No explanation, just some snafu. Had they called two minutes later, I'd have driven an hour to find this out, and an hour back. So the next week and the week after, I play telephone tag with my HMO and, after a few rounds, the request is okayed, or rather, it's okayed *again*. We set a time for mid-December.

I head out to the far side of L.A., find the hospital without too much trouble, find the sleep lab, and check in. While I'm doing the paperwork at the front desk, glancing through the questionnaire they'd sent me to fill out, my eye falls on the part Bob has filled out:

> Gayle simply never gets through a night of unbroken sleep. She sometimes falls asleep fairly quickly, but is nearly always awake when I wake up in the morning and often is awake if I wake up during the night. In fact, she frequently wakes me up with her tossing and turning. I generally sleep quite well on my own, but a week with Gayle can leave me sleepstarved as well. She does not show any particular symptoms of twitching, kicking, holding her breath, and the like. She falls asleep, but just can't stay asleep. Sometimes she seems to have a pretty good night; more often she'll complain about getting only a few hours.
>
> What's odd is that I've been unable to find any connection between Gayle's mood, the day's events, and whether she sleeps well.

Yeah, I know this woman. I sleep with her, too.

A technician appears, blond, brusque, fast-talking, introduces herself as Janine. She takes me down the hall to my room. It's a small room, fits only a bed and a night table, but it's not too dreary; the bed is a good size, and comfortable. Janine tells me I'll be having a "split-night-study," meaning that the first part of the night I'll be monitored for signs of apnea, and then I'll be fitted for a CPAP machine if it looks like I need it (a CPAP, pronounced "see-pap," is a *continuous positive airways pressure* machine, a mask fitted over your nose that delivers pressured air to keep the airways open as you sleep). She tells me if I'm not asleep in thirty to forty minutes, they'll give me a sleeping pill, which seems kind of crazy to me: that's what I'm here to get off of, and from what I've read, all hypnotics affect the architecture of sleep. I guess they figure, since they're here to measure my sleep, I'd better get some sleep for them to measure, however compromised. I guess I look dubious, because she adds, "You can refuse it, if you like."

"No, no, that's fine," I say. "It's just that I'm not likely to get to sleep until 3 A.M.—that's when I usually go to bed."

"Oh, you'd be surprised," she says; "most people come in here and sleep like babies. There are hardly any true insomniacs. We hardly ever get a real one. You may have heard of sleep state misperception?" I say, "Yes, but I doubt . . . ," but she's out the door.

I mull this over. Apparently there are "real" insomniacs and insomniacs who are not—real? Who are "unreal"? "inauthentic"? "fake"? Sleep, on the other hand, is sleep, whether drugged or undrugged. Though from what I've read—and experienced—it is not.

The clinic is full. It's full every night, but this night there seems to be some confusion. Janine pokes her head in the door and apologizes that they're taking so long getting to me. "No problem," I say. "It's hours till my usual bedtime." I change into my nightgown and stretch out for a read. My room is just across from the technicians' work station, and, drawn by the sound of the talk and laughter, I wander out into the hall and peek in. There's a formidable bank of computers, screens, diagnostic equipment; it emits a kind of low humming, as though it were alive. On the screens are the interiors of the sleep rooms, which answers one of my questions—yes, I'll be observed; though I see no camera in my room.

I feel strange, suddenly, sleeping with strangers, having my sleep observed by people I don't know. It makes me realize what a closed, private function sleep is, that's about to be displayed now for strangers to see. Oh well, they're friendly strangers; they have my best interest at heart. I think.

Finally around 11:30, a woman who introduces herself as Maria comes in to hook me up. It's an elaborate process, getting all rigged up; it takes over a half hour for her to attach the tangle of wires to the right parts of my body, fastening each on carefully with sticky tape. "What's this?" I ask, as she fixes the wires under my chin, on my calves and chest, on my temples, and at points on my skull. Maria finds my curiosity amusing, as I piece together a picture of what all these wires to chest, legs, and face are for. A polysomnogram includes the EMG, or *electromyograph,* which measures muscle activity in the limbs and under the chin; the ECG, or *electrocardiograph,* which monitors heart rate and rhythm; the EOG, or *electrooculograph,* which measures eye movements. And, of course, the main event, the EEG, or *electroencephalogram,* consisting of electrodes fastened at points on the skull that pick up electrochemical impulses produced by neurons as they transmit and receive messages, impulses that become slower and synchronized as we enter sleep and move into deeper stages. This is the device that tracks our progress through nonREM and REM stages and back again through the cycles, measuring the architecture of sleep across the night.

I'm particularly intrigued by the fat felt pen with the squishy tip that Maria is using to mark my temples and skull. It looks like one of those pens you use to address parcel post, a Marks-A-Lot, only the ink is bright turquoise. She is marking the places where she'll fasten the electrodes.

"How do you know where to put the electrodes?" I ask.

"It's where I made the marks."

"Yeah, but how do you know where to make the marks?"

"Well, we learn that in school." Then she laughs and says, "I guess I never thought of that. Yeah, I really wonder, too—now that you ask." She tells me if you put them in the wrong place, you get scrambled stuff, like computer garbage. (Peter Hauri told me it was through trial and error that they found where to place them; in the beginning they used a full montage of eighteen; now there are about a half dozen.) The information from these electrodes is transmitted through the wires to the box on the nightstand, and from there to the bank of computers in the other room, where it will be processed digitally. Back in the old days, when Dement and Aserinsky were studying sleep at Chicago, it took twelve hundred to fifteen hundred feet of expensive graph paper to record a night's sleep, so they'd turn the machines off to save paper—which is why they didn't pick up REM. It makes you wonder what sorts of things today's technology might not be picking up.

"Ta-dah," I say, displaying my headdress, a bird's nest of red, blue, and yellow wires. We are giggling like schoolgirls at a pajama party, up to some outrageous prank. "Smile, you're on *Candid Camera,*" I say, mugging for the hidden camera, which, she indicates, is in the wall to the left of the bed. "But," she says, "you're not supposed to know that." She then fastens a belt around my stomach and another around my chest, to measure breathing. She clamps a clip to the tip of my right ring finger, which she tells me is for measuring the oxygen content of the blood. Under my nose, she fits a plastic tube with extensions into my nostrils. It looks like one of those devices they use in hospitals to give oxygen, but it's a sensor that measures the flow of air. I'm afraid it will set me sneezing, but it doesn't.

The spaghetti weave of wires is then attached to the small box on the night table. But before Maria hooks me up to the box, I tell her I need to use the bathroom. She shows me how to hold the wires, and I carry them gingerly as I make my way down the hall. The face in the mirror is amazing, smudges of blue-green war paint on the temples, parti-colored wires sticking out of the hair—a sci-fi Medusa with headgear set to receive messages from outer space, a figure Salvador Dali could have hallucinated on a bad night.

"Have a good night," Maria says, as she closes my door. I look at my watch (there are no clocks in my room). It's 12:30.

Maria has told me I should sleep on my back, because they want to see how I breathe. So I try. But can't sleep on my back: usually I start out on my back and then, when I hear the beginning of a snore, turn over on my stomach—but that's out of the question with this snarl of wires. So I lie obediently on my back and wait for sleep to come. And wait. And sleep doesn't come, not even the telltale snore that signals sleep is near—no surprise, I'm not usually in bed at this hour. It is god-awful boring. No books on tape. Time passes, more time, a very long time, and I wonder why they don't come and offer me that sleeping pill, which I'd gladly take at this point. It's too light in this room—there's a nightlight kept on—and it's too warm, especially with the nightgown decency requires; and I feel constrained by the wires. So I lie there and think, Well, I guess you'll see you've got "a real one," I am *really* not asleep, the EEG will tell you that. I am thinking about hospitals, being here in a hospital, how I don't actually hate hospitals, how I find them sort of comforting, probably because I (knock wood) haven't had much contact with them, how I even have fond memories of hospitals, my father taking me on his "rounds" when I was a little girl, going around checking on his patients. A few times I feel like I'm drifting off, but then I'm wide awake again, aware of the nightlight, aware of the god-awful boredom, mainly the boredom.

After what seems a very long time, I need to pee, so I ring the bell. Maria comes and unhooks me from the box, I make my way down the hall and back, and then, as I'm getting into bed, Janine pokes her head in and asks, "In your opinion, have you been asleep?"

"No," I say.

"Were you aware I came into the room?"

"No. I must have dropped off. Shallow sleep, then? Stage one or two?"

She does a double take, then says, huffy, "Well, you're right where you're supposed to be" (putting Miss Smarty-Pants in her place), and shuts the door. She's said more than she's supposed to say: Maria's told me they aren't supposed to tell me anything, they're only technicians, they can't do the interpreting—"there are legal issues." *(Legal issues?)* There's this aura of hush-hush about it all that I find very infantilizing and frustrating—nobody will talk to me about what's going on. They don't even want me to know what time it is (but they can't keep me from looking at my watch). But Janine couldn't resist letting this much cat out of the bag, as if to say, "See, I told you, you're not a real one." And that was the only information I was to get out of anyone—for a long time.

So that's why nobody had come in with a sleeping pill—the EEG said I was asleep. But I was not asleep. I was truly awake. What in the world was it recording? I may have been in a state of deep relaxation, semi-meditative, I usually am when I lie there, and I may have dropped off, but I was aware of all those thoughts, the feel and look of the room, the long drawn-out boredom of lying there without a book to listen to—it felt like consciousness to me. How could I be aware of all that if I hadn't been awake?

Sleep state misperception. I have heard of it, have known I had a touch of it, from listening to books on tape: I'll hear the first ten minutes of a tape and have the sense I'm still awake when it clicks off at the end, but have no idea how we got to this part of the story, who these characters are, or what they're talking about. But I hadn't paid it much attention, had skipped over those parts in my reading, sure that my insomnia was no misperception. But now, to be told I was asleep for those two hours, when I was aware of all this going on around me and all these thoughts going through my head—this is amazing. Now, suddenly, sleep state misperception seems very interesting, like something I need to go back and read about.

After I settle down again, I find I can turn on my left side without disturbing the hookup. Since it's about 3 A.M., the time I usually go to sleep, I'm able to drift off (into *real* sleep) and into a dream: I am in England, having a sleep study, and the young doctor administering the study tells me in a clipped British accent that he's an insomniac and isn't it awful how little insomnia is understood, and I think, *Aha!* Finally, a doctor who gets it, and I tell him, "This perception is a misperception," and I come out of the dream feeling better: the dream sets things straight, in that weird way dreams do. It reminds me that I do have a doctor who's on my side.

It's about 5:30 when I wake up, but I feel like I've slept and I'll be okay to drive home, which had been a worry. I know I'm not going to get back to sleep again, and I don't (whatever the EEG says). Around 7, Maria comes in and unhooks me from the nest of wires. I fill out the morning-after questionnaire, get dressed, brush my hair and teeth, wash the blue marks off my face, and find my way out.

The questionnaire I filled out asked me, how did I think I'd slept, did I have dreams, and if I did, what were they, and would I recommend this sleep lab—and I answered, truthfully, yes, I would, everyone was friendly, efficient, it was comfortable and pleasant.

But then, when I got outside, I thought—whoa, what'd I say?

Follow-Through

Two weeks later I have an appointment with my doctor to go over the results. When I get to his office, he tells me he's sorry, he hasn't received the report (which was the sole point of our getting together). He calls the clinic and they tell him there's no way they can fax it to him on such short notice (two weeks?). I put it out of my mind and decide I'd better read up on sleep state misperception.

Early in February, I get an e-mail from my doctor: "Have you got the results of your sleep study yet?" No, I haven't. He has received the report, he tells me—it took some telephoning and cajoling—"but I don't find it consistent. They say you have *upper airway resistance syndrome*." UARS is a type of *obstructive apnea* that occurs when the passages of the upper respiratory system (nose, mouth, throat) obstruct the flow of air because they're too small or shaped wrong or have become flabby with age; this leaves you struggling for air (the word *apnea* means "without breath").

My doctor e-mails me the memo he's sent to the clinic, which reads:

> I thought the conclusion of Upper Airway Resistance Syndrome was not supported by the data, which did not show any respiratory events whatsoever. I called and spoke with someone there, who told me the MD who read the study was on leave. She told me she'd have Dr. P. call me to address my concerns, which I explained to her in detail. Though Dr. P. called, he did not connect with me. He did not leave a message that addressed any of my concerns. He called this past Wednesday and said he would try again on Monday, but did not. Do you not have any other physicians on your staff who are able to address physician and patient concerns? Meanwhile, what about the patient, who has now waited 2 MONTHS for her result?

He adds in a note to me, "This whole thing makes me tired, and I sure don't need that."

He and I finally connect at the end of the following week. He shows me the report, which describes sleep that's "very fragmented with multiple awakenings and two awakenings lasting more than an hour." There are nine arousals an hour (normal is none to five). There are nine minutes of deep sleep (normal is 20 to 25 percent) and very little REM (the report doesn't say how many minutes, exactly, and it doesn't say what total sleep time is, but it says I have 5.4 percent REM, when normal is 20 to 25 percent). I took ten minutes to fall asleep, according to the report (normal is ten to twenty), contrary to my certainty that I was awake the whole two hours before I rang the bell to pee. Sleep state misperception is not mentioned in the report; Janine's question, "Have you been asleep?" was off record—officially, nobody was interested in whether I thought I was asleep or awake. There is mention of higher temperature and faster heartbeat. No wonder, what with the nightgown and the warmth of the room, and the fact that I was, or felt I was, awake most of the night. But it's interesting that, even with my "misperception," I have 51 percent *sleep efficiency,* that is, time asleep in proportion to time in bed. A flunking grade—normal is 90 to 95 percent.

Does this make me a "real" insomniac? No. It means I have apnea: "All are symptoms of UARS."

"No way," says my doctor. "Look here: under 'respiratory events'—apneas, one; hypopneas, three; UARS events, none. That doesn't add up to UARS."

(His reading was later corroborated by an eminent sleep researcher I showed the report to, who agreed that it did not show evidence of a breathing disorder and confirmed my sense that "you cannot tell anything from one night, and you especially can't tell anything about *your* sleep, which, from what you tell me, does not normally take place during these hours." I asked him what he thought about giving a patient a sleeping pill, if he thought that interfered with the sleep architecture. "Of course it does," he replied. "But the HMO will only pay for one night; they have to get a sleep recording in one night, they have to get you out by 7 A.M., so they give you a pill." Sure enough, I come across a study that says administering ten milligrams of Ambien results in "a decreased need to restudy," in a "nearly 20% reduction in total studies needing to be performed," which yields "greater efficiency and lower cost for sleep laboratories.")

My doctor stands firm in his position that my report shows no evidence of a breathing disorder. "They turn everything into a breathing disorder," he says, and tells me that the clinic he went to tried to tell him his daytime sleepiness was due to apnea. "Everything is apnea to them. That's how they make their money. That's what they know how to treat."

"Well, if you've got a hammer, everything looks like a nail. But if they thought I had apnea, why didn't they come in with a CPAP machine?

They said they would. But you know, I wouldn't be surprised if I have a breathing problem"—and I told him about the snore I get that signals sleep is near. "I also have allergies—sometimes I wake up all runny and sneezy."

"Yes, but UARS is something that comes on in middle age, and you've had this condition a long time, so I don't think it's going to be the answer. Besides, it says here, 'mild snoring.' UARS is associated with heavy snoring."

"Yeah, Bob says he sometimes hears light snoring. I guess he'd know, after all these years. But I still don't think they saw enough of my sleep to know whether I have a breathing problem or not. I don't think I was actually asleep that whole first part—I never did get that snore."

"I think you should make an appointment with the head of this clinic. See what he says."

So I call and try to make an appointment, and I hit a wall—you want an appointment with *who?* And you say you are *who?* I see I'm not going to get far on my own, so I e-mail my doc to put in a call for me. Sure enough, he has to submit a whole new request, and my HMO has to pay extra to have the report interpreted. So my doctor spends more time on the phone, negotiating, cajoling, putting in another requisition, to get me a consultation. Odd, because when you read the literature the clinics put out, their procedures sound so neat and orderly—on-the-spot interviews with physicians, follow-ups within forty-eight hours, that sort of thing. Maybe this clinic really doesn't have its act together, or maybe my HMO doesn't have its act together, I don't know, but the two together are a marvel of inefficiency. Or maybe they figure if they make it difficult enough, we'll just give up and go away.

Finally I get a call back from the clinic telling me I can make an appointment with the head honcho. I ask for something on a Monday or Friday. I'm told that he sees patients only on Tuesdays. I teach all day Tuesday. I look at my calendar to see when my semester ends. How about May?

So on a day in May, almost a calendar year after my doctor initiated the process that got me my night at the sleep clinic, I head out to the far side of Los Angeles for my long-awaited meeting with the expert who's going to tell me what the report means. He is on the phone when I get there. I sit in the hall for fifteen minutes while he finishes his conversation (which does not seem to be with a patient, from the bits I hear through the open door). When I finally get in to see him, he is super-friendly, public-relations polite, all handshakes and smiles and warm eye contact. Probably after that fuss my doctor made, I spell trouble, and he is determined to head it off. He readily admits that upper airway resistance is not likely to account for the problem—"We can't exclude it 100 percent, but it's unlikely." He tells me that I have psychophysiological insomnia, and I should restrict the number of hours in bed to the number of hours I sleep: "If you estimate you're sleeping five hours, take yourself down to five . . . and get up at the same time every morning."

"Yes, I know, but when I wake up after a few hours' sleep—what about hormones, what about thyroid levels, and cortisol?" ("Faulty causal attribution," the behaviorist voice gnaws at me, "trying to blame it on physiology.") I'd just got back the results of a spit test that indicated slightly elevated levels of cortisol, and I take them out of my purse to show him. He does not reach across the desk for the paper.

"It doesn't jump out at me that we are looking at a physical ailment."

But you haven't looked, I want to say. You've looked at nothing, you've asked me nothing. I say, instead, "So, if it's *psychophysiological* insomnia, what exactly does the *physio* refer to?"

He says, "It's a problem that's become physiological. You need to reset your biological function, rebuild it in a more controlled manner." There it is again, the physio as a *consequence* of conditioning, never as an entity that might play a part on its own. How can they be so sure? How can they be so uninterested in the particulars—in our *hormones,* for example?

Then he adds, "I recognize where you're going with this. You're going to ask me to give you sleeping pills."

"Actually, I was hoping to get off sleeping pills."

"You need to regularize and restrict your sleep day in and day out for several weeks," he said. "You haven't tried."

"Okay, so I'll try," I said. (And I did try, as we saw in the last chapter.) But I wanted to say—I wish I had said—"Neither have you!"

Profits in Snore

It's "a super booming industry." It's "on the sizzling size of hot." "It's a monster market; it's bigger than *Ben-Hur.*" These are the things I read. There are "a large number of patients with significant sleep disorders, and not enough facilities available to them," says a pulmonologist who is part owner of Pacific Sleep Medicine, a small chain of sleep centers that "now boasts eight freestanding sleep centers in southern California." A founder of Pacific Sleep Medicine who chipped in an undisclosed amount in 1998 saw his ante jump a hundredfold. ResMed, which makes CPAPs, face masks, humidifiers, nasal devices, had profits in 2006 about half again as large as they were in 2003. For Respironics, the other major company that makes sleep equipment, the "haul about doubled" during those same years, according to SmartMoney.com, which comments that the "machines have slimmed down somewhat, while profits for their makers have plumped up nicely." There are "profits in snore."

And there are sure to be more profits. By some reckonings, a third of the U.S. population suffers from a sleep disorder, around 70 million people, and yet fewer than 15 percent of these have been diagnosed or treated. A business analyst says that "revenue in the sleep therapeutic market is expected to pass . . . the $2 billion mark by 2012," up from the 2005 figure of $800 million. Another analyst estimates that the untapped market for treating and diagnosing sleep disorders is more than $15 billion annually in the United States.

And all this has come about very recently. Throughout most of the 1970s, there were only three clinics. The first was founded in the mid-1960s by Anthony Kales at UCLA; the second, also in the 1960s, by William Dement at Stanford; and the third, in 1971, by Peter Hauri at Dartmouth. They studied patients as well as treated them, and they weren't moneymakers. By the end of the 1970s, there were thirty clinics. Today, there's a sleep center for every 113,000 people in the United States. "The number of accredited sleep centers increases by over 200 per year," reports the American Academy of Sleep Medicine. There's now a clinic within 150 miles of you, wherever you are in the United States, though only a third or so are accredited by the American Academy of Sleep Medicine. Their rooms are full five nights a week, all year round. Most have waiting lists of one to three months, with longer waits in Canada. Business is so thriving that some clinics rent blocks of hotel rooms at discount, for the overflow. Their focus has shifted almost entirely from research to treatment.

"The number of sleep specialists grows by over 350 a year," according to the American Academy of Sleep Medicine. Sleep has a lot of things going for it as a medical specialty. The hours are good; there's "less burnout" than in other branches of medicine, as I heard at the conferences. The procedures are mainly noninvasive and nonemergency, so patients tend to be in a better mood for them than they are when they're facing, say, cancer surgery. There's not the high risk of liability that's associated with other areas of medicine. Clinics have to protect themselves against someone's slipping in the shower or falling asleep at the wheel on the drive

home, but that's not much, compared to the risks other medical specialties have to cover themselves for.

The sleep business is keenly aware of itself as a business, intent on
"*managing* its growth," on "positioning and promoting itself" so as to
"fulfill its growth potential." (These are the terms I hear.) A "Sleep Center Management Institute," a sort of trade association, helps "develop
business protocols, marketing campaigns, and tools for sleep centers"
and provides "consulting services to physicians to help improve the efficiency and profitability of their sleep laboratories." It publishes a manual, *How to Successfully Market Your Sleep Center or Lab,* that offers
"over 200 pages of marketing techniques" and information about "how
to leverage marketing to reach, inspire and influence patients, referral
sources, insurance carriers, and the business community that will increase your bottom line." It sells for $395. *Sleep Lab Compliance and the
Law,* also priced at $395, has a preface that reads like "a promotional
message for physicians considering new involvement in sleep labs." Physicians are encouraged to make "ground-floor investments."

There are catalogues for products, so many products, I couldn't begin
to tell you what these things are for, all that equipment used on me that
night: the nasal airway measure, the oximeter that measures oxygen saturation from the finger, the parti-colored wires, the box for the wires, the
systems and software programs to score the tests and manage the data,
the devices to measure heart rate and breathing, not to mention the
CPAP machine and all that goes into it—silicone gel cushions used to seal
the masks, hoses, and pillows (not the kind of pillows you rest your head
on, but little rubber things that go into the nose). There's a world of
products out there. They'd work great in those parlor games where you
produce an object and challenge the other players to tell you what it is
and what it does. The manufacturers of these products are often closely
allied with the treatment centers: they are sometimes, even, one and the
same. In 2004, Medcare, a leading manufacturer of diagnostic equipment for sleep clinics, announced that it had acquired SleepTech, a major
manager of hospital-owned sleep centers, making the new entity, SleepTech
Solutions, "the largest company to focus on the needs of the rapidly growing field of sleep diagnostic medicine in North America, which is projected
to more than double in the next several years," according to a press release
by SleepTech.com.

The clinics tend not to be profitable in the first years. "The first couple of years are often a financial struggle for sleep clinics, as they attempt
to make up the money invested in equipment and the technology needed

to run the center. . . . 'You have a sizable up-front investment, and you have to bankroll that,'" says Dr. Lawrence Epstein, a pulmonary care and sleep specialist and regional medical director of Sleep HealthCenters, a privately owned company that runs several centers in the Boston area. Opening a clinic, then, means that you need to see a lot of patients, generate a lot of business, to make good on the initial investment. "This business is very much like a hotel business," says Paul Valentine, hired as head of Sleep HealthCenters in 2002. "Our job is to keep the beds full." Since the initial outlay may be difficult to come up with, this has encouraged the formation of companies like Sleep HealthCenters, cofounded by Israeli entrepreneur David Barone, a design engineer at the Ministry of Defense in Haifa. Sleep HealthCenters describes itself as providing coordinated care, as a kind of "one-stop shop for sleep disorders." Whereas other clinics refer patients elsewhere for treatment, this clinic offers everything: an initial screening interview, a physical exam, follow-up visits with a respiratory therapist. It sounds terrific—except that it lists its specialties as apnea, nocturnal eating disorders, and "sleep disorders associated with psychiatric disease." No mention of insomnia, unless you count insomnia as a "sleep disorder associated with psychiatric disease." The treatments it offers are medication and "lifestyle changes."

Medication and advice about lifestyle are things that we can, with all due respect, get elsewhere, for a lot less money. The clinics boast many successes and the Web is full of glowing testimonials—but they're all about apnea.

All about Apnea

A conversation overheard at a sleep conference:

"I'm looking for a job."

"At a sleep clinic or a sleep apnea clinic?" (There are clinics that call themselves "sleep apnea clinics.")

"Why, you know that every sleep clinic in this country is a sleep apnea clinic."

I whipped around and said, "May I quote you?"

"Sure," he said.

"By name?"

"Sure," said Don Watenpaugh.

One of the biggest surprises I had, researching this book, was that the clinics aren't really there for insomniacs. Michael Bonnet told me, early on, that sleep studies aren't recommended for insomnia, and so they're not covered by insurance. Sleep studies are only recommended if apnea or some other problem, like restless legs syndrome, is suspected. "Not that many insomniacs are seen by the clinics."

Sleep clinics diagnose 93 to 95 percent of the people they see as having sleep-disordered breathing, which is not surprising, considering that this is who usually gets referred to them, and considering that this is what they know how to treat. Most of the people who run the clinics, most of the doctors on the staff, are pulmonary specialists.

Apnea is "where their bread is buttered," as I hear from more than one researcher. A press release from Medicalnewstoday.com boasts, "What helps private companies improve their bottom line is the ability to sell CPAP equipment and other treatment devices." CPAP machines cost $1,500 to $2,200, with a "possible net profit of between $800 and $1,000." According to one survey, "15% of sleep centers sell masks and flow generators directly to patients," and another 15 percent "plan to start selling equipment directly within the next twelve months." "If you don't have apnea when you check in, you'll have it when you check out," said a researcher I talked to. "They'll find it, one way or another." Columnist Mark Hayter observes, "I've never heard of anyone walking away from a sleep clinic without a sleeping disorder." Apnea is replacing attention deficit hyperactivity disorder as "the most popular ailment."

It's good that there are places that diagnose and treat apnea. Apnea is a serious condition, and seriously underdiagnosed. People with apnea may wake up hundreds of times in the course of a night, gasping for breath, and though they don't usually remember waking up, their bodies register the effects of sleep loss: daytime sleepiness, depression, memory impairment, weight gain. Apnea can take years off a person's life, putting him at greater risk for stroke, heart attack, and high blood pressure; treatment with CPAP can save lives. I hear, on the Web and from people I talk to, things like this: "I'm a new woman now. I wake up refreshed and I'm energetic throughout my day." "I had no energy, no motivation, no desire to do anything," said Sean O'Brien, who would fall asleep while stopped at a traffic light. (Scary to think how many truck drivers have apnea, how many of those eighteen-wheelers hurtling down the highways are driven by guys who are half asleep.) After O'Brien got a CPAP, "My wife didn't know I was the same person. I don't snore a peep. My blood pressure has gone down. I'm less irritable."

I know people whose mood and energy have been so improved by these machines that they schlep them everywhere. I met a guy who came to a sleep conference without his CPAP, thinking he could make do for a few days, but he felt so pepless after one night that he broke into the exhibits to borrow one. Of course there are also many people who give up after the first week, saying it's like trying to sleep with a vacuum cleaner fastened to their nose. (CPAP compliance is, by some accounts, "very low." "What nobody's talking about," says the doctor who got me my night at the sleep clinic, "is that most of these clinics don't keep tabs on whether you're actually using the machine—they just let you go with no follow-up, figuring compliance is not their problem.")

So, yes, it's terrific that people with apnea have places to go for help—but what about insomniacs? And what about women? Since the clinics treat mainly apnea, the number of women they treat tends to be small, one in eight or nine, estimates James Rowley of Wayne State University School of Medicine.

"Pulmonary specialists are taking over the field, in a big way," I hear from a psychologist I sat next to at a conference breakfast. "The pulmonary docs wanted to get out of work with the elderly because Medicare reimbursements went down, so they suddenly all became fascinated by sleep."

"Along came sleep to breathe new life into the field—it was kind of nowhere before apnea, now everybody wants in on the act." I hear this from a sleep researcher who takes a dim view of the trend.

"Everybody wants to work on apnea," I hear from Michael Bonnet. "Apnea's simple; it's basically a plumbing problem. Apnea patients are easy to deal with: they get better. Insomnia is hard to treat, hard to identify; insomniacs are perceived as chronic complainers. Why should I spend hours and hours with one insomniac, when I could see and help ten people with apnea?" The sigh he gave was heartfelt, earned by years of working with insomniacs.

"Apnea is where the money is," I hear from Peter Hauri. "It's where you find the quick cures. It's a wow kind of thing—you get CPAP and you're cured. Insomnia is not that kind of fish. It's chronic, difficult to treat. It depends on basic research, figuring out how the sleep system works. It's hard to get grants for this kind of thing."

"Apnea is where the career opportunities are," I hear from Dement. "You could go broke if you saw only insomniacs." "Insomnia has not become a well-established, mainstream activity of sleep disorders medicine," he writes. "The marked success in the diagnosis and treatment of sleep apnea has maintained this clinical activity as the focus of most sleep centers." Though there are many more people with insomnia than with apnea, "the percentage of insomnia patients seen in most centers ranges from less than 10% to rarely over 25%." An effort should be made, Dement urges, to bring insomnia "into the mainstream of sleep disorders medicine."

The sleep field is tilting steeply toward pulmonary. This is where the revenue is, the funding, the career opportunities. "In 1999, the majority of individuals who sought American Board of Sleep Medicine certification and who directed sleep laboratories were chest specialists." This is where the research is: between 1994 and 1999, there were almost *twice as many publications about apnea* as about insomnia, even though there are about *ten times* as many insomniacs as people with apnea, as Gary Richardson and Tom Roth point out. "It would appear," they conclude, "that insomnia would benefit from substantially greater attention from the research community." The National Center on Sleep Disorders Research is lodged, at the NIH, within the National Heart, Lung, and Blood Institute. When it was founded, in the early 1990s, it needed a home, and there weren't a lot of places that wanted to take it in. Heart, Lung, and Blood gave it a home. If the arrangement had been made in heaven rather than in history and serendipity, pulmonary sleep disorders would be contained within the larger and more encompassing rubric of sleep disorders. But instead, sleep is contained within pulmonary, which is emblematic of its subordination.

There are many excellent sleep doctors in pulmonary medicine. Some of the people I talked to who expressed the most passion about sleep, the most compassion for me as an insomniac, were in pulmonary. It's just that most of them are, naturally, more interested in apnea than insomnia. At an interactive session at a recent annual meeting of chest physicians, sixty chest physicians, asked to respond to questions, did better on questions about sleep-disordered breathing: "Performance on questions about nonpulmonary sleep disorders was not good" (and 65 percent of these respondents either directed or were on the staff of a sleep lab). "The end result is that many patients who are referred to a 'sleep specialist' do not receive effective treatment if they have a nonpulmonary sleep disorder," concludes the report on this session.

Insomnia used to be ignored because sleep was ignored. Now it gets ignored because it's not apnea.

The clinics perform a useful screening function, to make sure insomniacs don't have apnea or restless legs syndrome or periodic limb movement disorder (jerky movements or muscle twitches in the legs or feet). However, one researcher I talked to denied that they're necessary even for this, claiming that you don't need the whole elaborate apparatus of a clinic to diagnose apnea: "You just put on an oximeter [the clamp on the finger that measures oxygen content of the blood] and let patients sleep, and if oxygen falls beneath a certain level, they're not getting enough oxygen to their lungs; then you know they have a problem. In Japan they charge a hundred dollars a night. The U.S. centers have huge economic incentives to drum up business. They're tremendously inefficient, useless, really." I don't know, it seems to me that the clinics are useful for screening. But there is a way they're doing insomniacs a disservice, by creating a general impression in the public mind that insomnia is being dealt with, taken care of, under control. I can't tell you how many people have said to me, when I tell them I'm an insomniac, "Oh, you should go to one of those what-do-you-call-ems, sleep clinics," as though the solution to my problem lay that way. I can't tell you how many insomniacs I've heard say, "One of these days, I'll get it together to go to a clinic," as though the solution to *their* problem lay that way.

What Insomniacs Say

Do insomniacs feel they are well served by this industry? From what I hear and read, my experience was not unusual.

First of all, I'm used to going to bed at 12:30 or 1, so I don't think it was at all useful. Then, what the doctor said when he read my test results to me (which were bad, by the way), was go home and try not to worry about it so much. The one thing I did find out is I don't have apnea or leg movements.

They only had me sleep on my back during the whole thing, when in reality I usually . . . sleep most of the night on my side. . . . Could that make my results worse than [my apnea] really is? . . . I had a very high amount of apneas, but this was on my back. I have no idea how many, if any, I have on my side.

I got told I was going to have to live with it. Like, good-bye and good luck.

What I wanted was the research, to learn about my hormone levels. They don't even look at hormones. There was a lot of borderline psychobabble and new age talk: make yourself comfortable, turn the lights off. I got told about sleep hygiene, told to get more exercise.

They gave me a pamphlet on sleep hygiene. You can read about sleep hygiene anywhere.

If you don't have apnea, forget it. They have nothing for you. That didn't stop them from taking my money. I was using my own money, and it cost quite a lot.

My doc said he'd refer me to a clinic if I wanted, but he said nobody he'd ever referred had got much out of them.

Some people describe experiences worse than mine:

It was awful. I went in saying, "I think this has something to do with hormones," and the sleep "expert" totally dismissed that, and his final recommendation was that I see a shrink. . . . I personally think they are a total waste of time and money unless you turn out to have apnea or restless legs syndrome.

They made me feel just horrible, blamed it all on me, said it was my lifestyle as a freelance artist that was making me not sleep.

Daniel Kaufman, one of the authors of *Natural Sleep,* was told, after a night at the Sleep-Wake Disorders Unit at Montefiore Hospital, the Bronx, in 1978, "Your sleep pattern indicates excessive arousal processes during sleep. And that is consistent with your personality. You tend to be somewhat self-critical, somewhat compulsive, easily agitated. You ruminate a lot, and worry too much." Bill Hayes, author of *Sleep Demons,* was told by Stanford doctors twenty-four years later, "You have psychophysiological insomnia. . . . Insomnia is part of your psychological makeup. . . . Disturbed sleep is a sign of unrest—of stress, anxiety, depression. . . . There isn't a cure." Despite the leaps and bounds sleep research has made in the quarter century between these two accounts, the diagnosis for insomnia remains the same: worry, stress, anxiety, depression. The therapy is the same, too: Kaufman and Hayes were both told to regularize their sleep.

The one big change is the fixation, on the part of Hayes's doctors, with apnea. "'A big uvula [the dangling flesh at the back of the throat], a steep, narrow palate, a tongue that's a bit too big for your jaw.' He looked positively ecstatic. 'Do you snore a lot?'" Informed that Hayes does, the doctor says, "You are a prime candidate for obstructive sleep apnea." Now there's the assumption that within every insomniac lurks a troubled breather. Apnea is us.

Are more insomniacs dissatisfied by their experience with sleep clinics than are satisfied? Nobody seems to have made an effort to find out, to ask how *we* feel, whether we find the clinics useful—nobody, that is, except Peter Hauri. Hauri did a nine-month follow-up study of his center in 1982 which was, as he said, "to our knowledge, . . . the only factual evidence currently available concerning the utility of sleep disorders centers." (To my knowledge, it is still the only study of this sort.) He reports that after nine months, "about 30% of the patients with long-term, serious insomnia seemed to benefit markedly from the sleep center evaluation," which was, he says, "not as strong as one might have wished." His general assessment is that "a few get dramatically better, most are helped somewhat, and a percentage are not helped in the slightest." He admits, with characteristic honesty, that a principle of suggestibility may be at work that puts a positive spin on patients' evaluations: patients are more likely to exaggerate their insomnia when seeking help, to convince the interviewer that it's serious; later, having spent money and effort on their problem, they're more likely to report positive effects, either to please the interviewer or make themselves feel better. The desire to please can be a powerful factor in people's reports (as I saw when I filled out the evaluation form at my clinic, checking "yes," I "would recommend this clinic to others"). Harvard sleep researcher Allan Hobson describes how, when he volunteered himself as a subject at his own sleep lab, he became aware of a strong desire "to please the experimenter." If this Harvard professor and head of a neurophysiology laboratory was "so eager to please," imagine how the rest of us feel.

I don't know how many insomniacs feel as I do about their experiences with clinics, but I come across quite a few people who say that they'd hoped to learn more about their problem, but they hadn't got anything by way of advice or medication that they couldn't have got elsewhere, for a lot less money. When I first heard, from Bonnet, that insurance doesn't usually cover a sleep study for insomnia, when I was told by my doctor that my HMO probably wouldn't "go for it," I was outraged that a person with a lifelong sleep problem could not get a referral to a sleep clinic. But now I think my HMO would have been right to stick by its refusal of my request. The only thing I got for the nearly two thousand dollars it forked over was material for this chapter. I don't pretend to understand the economics of health care in our country, but I can't think that this is a way to keep health costs down. If the clinics really are sleep apnea clinics, if apnea is what they do, then they should tell us that and not try to make every case of insomnia into a breathing disorder. If they have nothing to offer insomniacs, they should tell us to go elsewhere with our problem. Where else I don't know, but somewhere.

It's important to say that not all sleep clinics are alike. They differ widely in the ways they're owned, organized, managed. Some are adjuncts to hospitals, some are freestanding and privately owned by doctors or entrepreneurs. I suspect there's huge variability in terms of profits, that some clinics are real cash cows while others barely squeak by. I'm sure there's enormous variability when it comes to what they deliver.

A psychologist I met at a conference, who works in a clinic, tells me it's the "fly-by-nights" (I like that term, for slapdash sleep clinics)—the clinics that are not accredited, that send their scoring out to be done elsewhere, that do "unattended studies" or rely on untrained technicians—that rake in the profits. "It costs money to run a good sleep clinic," she says. But the clinic I went to did have accreditation, meaning that it had met certain requirements specified by the American Academy of Sleep Medicine, the professional organization representing sleep specialists. I'd bet that the difference between clinics has less to do with accreditation and more with the dedication and know-how of the doctors and staff.

Atul Gawande, a surgeon and professor at the Harvard School of Public Health, makes the disconcerting point that differences among doctors, procedures, and treatment centers tend to fall into a bell curve, with some very good and some very bad at either extreme, and the majority in the middle—and this goes for everything in which outcomes have been measured, whether it's hernia operations or heart bypasses. However, most specialties and doctors do not measure outcomes: "Baseball teams have win-loss records. Businesses have quarterly earnings reports. What about doctors?" Cystic fibrosis (CF), a genetic disease in which a mutant protein "thickens secretions throughout the body" and causes the lungs to fill gradually with mucus, has been way ahead, in terms of measuring outcomes and keeping track of the results of the 117 cystic fibrosis centers across the country, thanks to the efforts of the Cystic Fibrosis Foundation. All these centers, reports Gawande, are "ultra-specialized, undergo a rigorous certification process, and have lots of experience in caring for people with CF. They follow the same detailed guidelines for CF treatment. . . . You would think therefore that their results would be much the same. Yet the difference is enormous" between an average life expectancy of thirty-three years across the board and forty-seven at the best center, where "the oldest patient is now 64" and "not a single child or teenager . . . has died in years." The center that's achieved these outcomes is the creation of Dr. Warren Warwick. "The secret . . . is simple," he told Gawande: "you do whatever you can to keep your patients' lungs as open as possible." Gawande describes the "focus, aggressiveness, and inventiveness," the "intense drive and constant experimenting" that makes this doctor extraordinary. "He thinks hard about his patients, he pushes them, and he does not hesitate to improvise."

It would be more difficult to track the outcomes of sleep clinics than to track survival records of people with CF, but it would be interesting to try, and I'll bet if you did, you'd find that same bell curve, "a handful of teams with disturbingly poor outcomes for their patients, a handful with remarkably good results, and a great undistinguished middle." I bet you'd find that the difference is made by the vision and dedication of the doctors and staff, their willingness to "do whatever they can."

I hear from some insomniacs who've been helped by clinics.

> My doc really went the extra mile—once we'd ruled out apnea, he spent time talking with me about my lifestyle and what I could do that would be better for my sleep; and when that didn't help, he worked with me on medications until we found something that helped. I now take one hundred milligrams of trazodone and an occasional Ambien. I still wake up at night, but I can usually get back to sleep.

Bill Hayes came away satisfied with his experience: "I can't say for certain that the *amount* I slept changed, yet my view of sleep gradually did. I came to feel, more often than not, that I was in control of sleep rather than controlled by sleeplessness." I read interviews with heads of clinics who sound like they "go the extra mile." Dr. Vipin Garg, head of a sleep disorders clinic in Elizabeth, New Jersey, told Sleepreviewmag.com, "Anybody can make money doing sleep studies, but we have a mission—better health because of our treatments." His group is committed to serving a community that's 70 percent Latino or African American, many of whom do not have insurance. He does rigorous follow-ups to assure CPAP compliance. "We hear from patients that quality testing varies greatly from place to place," he says, adding that he'd like to see stricter controls. "What are the standards? As far as I know, there are none. If [patients] go to a bad center, they will lose trust in sleep medicine."

Here's a thought: why not base standards on the outcomes of treatment?

Subjective and "Objective" Insomniacs

The American Academy of Sleep Medicine explains in a 2003 report why it does not recommend routine use of sleep studies for insomniacs. For one thing, you can't tell much on the basis of only one night: "Patients with psychophysiological insomnia often, paradoxically, sleep well on their first night in the laboratory." (Not this one: if I slept as badly as I did that night in the clinic, I'd be dead.)

But the crux of the matter is that the EEG, the gold standard for measuring whether a person is asleep or awake and for gauging what stage of sleep that person is in, fails to corroborate what insomniacs report. It tells us that we're asleep when we think we're awake, and that what feels like a bad night may actually be a good night in terms of length and quality of sleep. "Some patients with insomnia have sleep state misperception," says the report. Quite a few have it, actually—well over half: in a group of 121 subjects reporting chronic insomnia, the EEG picked up sleep disturbance "less than 22% of the time," report Roger Rosa and Michael Bonnet, who found that this group "was no more or less likely" to have a poor night, according to the EEG, than a group who had no sleep complaints.

But with some insomniacs, the EEG does register sleep disturbances. What to make of this difference? Researchers use the term *objective insomnia* for insomnia that's confirmed by polysomnogram and *subjective insomnia* for sleep state misperception. *Pseudoinsomnia* is another term sometimes used—"we called them pseudo insomniacs and said they complained a lot," Hauri told me. The usual explanation is that insomniacs who complain about their sleep in the absence of objective evidence are more neurotic than the others. Quality of sleep, explain Jack Edinger and his colleagues, is "in the eye of the beholder." Since mood, anxiety, attitudes, and beliefs affect the way we perceive our sleep, it follows that if you're depressed, anxious, negative, you'll have complaints about your sleep, and if you're not, you won't. The noncomplainers are congratulated for having a better attitude.

Also congratulated for their attitudes are the people who think they sleep well but whose EEGs register sleep disturbances—for it turns out that "normal" sleepers often "misperceive," too, thinking that they've had a good night's sleep when the EEG says they have not. A. Alvarez, author of *Night*, describes a night he spent in a sleep clinic when he thought he'd "slept like a baby," though the EEG reported he'd slept five hours and forty-nine minutes, with twenty-three awakenings: "The scientifically

recorded reality of my night's sleep bore no relationship at all to my subjective experience of it. . . . I felt I'd slept well, the machines said I hadn't;
one of us had to be wrong." Puzzled by this discrepancy, Alvarez insists,
"Yet I wasn't imagining how I felt. A good night's sleep is restorative."
Puzzling, indeed: sleepers' perceptions and the EEG are often miles apart.

Sleep doctors used to show insomniacs their EEGs, assure them that
their sleep was normal, and assume that there would be an end to the
problem—sleep doctors as illustrious as Dement, I'm afraid: "I sat down
with her and went over the EEG recordings. . . . In my most comforting
and reassuring, yet authoritative manner, I said, . . . 'your tests show absolutely perfect, normal sleep.' . . . The patient flew back East and had
no further problems with insomnia." (I can imagine this woman, in the
presence of an eminence like Dement, nodding, smiling, saying thank
you, my mistake, and returning home—to her insomnia.) "It's very calming, very soothing, for insomniacs to know they may actually be asleep,"
said a speaker at a sleep conference. It may be soothing to some insomniacs, but it's not to others. One woman wrote me, *It made my blood
boil to be told i was getting sleep when i knew i wasn't.* Another insomniac told me: *I know the difference between being asleep and awake.
I had a horrible night, I have so many horrible nights I can't hold a job or
even follow a conversation anymore.* And another: *He told me there was
no problem. It's always got to be your error, like it couldn't possibly be
theirs. See, it says here you were asleep—what's wrong with you, that
you think you were not?*

But when researchers look more closely at the "pseudo insomniacs,"
they find that they are actually quite similar to the "real" ones. "They feel
groggy, they do poorly on some performance tests requiring attention,
and they have elevated metabolism, just like 'regular' insomniacs," Hauri
reports. Other investigators find that subjective insomniacs show "impairment in waking function" that is *worse* than "regular" insomniacs',
suggesting that though they're "occasionally dismissed as neurotic complainers," they ought not to be. Hauri also finds that the "misperceivers"
have more motor activity, more restlessness during sleep, more wakefulness than those insomniacs whose EEG registers sleep disturbance.

Something I'd like to know, which I don't see addressed, is what our
hormones are up to while we're "misperceiving": are they acting as
though we're asleep or awake? I'd bet also that there are lots of insomniacs like me who do not fall neatly into one category or the other, but
whose sleep is a messy mixture of both subjective and objective insomnia, who have some "misperception" but also have overall lousy sleep.

But the discrepancy between the subjective account and the "objective" measurement has been used to dismiss us: see, you're making mountains of molehills—you're "not a real one." "The physician should always be on guard when listening to reports of insomniacs, because they're usually exaggerated," advises a 1950s textbook. "Hence one viewpoint is that such individuals do not actually require medical help," writes a researcher in 2005. It doesn't help that we "misperceivers" are so often female: women complain more than men about their sleep, yet the EEG shows that they sleep better than men at every stage of life. This lends support to the stereotype of the hysterical female, prone to hypochondria and to exaggerating every little thing—women! what can you expect? A more nuanced view might consider recent findings that there's enormous variability in the way people respond to sleep loss, and that women take it harder than men do—we may be *experiencing* our sleep disturbances more acutely. But this takes us into the sticky wicket of the subjective, an area researchers would rather avoid. As Harvard sleep researcher Allan Hobson says, "Subjective experience is so problematical that all but the bravest scientists have been discouraged."

If it's attitude that makes the difference between those who experience their sleep disturbances and those who do not, then Alvarez is to be congratulated for his attitude. So are all those people with apnea who snort and splutter themselves awake, sometimes as often as twice a minute, but who have no memory of their awakenings. (Seventy percent of people with apnea are not conscious of waking up—the other 30 percent are insomniacs.) So, too, are the many people with restless legs syndrome who don't notice they have it—they also have a good attitude. However, I and all those insomniacs whose EEGs say we sleep more than we say we do, and those 30 percent of apnea patients who are conscious of their awakenings—we do not.

Maybe something more complicated is going on.

The EEG and Its Discontents

Let's look more closely at the EEG and what it does. The EEG measures the sleeper's progress from nonREM sleep stages 1 through 4 (deep sleep), through REM sleep, and back through nonREM. When we're alert and attentive to the environment, when we're thinking, the brain makes fast, random waves called *beta* waves. As we relax and move into *alpha,* the waves become slower, more regular, and more synchronized;

these look, on the EEG, like the teeth of a comb. As the cycles become slower still, we enter *theta:* it's here that the sensory gate to the outside drops down and we move into sleep stage 1, then 2. Stages 3 and 4, also called *slow wave sleep* (sometimes called *delta* for the delta waves that appear, waves that are slower and larger and more regular than theta waves, like "great ocean swells," as Dement says)—this is where deep sleep occurs, where breathing and heart rate become slow and regular and muscle relaxation becomes complete. Then, when we enter REM, choppy theta waves appear again, along with short bursts of alpha and beta like those that characterize wakefulness. In REM, the heart beats faster and blood pressure goes up, yet paradoxically, despite all this commotion, the body is in a state of near total paralysis (which is why Michel Jouvet termed REM *paradoxical sleep,* describing it as a "third state . . . as different from sleep as sleep is from wakefulness").

Normally, then, the sleeper begins in beta, awake, proceeds through alpha, a state of calm wakefulness, and then moves on to theta. At the moment that alpha yields to theta, the sensory curtain drops, the mind is cut off from the outside world, and reactivity is diminished. At this point, memory recall systems go off line. If you show normal sleepers pictures or tell them words just before they go to sleep, they won't remember them. Nor do they generally recall waking during the night, though everyone does wake up periodically. For most people, sleep is profoundly amnesic; there is something about sleep that "prevents memories from being stored in the normal way," writes Jacob Empson. This is why, unless we make special efforts to fix a dream in our consciousness, by writing it down or telling it to someone, it vanishes without a trace. And this is why most people with apnea and many with RLS do not remember their numerous awakenings.

But insomniacs do remember. Not only do we have better recall of information presented to us at sleep onset, we have, when awakened from nonREM, more thoughts, more dreamlike fragments and dreams, and more recollection of mental activity than normal sleepers. When awakened from REM, we are more likely to tell you that we've been awake, and are "more likely to identify REM sleep as 'light' sleep.'" Awareness of ongoing mental processes, of the continuous stream of mental activity that researchers say never ceases but is not remembered by most people, seems not to be diminished in us.

In 1982, Irwin Feinberg and T.C. Floyd suggested that "incomplete shutdown of memory control systems" might account for both idiopathic insomnia and sleep state misperception. They hypothesized that there might be a failure of "those control mechanisms which suppress memory consolidation," and which screen out awareness of the mentation that's now known to continue through all stages of sleep. They speculated that it might be the amnesic powers of benzodiazepines that explain why insomniacs think that they improve their sleep, when, according to the EEG, they don't increase sleep time by all that much: they simply wipe out *memory* of sleep disturbances.

Perhaps, then, insomnia is a *remembering* of things other people forget. A remembering of things better left forgotten.

Researchers have recently used *spectral power analysis,* a finer-grained, computer-aided type of analysis, to look at the microstructure of insomniacs' sleep, and have found that more beta persists in our sleep—that is, more high-frequency activity and less slow-wave activity—and the more beta there is, the worse the sleeper perceives the sleep to have been. Since beta is associated with attention, perception, and information processing, the persistence of beta indicates a level of brain activity closer to wakefulness. This suggests that some part of the insomniac's brain remains abnormally activated during sleep. Brain scans confirm this: Nofzinger's neuroimaging of sleeping insomniacs shows, as we saw, that "some regions of the brain aren't deactivating to the same extent. Insomniacs' brains do seem to be metabolically overactive, as they tell us subjectively. This might explain sleep state misperception." As Nofzinger suggests, "Maybe they aren't crazy." It's important to remember that his subjects *had normal EEGs.*

Insomniacs, then, are not *misperceiving.* They have the feeling of being awake because some part of their brain is actually awake.

What is certain is that there is often a "weak fit," as sleep researcher Deborah Sewitch says, between subjective report and "conventional polygraphic definitions of sleep and waking," a discrepancy that's "a feature of sleep-wake perception in general." The EEG, says Hauri, "doesn't tell the whole story." "It's hubris," remarks a speaker at one of the conferences, "to imagine that a few electrodes attached to a person's head is going tell you what's going on inside." When you think of the fantastically complex processes that take place during sleep, the billions of neurons signaling back and forth, the elaborate dance of neurotransmitters, it's no wonder that the EEG doesn't tell us more. It's like trying to figure out what goes on under the hood of a car from the heat the engine gives off.

There's a kind of closed, circular logic in the way the issue has been approached: sleep is what is measured by the EEG; the EEG says you're asleep; therefore you must be asleep, since sleep is what is measured by the EEG. It's like what my sleep technician told me as she fastened the electrodes on my skull: "The electrodes belong here because here is where I made the marks." When there's a discrepancy between what the EEG says and what you feel, that's *your* problem—you have "a sleep/wake discrimination difficulty," you need to be taught to improve the accuracy of your perceptions. Sleeping pills, according to this view, help "improve insomniacs' accuracy in discriminating the subjective experience of sleep from wakefulness"—which is a rationale for giving them in sleep studies. Drugged sleep, by this logic, is more "real" than undrugged sleep.

Researchers are now acknowledging that *they* may be the ones who've been misperceiving, that "the misperception," as Daniel Buysse says, "may be more in our tools than in our patients." This understanding received official recognition in 2004, when the term *sleep state misperception* was changed to *paradoxical insomnia*—"so as not to imply that it's the patient's fault," as Buysse says. This is a big step. It allows for a *paradox,* the coexistence of two truths that cannot logically coexist, but do anyway, and have equal weight; it allows that subjective perceptions and objective measurements may both be valid even when they contradict one another. However, the term was changed only in the *International Classification of Sleep Disorders*, the system used by sleep specialists, and not in the more widely used DSM-IV. Still, this is progress. It suggests that something may be learned by hearing insomniacs out, rather than ruling us out.

"Do I Wake or Sleep?"

"There is for me a state which may be technically sleep to you," says a subjective insomniac quoted by Sewitch, "but is wakefulness to me and uhhh—it's an intermediate state—it's very hard to define, uhh—but I definitely felt that it's there."

Sleep turns out to be, again, more complex than our categories for it, larger than our conceptualizations of it or our means of measuring it. If sleep is more than what is measured, what is that "more" that is not being measured? So great are the mysteries of sleep that scientists have resorted to paradox, the language of logical impossibility, the language of poetry, to allow for this coexistence of contradictions. Paradox has long been a part of the language of those who study sleep. Michel Jouvet described REM sleep as paradoxical sleep to suggest the intermingling of sleep and wakefulness that occurs with dreams, where the brain is as active as it is during consciousness though the body is immobilized. Now we have "paradoxical insomnia."

Nor are these the only in-between states where sleep and wakefulness curiously intermingle. In cataplexy, the sleep attacks that afflict some narcoleptics, the muscles go limp and the person is plunged, while still conscious, into the sleep paralysis and dream state of REM, sometimes experiencing images and fantasies so lifelike that he or she can barely distinguish them from reality. Sleepwalking and sleep-talking, the so-called *parasomnias* (Latin for "near sleep"), also show dramatic comminglings. Sleepwalkers, as Dement says, "wake up enough to get the most primitive parts of the brain working—the emotional brain and the basic motor centers—without engaging the brain's more reflective and self-aware functions"; the sleepwalker may recognize a door but not know how to get it open.

But normal sleepers experience confusions, too. Hobson describes how, when he volunteered himself as a subject in the sleep lab, "I was so eager to please the experimenter it was hard to say, when feeling confused upon being awakened, 'I really don't have any idea what was going on.'" Most people have experienced states that are, in Shakespeare's words, "tween sleep and wake" (Shakespeare's word *wake* is so much more vivid than our word *wakefulness,* but modern grammar forbids us to use this word as a noun; lucky Shakespeare, to have written before the rules). We mostly experience these kinds of in-between states as we're drifting off to sleep or coming awake. As with *hypnagogia,* for example, those wild, wacky images that dance on the insides of the eyelids when sleep is near: a human face sprouts the trunk of an elephant, then you're flying through a canyon, skimming the river's surface, then a valley opens up, and a woman, arms held out in supplication, is led captive through the smoking ruins of a city. This "kaleidoscopic sequence of rapidly morphing images, merging and dissolving" (as Rubin Naiman describes it in *Healing Night*), "unsettles our waking hold on the world." I get such images only when I'm totally exhausted and have had a day filled with new experiences, as when I'm traveling or at a conference. Bob gets them all the time. His are filled with geometrical shapes, mine are filled with faces, faces of people I've never seen, laughing, crying, raging. I love these images; they're intensely interesting and strangely affectless, even when the faces are crying or raging; they lack the emotional charge of dreams. They're the harbingers of sleep.

Waking up also sometimes puts people in a weird in-between state: you come suddenly out of a deep sleep and have the feeling of disorientation where sleep refuses to let go; this is called *sleep inertia*. I don't get this, but I do sometimes get caught in a dream that won't let go, and it takes me a while to figure out that the earthquake that's shaking the bed is really my dog on the bed, scratching a flea.

"Do I wake or sleep?" asks Keats, rousing himself from reverie in his famous *Ode to a Nightingale*. It may be that the poets are more fascinated by these weird in-between states than the scientists, and you'll find more descriptions of them in creative than in scientific literature. The more you lie in bed, the more aware of them you become. Proust, who spent a great deal of time in bed the fifteen years he wrote *Remembrance of Things Past,* was intensely aware of them. "I had been thinking all the time, while I was asleep, of what I had just been reading," he writes, as though this is a perfectly ordinary occurrence. You might also find reference to them in writings of mystics, since meditation is a sort of hovering-between state. Transcendental meditation, when I used to do it, put me into a state of total relaxation, heart and breathing slowed down as in sleep, yet I was fully aware of everything going on around me, conscious, except that my mind was—as it is not otherwise—perfectly still.

Such states tell us that the line between sleep and wakefulness is not a clear demarcation, as between noon and midnight, but that it's more like the shades of gray at dusk and dawn, though the gradations are less predictable than those between twilight and darkness or sunrise and full morning, since there may be this toggling back and forth, this interlacing of each with the other. There are, of course, those sleepers who go "out like a light" and come to just as easily, no hovering in between. That flip-flop switch described in chapter 5, that switch that flips decisively from one position to the other, may be the ideal, optimal way the system works (I bet the scientists who described it are good sleepers who don't spend a lot of time lolling around in bed), and the toggling between may be the experience of those of us whose systems are in not such great shape. But there are so many of us for whom that binary mode of sleep and wakefulness doesn't tell the whole truth that it makes me wonder, again, about the norm, and wonder about people in non-Western cultures, where boundaries between sleep and wakefulness are more fluid—what might they have to say? Or what might our ancestors say, since that stretch between first and second sleep that Thomas Wehr's subjects entered into, that seems to have been commonplace to the millions who lived before electricity dispelled the long darkness of night, is another of those hovering-between stages, with an endocrinal state all its own.

You might say that sleep itself, any sleep, all sleep, is a kind of paradox, in that it is, in the words of a seventeenth-century poet, "living without life and dying without death." The biggest paradox of all is how a state so life-denying, so like death that it was represented mythologically as the twin brother to death, can be so essential to feeling alive and to being alive.

I Have a Dream

I naively imagined, before I started this book, that the clinics were doing research, that they were places where researchers were studying sleep disorders and collecting data, as the older clinics were. I thought someone was keeping track. But no.

When I asked Dement if he thought clinics ought to be collecting information, he said, "I always thought we should." He went on to say, "You're getting me frustrated—we used to do that at Stanford. We started a lot of good things, but we couldn't keep them going. We had a lot of good ideas for studies, we even had some going—but somebody has to enter the results, somebody has to pay that salary, and we didn't have enough funding after a while." He describes how, in 1975, an NIH grant was not renewed: "The Stanford Sleep Center was in its glory years of sleep research, having just made major discoveries in sleep disorders and basic sleep research. . . . I was stunned, and deeply pained that I had to lay off all but a few of my twenty employees."

The clinics are in an ideal position to be gathering data, since many insomniacs pass through their hands. They could collect information about diet, habits, family histories, hormonal profiles, people's hunches about where their insomnia comes from—just collect the information and stash it away. If they don't have the resources to do a study, keep it on file, or send it to a central database for someone else to look at later. Who knows what patterns might emerge? Maybe insomniacs who come from families of insomniacs also have no stage 4 sleep, or maybe insomniacs with sleep state misperception have peculiar patterns of hormonal secretion. And follow us up: see which treatments work with what kind of insomnia. And which do not.

I imagined the clinics were engaged in research because I wasn't aware of the widening division between research and clinical treatment that Jouvet describes: "The evolution of sleep research in the last decade has been marked by a relative decrease in interest in fundamental problems and more emphasis on clinical applications. The domain of sleep research has been invaded by 'sleep medicine.'" Jouvet applauds sleep medicine for taking "giant steps forward," especially with apnea, but regrets that "basic researchers, looking for the mechanisms and functions of sleeping and dreaming, are less numerous." I get a sense, talking to researchers, that they feel outnumbered by "the techies" and impoverished by comparison; I sense that basic research is being starved of funding, while the clinics are "fat cats." Some suggest that the clinics have raked in the benefits of the research and are giving nothing back in return, are failing to reseed the ground from which they grew. "There are far more technicians than scientists, these days," says one researcher. "They've sort of taken over the field. They're prosperous, while we're barely able to carry on our work."

On the basis of the way my sleep clinic failed to work for me, I've thought about the way a clinic might work for us, as a place where we—insomniacs and researchers—might actually learn something about our sleep. It would study our sleep for the hours we actually sleep, and for more than one night—since insomniacs' sleep is so erratic, you'd need several nights in a lab to identify anything with confidence. It would use spectral analysis and neuroimaging as a matter of course. It would take a full history. The questionnaire at my clinic asked nothing about family. It asked about my general health, nasal congestion, snoring, morning headaches, medications; it asked whether I'm afraid of the dark, whether I experience pain or discomfort, whether I wake up screaming or grind my teeth or wake up with a headache or a dry mouth, whether I take naps, and how much caffeine and alcohol I consume (that was all it asked about anything I ingest). It asked whether I have racing thoughts, and do I feel sad or depressed or anxious (which I never know how to answer: doesn't everybody? how often? compared to whom?). It also asked, "Why do you think you have the problem?" which I was glad to see, but it gave me only three lines to answer. And that questionnaire was the sum total of what this clinic knew about me—and it was never referred to. In my ideal clinic, trained professionals would talk to patients, hear what we have to say, keep an open mind about what we know, question us as though we might actually have some understanding of what goes on in our bodies.

I'd like a place where somebody would hear me when I say, I think this has to do with hormones. I'd like to know about my cortisol and thyroid levels (thyroid is complicated: too much can make sleep worse, too little can make it worse, and levels can also be affected by sleep deprivation—more on this in the next chapter). And somebody, somewhere, please tell me why I slept so beautifully when I was pregnant, or at least pick up on the fact that I had this powerful response to pregnancy hormones and consider that this might be a clue to something about my problem and possibly a clue to what might help.

And, while I'm making my wish list—why not have clinics that specialize in insomnia? If there are sleep apnea clinics, why not insomnia clinics?

Above all, somebody, register me as a person with my own physical and psychological peculiarities and work out a plan of action tailored to those peculiarities, rather than giving me the same old one-size-fits-all bromides. Get on the case and stay on it, follow up every hint and hunch, do whatever is necessary—like Dr. Warren Warwick, who's had such success with cystic fibrosis.

Dream on. What we have instead is the nightmare of managed care, which is all about haste and mass production and cutting costs. Okay, so why doesn't somebody step outside the system of reimbursements and build a clinic that at least rich people can afford? Better that somebody be helped than nobody. As the market analysts know, as the pharmaceutical companies know, as entrepreneurs and investors know, people will pay for sleep, and pay dearly. "People with problems sleeping are easy targets," to quote the head of a sleep lab. "They've tried everything. They're really a desperate group."

I at times would have sold my soul.

CHAPTER 10

Alternatives

Dr. Andrew Weil advises, "Successful patients search out possibilities for treatments and cures and follow up every lead they come across. They ask questions, read books and articles, go to libraries, write to authors, ask friends and neighbors for ideas, and travel to meet with practitioners who seem promising. Such behavior leads some doctors to label these patients difficult, noncompliant, or simply obnoxious, but there is reason to think that difficult patients are more likely to get better while nice ones finish last." Excellent advice: read everything, talk to everyone, follow every lead. More than one insomniac I've talked to has come to this same conclusion: *You just have to pay attention and try everything and maybe there's something out there that will work for you. I say, read the books and get on the bulletin boards and ask people their experience.*

But this is one of those places I get cross. Once upon a time I had the energy, resources, and spirit to track down anything anybody ever told me worked. I'd try it all. But lately, I'm not so eager to chase after yet another time-consuming, costly therapy. I got tired. There is so little known about alternative approaches to insomnia that we are, once we venture off the well-worn path of drugs and behavioral modification, left wandering without a map. As useful as anecdote is, I'd like more help when it comes to what I put in my body, where I put my time and energy. I'd like more research.

Alternative medicine, sometimes called *holistic* or *complementary medicine,* embraces a wide range of methods, from ancient techniques such as acupuncture and herbal remedies to new-age metaphysical-spiritual approaches. These approaches differ widely in assumptions and technique, though all have in common an emphasis on the body's natural powers of healing. They are holistic in that they consider the whole person—mind, body, lifestyle, spirit—and look at the body as a whole, not organ by organ or system by system. They aim to reestablish balance among the body's systems, thereby allowing our innate healing capacities to work.

Unlike mainstream medicine, which sees illness as an invasion from without and makes war on the invaders, alternative approaches try to increase the body's resistance to harmful influences, to prevent illness by keeping the body fit. Conventional medicine is "all about fixing," as a doctor friend says. "When you break a bone, when your appendix bursts, you want conventional medicine, not herbs. But chronic conditions—arthritis, headaches, allergies, fatigue, insomnia—are, by definition, conditions that can't be fixed, and for these, we in mainstream medicine have nothing." It is for these kinds of problems that people seek out alternative approaches—and we do not usually inform our doctors, knowing how dismissive they're likely to be. ("Snake oil, quackery, charlatans, witch doctors," I hear my father snort.) Critics object that there's no proof that any of these approaches work; defenders point out that absence of proof is not proof of absence, when there has been so little research.

About half of all Americans turn to some form of alternative medicine, and the rate is this high in other developed countries. People pay out of pocket, since these methods are not usually reimbursed by insurance, and they pay handsomely—more than $27 billion annually in America. The number of people turning to alternatives grew steadily throughout the 1980s and 1990s, as mainstream medicine plummeted in prestige. Consumer satisfaction "tends to be very high," says Dylan Evans in *Placebo*. Alternative practitioners spend on average forty minutes with each patient, as compared to the seven or so minutes we get from most mainstream doctors, and they take more complete histories. They listen and make efforts to establish a relationship with the patient. Unlike mainstream practitioners, who tend to view the informed patient as a bother rather than an ally, they welcome patients as active collaborators—and it's well documented that the more actively involved people are in their care, the more likely they are to improve. Alternative practitioners enlist touch as a source of both information and comfort—they probe, feel, tap, prod, pummel parts of the body—whereas mainstream order a battery of tests and read what the numbers say. "Modern care . . . lacks the human touch," as Atul Gawande says.

Considering how many millions of people turn to alternative methods, the lack of interest the scientific community accords them is extraordinary. In all the sleep conferences I attend, I come across maybe three papers on the herbals and supplements people commonly take for sleep. University of Toronto researcher Leonid Kayumov was a lone voice at these conferences. An affable young man with a thick Russian accent, Kayumov showed up at several conferences with posters on yoga, aromatherapy, and most intriguingly, "brain music," studies that were subsequently published in reputable journals but were not presented at any of the sessions. "There's no money for this kind of research," he told me. "It's a terrible drain on our lab." There is no funding because there are no big profits: nobody can own the exclusive right to naturally occurring substances such as herbs, foods, and vitamins. As pioneer sleep researcher Eliot Weitzman said, "There have not been really good studies [on nutrition and sleep], because in order to do them, somebody has to pay for them. Drug companies won't, because they can't make any money on it. The companies that are making things like tryptophan are little companies. They're not about to do research." No patents, no profits, no research.

But some alternative approaches have been around for millennia, and it seems presumptuous to dismiss them without knowing more. In 1992, a center for research on alternative medicine was established at the NIH, committed to doing studies according to rigorous standards of control—that is, they were double-blind with placebos (*double-blind* means that neither the subjects nor the experimenters know which group is getting a placebo, so predispositions won't influence the outcome). Initially called the Office of Alternative Medicine, with an annual budget of $2 million, it was later designated the National Center for Complementary and Alternative Medicine. In 2005, it had an annual budget of $123.1 million, which is many times more than it started out with but still not a lot, when you think what it costs to do a study, and that this is the sum total for all alternative approaches to everything that can go wrong with the body. But it's a major step in terms of getting some validation for these approaches, and a step toward sorting out anecdote from evidence. Until you subject testimonials to controlled studies, you can't tell what's the effect of a treatment and what's coincidence.

On the basis of anecdote and such research as I can find, and on the basis of my own experience with an alternative doctor (an MD), I'd say that there may be some help for some insomniacs in some of these approaches. In this chapter I'll look briefly at the methods I've tried and heard and read about, and suggest areas for further exploration.

What We Eat

Most doctors give you a blank look if you mention diet, nutrition, vitamins, food allergies, whereas alternative practitioners, who aim to keep the body resistant against harmful influences, see these as matters of vital concern. It seems strange that mainstream medicine would turn over an area so basic as what we eat to practitioners it has little respect for, but this seems to be the case.

Yet "there is solid research evidence that your sleep may be affected by what you eat," writes Peter Hauri, whose *No More Sleepless Nights* is one of the few self-help books that has a chapter on foods. The diet best for sleep is the diet best for your health in general, he says: whole grains, lots of fruits and vegetables, and variety, with most of your calories consumed early in the day. I once saw such a diet work wonders. Bob's mother, in her late eighties, was living on TV dinners and junk food; she was a bag of bones, tired, jittery bones, until a woman came in and started cooking nourishing meals for her; within a few months, she'd put on weight, her color and mood were improved, and she was sleeping better, in spite of her Parkinson's.

But beyond this generally good advice, not a lot is known. It's easier to know what *not* to eat. For me, anything too rich or spicy or in too large a quantity consumed too close to bedtime leaves me lying awake, tracing its progress through my gut. Digestion is an active, intense, heat-generating process, not something you want to initiate close to sleep. It takes energy to break down the complex molecules of animal and vegetable that we ingest into the simpler molecules that feed our cells; it takes energy to shuttle the nutrients into the bloodstream, to the target cells. And like anything that generates energy, digestion generates heat. I shed sweaters when I eat, I fling open windows, the connection is that direct— and anything that raises temperature can wreck sleep. Of course there are also those people who conk out after a big meal; I think they're a different species from me.

Some experts say carbohydrates are best for sleep and some say proteins are best. The argument seems to hinge on tryptophan, an amino acid crucial to sleep. Tryptophan is not made by the body. It comes from high-protein foods, poultry, meats, fish, eggs, milk, nuts, pumpkin seeds, beans, soybeans, leafy green vegetables; the tryptophan in turkey is what makes people fall asleep after Thanksgiving dinner. It converts to 5-HTP (5-hydroxy-tryptophan), which converts to serotonin; melatonin is made from serotonin. Tryptophan is easily depleted by caffeine, alcohol, by the artificial sweetener aspartame, by lack of sunlight or exercise, and by stress. It has a hard time reaching the brain, since amino acids are large molecules that compete with other amino acids to get through the blood-brain barrier. Alternative practitioner Julia Ross, author of *The Mood Cure* and *The Diet Cure,* says you need to eat a lot of tryptophan-containing foods to get enough of it. Ross, who heads a clinic for nutritional therapy in Mill Valley, California, recommends a minimum of four ounces of protein food per meal, a chicken breast–size portion three times a day. But others claim that carbohydrates are what's essential, since these are converted to simpler glucose molecules that get to the brain more easily and escort the tryptophan molecule through.

It could be that carbohydrates work best for some people and protein works best for others. I've heard people say they started sleeping beautifully when they went on the Atkins diet, and I've heard people say that they stopped sleeping entirely when they went on this diet. We're as variable in our responses to foods as we are to drugs: one person's soporific is another's stimulant. Opinion leans more toward protein these days than it did in the 1980s and early 1990s, when everyone was pushing pasta as the complete meal (I never believed it). Now only the most complex carbohydrates are recommended, those found in whole grains, beans, and brown rice. The advice given to insomniacs in *Alternative Medicine: The Definitive Guide* states today's received wisdom: "Eat more protein in the form of moderate amounts of meat, nuts, beans, and avocados. Protein is digested more slowly and doesn't cause an insulin spike, which may interfere with sleep."

Simpler forms of carbohydrates are more rapidly converted to glucose and cause insulin to spike: the pancreas releases insulin, and after it has done its work breaking down glucose, there's a dip in blood sugar which may wake a person up. Complex carbohydrates take longer to break down and don't cause that insulin rush and dip. Insomniacs are advised to stay away from sugar, but here again, sensitivities range widely: some people's sleep is wrecked by sugar, other people are hardly fazed by it. Are these differences a matter of age—do our bodies deal less well with simple carbohydrates and the sugars they're converted to, as we grow older and become more insulin resistant? Or do our differences have to do with whether we have *hypoglycemia* (low blood sugar), a condition alternative practitioners associate with insomnia?

Hypoglycemia is one of those syndromes that alternative practitioners find everywhere and most mainstream doctors dismiss entirely. "Low blood sugar, or hypoglycemic distress, is by far the most common problem that we see at our clinic," says Julia Ross of her Mill Valley clinic. The alternative doctor I saw told me I am hypoglycemic, and I do seem to have a problem, whether you call it hypoglycemia or something else. I don't have the carrying capacity other people have; I get famished, faint, if I go without frequent infusions of calories. My alternative doctor explained that if you need constant calories through the day, you'll continue to need them through the long fast of sleep, and if you don't get them, your blood sugar dips and you wake up hungry. This makes sense, except that when I wake up after two, three, or four hours' sleep, I don't feel hungry. But hypoglycemia "does exist," says Peter Hauri, "and may relate to awakenings at night."

Health experts now tell us that it's good to graze, to take in calories in small amounts throughout the day, and my body has always told me so. It would be nice to think this is my "body wisdom," except that I don't trust my body, not for a minute: left to its own devices, it would live on candy, cookies, ice cream. When I was younger, I'd chow down bags of candy corn and malted milk balls. Alternative docs say a sweet tooth is a sign of hypoglycemia: sugarholics wear out their systems from too much sugar, and this makes their blood sugar erratic. Maybe so, but I had a sweet tooth before I was old enough to have possibly worn the system out. These days, I limit myself to the occasional pint of sorbet and try to confine my binges to popcorn or nuts. But I'm always at war with my appetite. What it wants for my body and what I want are different things. It's like having a juvenile delinquent in the house.

I probably have a touch of *night eating syndrome,* not the full-blown variety, because my appetite shuts down a few hours before sleep and stays shut down until the next afternoon, but I consume most of my calories at night. I've experimented with shifting my eating to the daytime, but when I do this, I eat at night anyway (and I have a horror of weight gain, since dieting destroys sleep: hunger and diet aids are anathema to the insomniac). Night eaters consume as much as 60 percent of their caloric intake after dinner, they have frequent nighttime awakenings, and their neuroendocrine profiles are askew. Grethe Birketvedt and her colleagues at the University of Tromsö, Norway, looked at the endocrinal profiles of twelve night eaters and found that they had lower levels of melatonin and leptin during the night. (Leptin levels normally rise during sleep, which may be what suppresses appetite while we sleep.) The researchers also found that night eaters' levels of cortisol were higher during the day but weaker in response to stressors: when the system is stressed all the time, the stress response is weakened. The adrenals are "worn out."

Adrenal fatigue is another syndrome that alternative practitioners find everywhere and conventional doctors barely acknowledge. Alternative doctors see a relation between adrenal fatigue and erratic or abnormal blood sugar levels: when blood sugar falls, the adrenals are mobilized to produce stress hormones that raise blood sugar and produce energy, and if this goes on too often, the adrenals become overwhelmed. "Bullshit," said a doctor I ran this by. That was his very word, and it pretty much sums up the mainstream view of the matter. But alternative practitioners see adrenal fatigue not only as central but as key to a constellation of other problems, including allergies, autoimmune conditions, rhinitis (all of which I have). They offer adrenal supplements—ground-up adrenal glands of animals—to beef up our ailing adrenals. I took these for several months, but if they had an effect, it was mainly on my pocketbook.

A hair-trigger response to alcohol (which I have) may also be part of the hypoglycemic profile. Alcohol "acts just like a sugar biochemically, only more so. It contains more calories per gram, and it gets into your bloodstream faster," says Julia Ross, who claims that more than 95 percent of alcoholics are hypoglycemic. The longing for alcohol may be a longing for the quick hit you get from sugar, says Ross, who treats alcoholism by treating hypoglycemia. I think it's true that when I long for a predinner drink, as I sometimes do, it's a pick-me-up that I really want. Sometimes grape juice will do the trick. And sometimes not.

Foods that are said to disturb sleep include the nightshade vegetables (tomatoes, eggplant, potatoes) and some leafy green vegetables, spinach in particular. Foods that contain *tyrosine* and *tyramine* (a metabolite of tyrosine) may also be problematic. Tyramine is formed in the breakdown of protein as food ages, so it's found in many cheeses, yogurt, sausage, and smoked meat and in fermented beverages, beer, and wine; it's also in nuts, lentils, and beans. Tyrosine is found in bananas, almonds, sesame seeds, and poultry. But this list of foods is confusing, because some of them—bananas, cheese, yogurt, nuts—are recommended as bedtime snacks. These also contain tryptophan (like that time-honored soporific milk); I've heard it said that if you eat them with carbohydrates, it frees up the tryptophan to get through to the brain. Celery is said to have relaxing properties, since it reduces adrenaline. Inspired by a friend's account, I bought a juicer and juiced celery by the bucket. Nothing.

If you consult an alternative practitioner, chances are that you'll be alerted to possible food allergies. The most common of these are to wheat, milk, egg whites, yeast, tomatoes, shellfish, peanuts, chocolate, soy, food dyes and additives. Alternative practitioners say that food allergies cause the release of histamines, as airborne allergies do, and these may have a wake-up effect. Antihistamines are taken to damp down the effect of airborne allergens, but the histamines released by food allergies aren't so easily counteracted. At the urging of an alternative doctor who ran a test that picked up milk and wheat reactions, I gave up both. It made no difference to my sleep, or my sneezing. I went back to the wheat, but stayed off the milk (to good effect, I think).

Calcium and magnesium are natural relaxants, so I and many insomniacs take these before sleep. Stress depletes them; so do alcohol, sugar, and white flour. Our ability to absorb calcium decreases with age, so that even if we think we're getting enough, we may not be. We need magnesium and vitamin D to absorb calcium—and we need calcium and magnesium to convert tryptophan to 5-HTP and serotonin. We also need the B vitamins, especially B6, for this conversion. Whole grains, bananas, sunflower seeds, blackstrap molasses, walnuts, peanuts, tuna, salmon, the omega-3 fatty acids are rich in B vitamins, and these are thought to be important for sleep. Brewer's yeast is, according to Philip Goldberg and Daniel Kaufman in *Natural Sleep,* "a virtual wonder food that has an excellent effect on sleep." I sometimes eat it before bed; nothing.

Our diets may be deficient in the nutrients we need to convert tryptophan to 5-HTP and serotonin, not only because we eat junk, but also because there is far less mineral and nutrient content in foods today than there was fifty years ago. This is a major reason to eat organic fruits and vegetables: not only are they free of pesticides, but the soil they grow from is not depleted or chemically treated, so they provide more nutrients, which, theoretically, ought to make for better sleep. But I eat organic, and I sleep the way I sleep; so I don't know. But they're better for you, and they taste better—once you get used to organic apples or bananas or carrots, you'll never want to go near that waxed, blanched, pulpy stuff that passes for produce in regular supermarkets.

Supplements

In the 1970s and 1980s, tryptophan was hailed as the miracle sleep supplement and was widely used. Peter Hauri found it to be effective "with about half of insomniacs." But in December 1989, the FDA pulled it off the market. It had been linked with a rare blood disorder and forty or more deaths. The problem was traced to a contaminated batch produced by a Japanese manufacturer, and though it seems to have been confined to that batch, the FDA kept tryptophan restricted; it is now available only by prescription. The scare put an end to research on it. Alternative health practitioners are bitter about this. Some say that the FDA is protecting the interests of drug companies that were threatened by a supplement so effective and easily available. But 5-HTP, a supplement that became available in the United States in 1997, is as good as or better than tryptophan. And 5-HTP is what tryptophan is converted into, on its way to serotonin; it's a more direct precursor to serotonin. Alternative docs say it's extremely effective for some people's sleep, but that it doesn't work for everyone. It didn't work for me (neither did tryptophan).

Alternative medicine advises that everyone's nutritional needs are unique and that some of us may need a lot more of some vitamins and minerals than others, either because we're born with a deficiency or because we've been made deficient by some sort of environmental assault. One study found that in a group of fifteen to twenty people, "there can be a range of nutritional requirements . . . that varies by as much as 700%"—which makes the search for a "recommended daily allowance" (RDA) "a bit like trying to determine the ideal shoe size for the population," says William Walsh, former research scientist at the Argonne National Laboratories and founder of the Health Research Institute at the Pfeiffer Treatment Center, Illinois.

This is the assumption of *orthomolecular medicine,* sometimes called *megavitamin therapy.* The term was coined in 1968 by Linus Pauling, winner of two Nobel prizes. *Ortho* means "correct" or "normal": Pauling was suggesting a type of treatment that aims to correct or normalize the biochemistry of our bodies by restoring the proper balance of vitamins, minerals, and amino acids. Orthomolecular medicine has been derided since Pauling coined the term, but recent understanding of the role of nutrients in the biochemistry of the brain has given it greater credibility. Neurotransmitters are made from amino acids: nutrients, minerals, vitamins, are their "biochemical building blocks." "The brain is a chemical factory which produces serotonin, dopamine, norepinephrine and other brain chemicals 24 hours a day," writes Walsh. If our diets are deficient in nutrients—as they may easily be—or if we've inherited a metabolism that gives us unusual requirements, the balance and working of neurotransmitters may be thrown off. A landmark study of bipolar depression in 1999, by Harvard psychiatrist Andrew Stoll, lent support to this idea. Stoll found that bipolar patients given large doses of omega-3s did significantly better than a matched group of patients who were given placebos.

Orthomolecular medicine has other distinguished proponents, like Carl Pfeiffer, former director of the Brain Bio Center in Princeton (now the Carl C. Pfeiffer Institute), who discovered that imbalances of trace metals could contribute to delinquent and violent behaviors. William Walsh founded the Pfeiffer Institute to further his work. It claims success in treating violent behaviors, learning disorders, hyperactivity, autism—and insomnia. I heard of one insomniac who was helped by this clinic, and of course its own literature makes glowing claims. Twenty years ago, I'd have checked it out. I intended to, and I almost did, but when faced with the travel logistics to central Illinois and the thousands of dollars it would have ended up costing, I backed off. As I say, I'm tired.

But my interest was rekindled when I read about a man who used megavitamin therapies to stave off the ravages of fatal familial insomnia (FFI). FFI is possibly, as D. T. Max says in *The Family That Couldn't Sleep,* the worst disease a person can get: as you stop sleeping, you start going to pieces, hallucinating and flailing about, all the while retaining awareness of what's happening to you. "DF," as he was called in the case study that got my attention, came down with this inherited disease at the age of fifty-two, which is the age when this affliction usually hits. However, his father and uncle had died of it at age seventy-six and seventy-four, respectively. Because the disease doesn't usually come on that late, "it is worth mentioning that DF's father was a prominent talk radio nutritionist who promoted the regular consumption of wheat germ and who richly supplemented his own diet with antioxidant vitamins": the possibility that this diet might have delayed onset "is worth considering." DF, when he was at the stage of the disease when he'd been enduring bouts of sleeplessness that went on for seventy-two to ninety-six hours, went on an intensive vitamin therapy, administered by the Clymer Institute for Alternative Health in Quakertown, Pennsylvania, taking, each night, a combination of high doses of antioxidants, niacin, brewer's yeast, a B complex, blue-green algae, zinc, magnesium, inositol, PABA, grape seed extract, Co-Q-10, choline, concentrated wheat germ oil, tryptophan, melatonin, and a nutrition bar—and, "within 30 minutes of this treatment reported that he fell into natural and restful sleep . . . ranging from 5 to 6.5 hours." He "exceeded the average survival time by nearly a year," during which time he wrote a book and "purchased a motor home and embarked on a solo tour of the U.S." The authors conclude that strategies that promote sleep "may alter the time course of the disease as well as the quality of life."

I plan to give that vitamin cocktail a try. Someday.

SAM-e, pronounced "sammy" (S-adenosylmethionine), is a neuro-transmitter that's widely taken as a supplement in Europe. Julia Ross describes it as "a chemical found naturally in every cell of our bodies and crucial to many cellular functions, including production of serotonin and other mood-regulating neurotransmitters in the brain." It's depleted in the course of aging, and since it requires vitamin B and folic acid for its production, it's also depleted by poor diet and alcohol. Some people use it for sleep, though others find that it speeds them up. I started taking it for arthritis one semester when I was having trouble getting up the four flights of stairs to my office; my knees were protesting alarmingly. Something made a radical improvement—in my knees, that is, not my sleep—but I don't know what it was: I unscientifically started taking glucosamine-chondroitin at the same time I started SAM-e. Also, I got off of Ativan and cut out milk (which is reportedly bad for arthritis), so I don't know what did what. But I twice cut out SAM-e, and both times the arthritis came back. I'm sticking with it for the time being, at half the recommended dose, though I read some alarming things. One study I came across said that the injection of SAM-e into certain parts of a rat's brain "caused neuronal degeneration" like that which occurs in Parkinson's disease. I hope I'm not swapping functioning knees for a functioning brain. I also read that SAM-e may break down into another amino acid, homocysteine, which is strongly correlated with heart disease, but that taking a B complex counteracts this.

Supplements can be a little scary.

Many insomniacs—and some researchers—swear by melatonin supplements. Melatonin is the hormone secreted by the pineal gland in response to darkness. Levels begin to rise a few hours before sleep, which is thought to precipitate the drop in body temperature which brings on sleep, and they remain elevated through the night, declining just prior to the termination of sleep. Melatonin is a powerful antioxidant that protects the brain and nervous system against free radical damage, and it may be involved in the synthesis and action of GABA and natural opioids. It is not something you want to lose, but you do lose it as you age. Caffeine, alcohol, and cortisol deplete it—and so does poor sleep. Too little light during the day or too much light at night, even from a computer monitor, may also interfere with it. So do anti-inflammatories such as aspirin, ibuprofen, and acetaminophen, and being within three feet of electrical appliances.

I heard about melatonin years before it hit the press. I came across mention of some Israeli doctors working on it, and a doctor friend pulled some strings and got it for me. What a disappointment. It then burst on the scene, the miracle drug of the 1990s, demand for it so high that vendors couldn't keep enough of it on the shelves. Books like *The Melatonin Miracle* and *Your Body's Natural Wonder Drug* described it as the miracle cure that slowed aging and countered cancer, heart disease, diabetes, migraines, autism, high blood pressure, and Parkinson's, with recommended doses that were all over the place, from 0.1 milligrams to 5 milligrams. Today the claims made for it are not so extravagant. Most researchers acknowledge that it helps with jet lag and that it may help insomnia when the problem is associated with a circadian problem or with difficulty initiating sleep; but evidence for its effectiveness with sleep maintenance insomnia is "mixed." This has not stopped Takeda from taking a big chance on it, developing their new pill Rozerem.

There may be some risk to taking melatonin on a regular basis. Since it seems to decrease sex hormone production, it is not recommended for adolescents. Also, it may constrict the coronary arteries, and may increase depression in those prone to it. It may promote immune response and inflammation, so it's probably just as well that it didn't work for me, since my immune system is already overzealous. An alternative to taking melatonin might be, especially if you do a lot of night work, to wear glasses or use lightbulbs that remove the blue component from light; this is said to promote the release of melatonin. On the other hand, if your pineal gland is calcified, as happens in many people past a certain age, you might not have much melatonin to release. I'd like to know if my pineal gland is calcified and whether it's worth my while to try those glasses. I suspect I'm not a melatonin responder, but I know many insomniacs who are, including one who claims that it enhances the effects of benzos, so he can get by on a lower dose.

You have to find your own way.

I found a GABA supplement that I thought helped once, twice, but the third time, not. I've since read that if you take this supplement with niacinamide (vitamin B3), pantothenic acid (vitamin B5—seven hundred milligrams), and inositol (also a B vitamin—five hundred milligrams), and combine these with three milligrams of melatonin, an hour before bedtime, it may have an effect, but I didn't go back and try. (Inositol is also recommended for sleep. Part of the B complex, it is present in wheat germ, brewer's yeast, lecithin, and unprocessed grains, as well as oranges, cantaloupe, unrefined molasses, lima beans, raisins, peanuts, cabbage, some nuts, and liver.) Phyllis Bronson, a nutritional-biochemical consultant in Aspen, Colorado, says that improvement from GABA supplements "can be quite dramatic," but cautions against using them without the supervision of a physician or nutritionist who can set up an individually prescribed program. I keep hearing this sort of warning. Walsh cautions against "nutrients in overload," which you can get even from multivitamins: "If you happen to have the wrong biochemistry, it might make you dramatically worse." This is sobering to someone like me who does a lot of self-prescribing, though I can't say it's stopped me doing it.

Herbal Remedies

Herbal medicine has a long and honorable past. Emperor Shennong of China, 3000 B.C., extolled the powers of medicinal herbs. Clay tablets of the ancient Assyrians and Sumerians, from forty-five hundred years ago, recorded the attributes of hundreds of herbs. First-century Roman writer Pliny the Elder, in *Natural History,* listed poppy, rose flowers and juice, valerian, saffron, iris, as soporific. Italian Renaissance writer Ficino advised a formula made of white poppy seeds, lettuce seeds, balsam, saffron, and sugar at bedtime, dissolved and cooked in poppy juice. Many of the old remedies—poppy, valerian, lettuce—do have a soporific effect. American Indians used nutmeg oil, which may also have an effect. Pueblo Indians eat large amounts of mushrooms, which are full of vitamin B. A current folk remedy, "a cup of hot milk with two teaspoons of the darkest molasses you can find," makes sense for the vitamin B and calcium in it.

Once upon a time, herbal remedies were all we had, and botany was part of medical school curricula. "Then scientists learned how to extract and synthesize the active constituents of medicinal herbs, and medical botany was replaced by modern pharmacology," writes Arnold Relman. Even today, about 70 percent of pharmaceuticals in use by mainstream doctors "are, or derive from, natural plants," and most of them are still used the ways they were traditionally used, according to Dylan Evans. In Europe and England, herbal remedies are sold in pharmacies alongside mainstream medicines. In the United States, a 1999 survey found that about 48 percent of people surveyed "had used herbs within the previous year and 24% admit to using herbs regularly."

Herbs known to help sleep include passionflower, also called helmet flower, hoodwort, and mad-dog weed; skullcap, a member of the mint family (mint also may have sedative properties); hops, rich in vitamin B; chamomile, kava kava, lemon balm, Reishi mushroom, and valerian. These are often combined in supplements available in health food stores.

I can't say I've heard rave reviews about any of these, but they do seem to have a mildly sedative effect, alone and combined. I have felt the effect of chamomile tea, a wave of sleepiness, pleasant unless I'm at a dinner party where I'm trying to hold up my end of the conversation, though it's nowhere strong enough to put me out. I never felt a thing from kava kava, which is perhaps just as well, since in 2002 the FDA warned that there is evidence it may do liver damage.

Valerian has been called an "odiferous root." That is an understatement. I'll never forget the gasp a roommate uttered as she leaped back from a kitchen cabinet she'd opened by mistake—"What's *that?*" I had to admit, it was impressive—the smell of rank gym socks forgotten in a closed locker over a long school break, of an overripe cheese left out way too long. My experience with valerian wasn't a happy one. The tea was too terrible, and the pills were so huge they lodged in my craw and burned all the way down. But if you can figure out a way of getting it down, some studies suggest that it helps with sleep. (Simmer it with a few pieces of licorice root or star anise, I've been told.) Dr. Andrew Weil recommends taking it by tincture, one teaspoon in a little warm water, and calls it "the safest sedative I know."

Some people swear by St. John's wort. In Germany, where it's been researched, it's said to outsell Prozac—66 million doses in 1994 alone, according to Herbert Ross in *Sleep Disorders*. It is thought to act something like an SSRI, to raise serotonin levels, and it takes about the same amount of time, two to three weeks, to kick in. I tried it twice and it seemed that both times, after a few weeks, I felt depressed. Maybe it just coincided with a bad time of the semester; or maybe it was consistent with the negative reactions I have to antidepressants.

The best supplement I ever bought at a health food store was made from poppies. People have known about the soporific effects of poppies for so long that representations of Hypnos, the god of sleep, depict poppies growing around the mouth of the cave where he sleeps. The supplement I chanced on was made from California poppies, not the opium poppies from which opiates are derived, which are illegal to grow in the United States, but that gorgeous golden flower that carpets the California hills in the spring. "Both are members of the Papaveraceae family, but they are members of different genera," I read. I had no idea that the California state flower had these powers, but "preliminary research suggests that the California poppy can prolong sleep time," states the Natural Medicines Comprehensive Database; one of its constituents, protopine, "seems to have benzodiazepine-like activity," and it "does not appear to be habit forming." I now take this supplement occasionally when I'm wound up and have nothing pressing the next day. I still wake up frequently, but I drift right off again, and I can sleep longer than I usually do; and I dream marvelously—that is, when it works, which it does not always do. I've found that it works well for one night, when I haven't taken it for awhile, and then it doesn't work again—until I've left it awhile. (This is a problem with herbals: they're less predictable than pharmaceuticals.) I am intrigued by this substance and wish I knew more.

A cautionary note. Herbals and vitamin supplements are not regulated, so you don't know what you're getting, how much of the substance the pill contains, where it comes from, what taint of pesticides or contaminants it may contain. The tryptophan story is a cautionary tale: people died. And even when substances are not tainted (and most of them are not), just because something is "natural" does not necessarily mean it is safe. Not that FDA regulation is an absolute guarantee of safety—many drugs that the FDA okays get taken off the market—but it does at least give some assurance of what's inside the bottle in terms of quantity and strength. When something comes from a health food store, you just have to hope the label tells what's inside and that it's harmless. The worst I ever got from my extensive sampling of health food products (that I know of) has been an occasional case of indigestion. I believe in a general way that we should experiment, but nothing I say in this chapter should be taken as an endorsement. The most I can say is that some of these things seemed to have worked for some people at some time. You should research any supplement you take as you'd research any drug, make sure you get it from reputable sources, and if you can find a doctor who is knowledgeable about these things, ask for advice.

A word about marijuana. Some people use it for sleep; some say it helps them quiet the babble (though I've also heard it doesn't work very long). I find this amazing. Marijuana, the last time I took it, about thirty years ago, made me intensely involved in my own babble; I'd get fascinated by my mental processes, go into my head and not come out, which made it useless for social occasions or for sleep. Also it sped up my heart. But then anything seems to speed up my heart.

Traditional Remedies

Ayurvedic medicine, the traditional medicine of ancient Hinduism, is over five thousand years old. Ayurveda, which means "knowledge of life" in Sanskrit, aims at restoring the balance between body, mind, and spirit. It makes use of herbal and dietary therapies and oils—coconut, sesame, mustard oil—applied topically to the head and feet. The oil has to be refined, I was told by an insomniac who swore by it: "then soak in a tub," she said. Somehow I missed the bit about the tub and got very greasy sheets. That is, sad to say, all I got out of it. But I didn't really give it a try. It is, as Weil says, "one of the oldest medical systems in the world," and is to this day an integral part of medical practice and daily life in India. Practitioners identify your "constitution" by ascertaining which medical humor, or *dosha* (air, fire, or water) dominates your behavior and physique. They diagnose by asking questions, touching, taking pulses, observing the way you move, walk, and behave; they then prescribe, on the basis of their diagnosis, an individual treatment plan. Yoga, a "sister discipline," is also enlisted, along with medication and massage. Some of these remedies, says Weil, "have great therapeutic value," and "might be worth exploring if you have a stubborn chronic disease that conventional medicine cannot cure."

Acupuncture originated in Chinese medical practice over five thousand years ago. Today, it is estimated that Americans make 9 to 12 million visits annually to acupuncturists and spend $500 million on treatments. Acupuncture is based on the premise that health depends on a balanced flow of qi, the vital life energy present in all living things. When the flow of qi is blocked, through trauma, stress, poor diet, or disease, problems develop. A Chinese practitioner looks for imbalances, through examination of the tongue, body odor, voice, general demeanor, and pulse (or pulses—there are several pulses; the system is quite elaborate). He or she then inserts needles, hair-thin, into the body along the energy pathways through which the energy flows, called *meridians,* leaving them in place for twenty to thirty minutes, to unblock the flow of qi.

"In conventional western medicine, two insomniacs who come to a physician with the same complaint . . . in all likelihood leave the office with the same prescription," explains Herbert Ross, whereas the traditional Chinese medical practitioner may find different patterns that require different acupuncture points and a different herbal formula. The acupuncturist will ask you if you have trouble falling asleep or staying asleep, and what time you wake up during the night, since "Chinese medicine recognizes an organ time clock—two-hour time periods in which certain organ systems are more active."

I gave it several tries, the first time for several months. It didn't help my sleep, but I realized, after a month or so of weekly visits, that I hadn't had a headache that whole time. The needles never hurt, not even a little, and I always felt relaxed and euphoric afterward. Studies have shown that endorphins, the brain's natural painkillers, are released during treatment, which may be why acupuncture is effective with pain. I liked the way the practitioners asked questions about my insomnia, wanted to know the particulars of whether I had problems in getting to sleep or staying asleep, what time I woke up and what happened then. I liked the way they looked at my tongue and sort of sniffed me over, and was reassured by the attention paid to my pulses: it felt right that a healer would have this kind of relation to a body. I gave it another try a few years later, but only for a few months; and then another try a year after that, for several weeks, less inclined, with each attempt, to hang in there. But I know insomniacs who swear by acupuncture, and there are studies that say it helps sleep, that it elevates nighttime levels of melatonin.

Homeopathy was founded in the early nineteenth century by the German physician Samuel Hahnemann. It is based on the principle that "like cures like," that "the same substance that in large doses produces the symptoms of an illness in very minute doses cures it": if you're treating an allergy, you introduce minute quantities of the suspected allergen into the body, and if you're treating insomnia, you introduce tiny amounts of coffee. This is the principle behind vaccines, except that the quantities are much more minute in homeopathy: they are potentized, which means "diluted," sometimes hundreds of times. There are more than three thousand remedies, derived from minerals, plants, and animals, and the more a remedy is potentized, the more powerful it is said to be: "the final remedy is diluted to such a degree that it contains no molecule of the original substance, only its energetic vibration." There is no known scientific principle by which this can happen.

Mainstream science debunks homeopathy because it has no scientific basis. The effect of herbals is understandable—they're another form of medicine—but homeopathy is something else. Yet it is practiced worldwide. In Germany, its birthplace, it's part of the required training of all medical students, and about 20 percent of physicians practice it; in France, 40 percent of physicians practice it, and pharmacies carry homeopathic remedies alongside conventional drugs; in Britain, homeopathic clinics are part of the national health system. The World Health Organization cites it as one of the systems of traditional medicine that should be integrated with conventional medicine. A 1991 study in the *British Medical Journal* reviewed 107 controlled clinical studies, 81 of which showed benefits. A colleague of mine who grew up on the site of a nuclear reactor, who has suffered serious health problems all her life, swears that homeopathy saved her. She became so interested in it that she learned to mix her own remedies. Judy Baxter, quoted in the first paragraph of this chapter, says, *It is definitely the most helpful thing I've found for my sleep—but unfortunately, it stops working.*

Placebo? Perhaps. Does it matter, if it helps you sleep?

People with transient insomnia are told to try one of several homeopathic remedies available in health food stores. I tried Coffea cruda, a remedy a friend found effective with her insomnia, made from coffee. It didn't put me to sleep that night, but the next day I was unusually sleepy, which made me wonder if it wasn't having some effect (or maybe I was just sleepy that day). People with chronic insomnia are advised to find a homeopath, who will take a thorough medical history, look for the patterns of feelings and behavior that produce the problem, and then prescribe a remedy. I found one and went to her for several months. She sent me home each week with a vial of something. Nothing. Several months and a few thousand dollars later, she told me she wasn't sure she could treat me if I stayed on thyroid supplements and hormone replacement therapy. There was no way I was going to go off these, so that was that. She may not have been the right homeopath for me. There's a Hahnemann Institute that's well reputed near where I live, but I didn't hear about it till later. I didn't have the heart to try again.

Tricks, Techniques, Devices

People find help in odd and interesting places, so it's good to keep an open mind.

I hear about success with aromatherapy, especially lavender and cedar. I hear about *a gizmo that tickles your scalp and makes you yawn,* a *shower with hard pounding nozzles in your back,* a Jacuzzi. I hear about what one woman delicately refers to as "self-organized orgasm." I hear about infrared sauna therapy, which raises the body temperature three degrees for at least ten minutes; this may have an effect for the same reason that twenty minutes of aerobic exercise does, by raising the temperature long enough so that, when it goes down again, it drops to lower than it was before. I hear of successes with craniosacral therapy (*cranio* meaning head, *sacral* meaning the base of the spine). This is a technique that is said to manipulate the sutures of the skull, where the bones meet, to ease pressure in the craniosacral system. (It's generally believed that the cranial bones don't move, but according to Dr. Weil, x rays confirm that the cranial bones do move.) A recent study suggests that it calms the sympathetic nervous system, though how it does this, nobody knows. Maybe for the same reason that tickling the scalp does—"simple touch," as one study described it.

I hear about a cathode ion collector dish: *Place it next to the head of your bed*—and if you don't have such a dish, *an anode generator, placed across the room from your bed and aimed where your head will be lying, will provide a sufficiently charged field for inducing sleep. But don't aim it directly at yourself unless there are at least 25 feet for the ionic field to disperse. Wait for about 15 minutes for a steady stream of ions to be flowing over the bed.* I hear about a magnetic pad that worked for six weeks but then had no further effect. I read about impulse magnetic-field therapy, "a matchbox-size device . . . placed near the patient's head, preferably under the pillow," that supposedly stimulates the pineal gland to release melatonin. One study that was double-blinded and placebo-controlled looked at one hundred subjects randomly assigned to treatment or placebo and found that 70 percent of those treated with the magnetic device "experienced very clear or even extremely clear relief of their complaints," whereas only 2 percent of placebo patients experienced very clear relief—a "highly significant" difference. I read about a silver lollipop, an aluminum-coated mouthpiece placed in the mouth twenty minutes before bedtime that emitted low-level doses of electromagnetic radiation. It sounded promising, but that was in 1991, and I never heard anything about it again.

Transcranial magnet stimulation (TMS), which uses electromagnetic pulses to stimulate neural activity in specific parts of the brain, is a fascinating technique that's drawn the attention of so many mainstream researchers and practitioners that I'm not sure it should be classified as "alternative." Alternative or not, it is innovative and exciting. Magnetic fields can pass easily through an insulator even as thick as the skull; with a TMS instrument, pulses are directed to specific areas of the brain to make them more or less active. The method has worked to dispel the "inner voices" of schizophrenics and has had success with clinical depression; researchers hope that it may someday replace electroconvulsive therapy. It has recently been used to produce what looks like slow wave sleep, the deepest kind. "With a single pulse, we were able to induce a wave that looks identical to the waves the brain makes normally during sleep," says Giulio Tononi, lead researcher on this study. The University of Wisconsin and University of Milan researchers involved in this project will now try to find out whether the artificially stimulated slow waves perform the same restorative functions that natural waves do. They have hopes that this work may cast light on the functions sleep actually performs.

At one of the conference exhibits, I came across a device that does cranial electrotherapy stimulation, a technique begun in the Soviet Union in the 1950s, the so-called sleep machine. In the version I found, you attach clips like earring clips to your ears; these are connected by wire to a box that emits a low-level current, sending pulses of electrical stimulation through the brain, which is claimed to produce an alpha state that helps with insomnia, depression, stress, pain, and learning. A study that administered twenty-four fifteen-minute treatments showed "significant improvement" in the time it took to get to sleep and time spent awake in bed, improvements maintained at the two- and three-year follow-up. Since it didn't take enormous expenditure of energy or time (and I could send it back within thirty days), I took one of these devices home and used it now and then—but not consistently enough to know whether it makes a difference (effects are said to be cumulative). Then the thirty days were up, and back it went.

Sorry to be such a disappointment. I'm not good at sticking these things out.

At the first sleep conference I attended, in Seattle, I made a beeline for a poster, "Brain Music Therapy for Treatment of Insomnia and Anxiety," where I met Dr. Leonid Kayumov. Kayumov explained that brain music is made with a special computer program and the patient's EEG. The EEG patterns are converted into music that's recorded on a compact disk, "and when you play it back, it influences the bioelectrical brain activity." He and his research team found that it made "a dramatic improvement in sleep quality," whereas the placebo, which was made from someone else's EEG, made "no significant difference." They also found that brain music increased melatonin. I asked him, if I got myself to Toronto, would he make my EEG music? He looked dubious.

I find work on brain music by other Russian researchers. Ya. I. Levin, of Moscow City Sleep Center, also found "positive effects in more than 80% of the insomniac patients, both from the point of view of subjective sensations and in terms of objective studies." This study found a 50 percent placebo effect, unusually large, which suggests that music of all sorts may be effective as a sleep tool—as other studies confirm. There are many kinds of music therapies available on the Web. I once fought back an anxiety attack while driving by singing camp songs at the top of my lungs, and I once fought back seasickness by humming loudly, but the only music I could ever sleep to was completely atonal, lots of gong sounds. I think it was Tibetan, but I don't know; a friend made the tape for me, and I played it until it wore out. It was pleasantly soothing.

Eye movement desensitization and reprocessing (EMDR) is a fascinating therapy that originated in 1987 for the treatment of posttraumatic stress disorder. Therapists use hand movements or a flashing light to provide side-to-side stimulus for the eyes to follow; sometimes they use auditory stimuli, tones or tapping, that are made to alternate from ear to ear. While this is going on, the patient talks about the traumatic events, and somehow, in the process, comes to see them in a less threatening light. Some say it's worth months of talk therapy. Some say it helps sleep. Nobody understands how it works, but results are sufficiently convincing that, by June 2002, there were forty thousand therapists around the world using it.

"Something about EMDR's oscillating stimulation does have a dramatic effect," writes Andrew Solomon. "I was flooded with incredibly powerful images from childhood, things I hadn't known were even in my brain. . . . It's a powerful process. I recommend it." On the basis of his description, I went to a therapist a friend raved about. This therapist didn't use visual stimuli—she said she found them distracting; she handed me two podlike things instead, to hold in my hands; she then made them vibrate, oscillating from one hand to the other, while I talked. Though she cautioned that EMDR was not about recovering memories, I guess that's what I was hoping for, but I did not get that flood of images Solomon describes, or anything, really, so I didn't go back. But there is an offshoot of this technique that I think I have found helpful for sleep. Clinical psychologist John Preston describes a two-minute technique involving back-and-forth eye movements to quiet the "busy brain." Hold your neck and head still and move your eyes from side to side, as though you're watching a game of table tennis. Do this about twenty times, then stop, relax, and take a reading of your body; then do it another twenty times, then stop, then do it again. Preston advises doing this while sitting up, though I've done it in bed: on nights when my mind shows no sign of showing down, I find a spot of light way over to the right of the room and another way over to the left, and move my eyes as Preston directs, trying to bring my breathing in synch with the eye movements, and I think I have sometimes noticed a quieting effect. I can definitely recommend this one: it can't hurt.

There is also a whole world of so-called mind machines, or sound-light machines—*buzzie blinkie thingies,* as a friend calls them. The version I bought (and used a half dozen times), the Proteus Mind Machine, which cost $229, consists of a pair of goggles and earphones that are attached to a box with controls that you can set to a range of different modes. The goggles flash pink, blue, purple, green lights, like strobe lights, strong enough to pulse through your closed eyelids; they seem to be coming from the inside of your eyelids, from deep within your brain. Meanwhile the earphones hum and thrum and throb, and the sound goes loud and outer-spacey, then soft and fading-out. It is quite powerful. You can't sustain a racing mind with all this going on; you can barely sustain a thought. (This is *not* for anyone at risk for seizures!) An insomniac friend describes his experience with the Proteus as "encouraging":

> *I put on the goggles and headphones, and fell asleep again in ten minutes, slept thru the night. Similar things have happened on other nights. . . .*
> *The subjective effect is similar to that of the eye-movement technique, except maybe stronger, and no effort is required. At alpha frequencies, internal chatter seems greatly diminished. One's usual worries become unwoven—they sort of fall apart. One has the occasional passing thought, perhaps an anxious one, but it seems soon forgotten.*

A few times when I've done it, my mind does go still—but not my heart: it speeds up. It speeds at anything, it seems. The overall effect on me is, well, energizing.

Some "mind machines" combine sound and light with biofeedback devices. Proponents of these claim they can put you into a "theta state," an associative, creative state where you have access to childhood memories, and that the machines can be truly mind-altering, improving memory, curing depression and insomnia, and even reversing the effects of head injury. A less high-tech version of what they do, which some people find helpful, is just staring at the TV "snow," or static, with the sound off. *Puts you in theta in ten seconds.* Worth a try.

Biofeedback devices give "feedback" on physiological processes through auditory tones or visual signals, so you can learn to consciously regulate unconscious functions such as heart rate, breathing, blood pressure, muscle tension; they teach you to bring the autonomic nervous system under voluntary control. Practitioners of biofeedback claim success with alcoholism, addiction, ADD, cancer, anxiety, depression, chronic pain, autism, schizophrenia, brain injury, migraines, asthma, gastrointestinal disorders, and incontinence—including urgency, or the feeling of needing to urinate when one doesn't (which might be useful to people whose insomnia is related to that problem). Hauri had success with biofeedback for insomnia, as we've seen. Neurotherapy, also called neurofeedback therapy, is a form of biofeedback that trains the brain to recognize and replicate alpha and theta. Electrodes placed on the scalp register what kind of brain waves you're producing, signals are fed into a computer, and when you've attained the desired brain wave, the computer responds with a light or sound signal that encourages your brain to continue what it's doing. The techniques are promising but mysterious, and need much more research.

My experience with biofeedback was confusing. It was a long time ago, in the early 1980s. There was, as I recall, a pretty crude device, a monitor with a screen and a needle that I was supposed to make move into a range designated as "alpha," by doing something with my mind. The instructor told me to use whatever technique I could—meditation, visualization, autosuggestion—to get the needle to move. I found that the mantra I used in meditation would make it move, so I'd sit and meditate for twenty minutes and be told I was getting the knack of it. But I already knew how to meditate, and I knew that, whatever its virtues, it didn't help me sleep, so I quit after a few sessions.

This stuff's *expensive*.

Transcendental Meditation and Hypnotherapy

Transcendental meditation (TM) is something I have had success with, but not for sleep. I learned it in 1970, when I was a graduate student teaching at Queens College. One semester when I had 8 A.M. classes, I bonded with a fellow insomniac, Bertie, down the hall, whose bloodshot, darkly ringed eyes told me she was as wrecked as I was by our schedules. At the end of the semester, she said she was going to take a TM course. It was all the rage. The Beatles had traveled to India to learn from Maharishi Mahesh Yogi at his ashram in the foothills of the Himalayas; the guru had appeared, beaming, on the Johnny Carson show, and suddenly everybody was doing it, from the Beach Boys to Mia Farrow. I'd never paid it much attention because I wasn't into Indian mysticism, and because I never had any ability to control my zinging mind. When people talk about meditation, they usually talk about controlling the attention and focusing the concentration in ways that make me want to run and hide under the bed. But TM is quick and easy, yet proponents say that it has effects "similar to those that have been observed in highly trained experts in yoga and in Zen monks who have had 15 to 20 years experience in meditation," though it requires nothing like that kind of discipline or time to learn. So when Bertie tried it for insomnia, I paid attention.

When I saw her at the beginning of the next term, I asked, "So, does it help your sleep?"

"No," she said, "but it helps me to get through the days I haven't slept."

That was good enough for me. The following summer, when I was at my mother's, I took a class at Stanford and learned the technique. You go to a few lectures, and then, if you decide to follow through, you make an appointment to meet one of the instructors. There's a small ceremony, to which you're asked to bring an "offering" of fruit and flowers. Some Indian words are muttered, some incense burned, and the teacher assigns you your own individual, personal mantra. The mantra is assigned on the basis of a questionnaire you fill out and your offering of fruits and flowers (mine was what I could pick from my mother's backyard). My instructor was a flower child with bright blue eyes and translucent skin; he looked like an angel. He told me my mantra and had me repeat it over and over, then told me to think it, say it silently, internalize it. Now it was wholly mine, and I was never to speak it out loud again. I never have.

In the very first session, I could tell something was happening, and meditation soon became a regular part of my life—in my modified version of it, that is, since I never could get it to work the way it's supposed to. You're supposed to meditate twice a day, but I never could get it to work in the morning, so I gave up on that and did it only in the late afternoon or early evening. You're supposed to meditate sitting in a chair, but I always did it lying down, because sometimes I lose consciousness for a few seconds or a few minutes and go into a quick nap—and when I come to, I'm good for hours. As I think the mantra, pronounce it internally, it's as though it becomes incorporated into my breathing and heartbeat and slows both down, and I can feel a quieting inside. It acts as a word repellent, sort of butts the words away, makes everything go still in there, and then it's as though I'm asleep but conscious too: I'm aware of everything going on around me, except that my mind is perfectly still—which makes me realize what a babbling is usually in there. (I'll say more in the next chapter about quieting the babble.)

Early on, I made the mistake of trying to use my mantra to get to sleep. I'd get relaxed and drift off, but then I'd come to twenty minutes later, energized and good to go for the rest of the night. Transcendental meditation is not a sleep tool, but it is a way of getting through the days you don't sleep, as Bertie said. In fact some of the same things happen in meditation that happen in sleep: oxygen consumption declines, heart rate slows, prolactin levels go up, and levels of lactate in the blood fall off (*lactate* is a metabolic waste product that builds up in the course of the day and dissipates with sleep). For years, I relied on TM as a way of getting through three-hour night classes. I'd meditate just before class, never had to set an alarm—even if I lost consciousness, I'd always snap to in twenty minutes. It worked like an instant nap. It worked like a charm. (Thank you, Bertie, wherever you are!)

If transcendental meditation can work for me, who hasn't a shred of mysticism or ability to control my thoughts, it can work for anyone, I figured, and I went around recommending it to everyone I knew. But two of my friends took the course, and it didn't do a thing for them. I asked them, after they'd given up on it, to tell me their mantras. One of them was *sheering* (emphasis on the -*ing*), and the other, I can't remember, but I remember that it also had two syllables and the *ng* sound (as mine does). It may be that the vibratory quality of the *ng* helps the sound synchronize with the heartbeat and breath. "The vibratory frequencies of these sounds, which have been handed down through an ancient and honorable tradition, are said to resonate harmoniously with the meditator's nervous system, producing different brain-wave effects than arbitrarily chosen sounds," write Goldberg and Kaufman in *Natural Sleep,* who had success with TM themselves. But some people say you need only repeat soothing words, like "come sleep" or "I sleep well." Dr. Herbert Benson, a cardiologist affiliated with Harvard Medical School, teaches "a demystified form of meditation" in which practitioners use a soothing word instead of a mantra. But I like my mantra. And I didn't mind the little bit of mysticism associated with the course; I thought the flowers and fruit were sweet, and the ceremony kind of charming.

Long-term effects claimed for TM include enhanced creativity and improved academic and job performance. Some studies find that it lowers blood pressure as effectively as antihypertensive drugs. I can well believe that if you did it regularly, as I have not, it might have amazing effects. I met a man a few years ago who'd been doing it about as long as I had, only he'd done it to the letter and "never missed a day" (I stopped it a few years ago). He looked disgustingly youthful, though he was my age. And who knows but it might, in the course of time, improve your sleep, if you were rigorous. There are testimonials that it does, and even some studies. It needs more research.

One study found that only eight sessions of meditation over an eight week period (this was "mindfulness meditation," which, I gather, requires more mind control or concentration than TM) produced activation of the left prefrontal cortex, the area associated with positive emotions (it becomes enlarged in monks who are experienced meditators). Researchers have found that people whose EEG shows greater activity in the left frontal cortex are generally more cheerful, outgoing, optimistic, and forward-looking than those who have more activity in the right hemisphere, who tend to be more inward-looking, pessimistic, fearful, anxious: when right frontal activity dominates, negativity may as well. There's an ancient yogi technique, breathing through the right nostril, that is said to activate the left hemisphere. Some say that lying on your right side will activate it, too. One study found that vigorously grinning or contorting the right side of your face may also do the trick. Probably it's best not to do this in a public place.

(Do insomniacs have greater right-brain activation? You'd think so, if we're as depressed, anxious, fearful, inward-looking, as we're said to be. I asked Eric Nofzinger if his neuroimaging studies were turning up any right-brain left-brain differences in his subjects, and he said he had noticed some differences but hadn't paid them attention, and yes, it would be interesting to look, and no, he knew of no one who was looking.)

I have heard insomniacs swear by hypnotherapy. The hypnotherapist I saw worked out of her home by the railroad tracks. The room was candlelit, pungent with incense, bead curtains draped the doors and windows. She wore a flowing purple robe and bangling bracelets. She tried to get me to visualize a man sitting on top of the world. I had no idea what she was talking about. She told me to tell myself, "I feel calm, relaxed, I sleep well," which seemed about as useful as telling myself to go to sleep. I shouldn't have gone back, but I didn't want to hurt her feelings, so back I went again, and again. Then the fourth time she put me into some sort of a state. Oh, good, I thought, relaxed into it, and stayed relaxed for a half hour or more. Then I went home and was wide awake the whole night.

Years later, after enough time had passed for me to forget this experience, I went to another hypnotist, but when he started sounding like the first, I ran for the door.

I wish I could say I've found something that's worked. I'm willing to believe I happened on the wrong hypnotist, the wrong homeopath, the wrong biofeedback man, and that there are right ones. I'm willing to believe that I just don't try hard enough: I don't sufficiently research things, don't stick them out, get easily discouraged, get put off by flakiness. Even my yoga was ill-starred. I got off to a great start, was greeting the day with salutations to the sun, but then one day, after a particularly energetic series of downward-facing dogs, I got flashers and floaters like giant spiderwebs in my right eye. My retina was on the way to detaching; it didn't detach, but it puckered badly, leaving me with a wrinkled retina. There are no longer any straight lines in my right field of vision. Maybe it would have happened anyway; or maybe, for a very nearsighted sixty-something person, a downward-facing position that sends a rush of blood to the head isn't such a great idea. I still do a few yoga exercises, but in a mild, never-downward-pointing way.

I know I'm not persistent enough, but I have tried, in my way, have sunk some money and time into these things. There's a box in my basement that's a graveyard for old pill bottles: valerian, melatonin, 5-HTP, GABA, Sleepwell, Staycalm, Calmdown, Calmforts, Sleepsound, Sound-sleep, all full except for the three or four or twenty pills I took before ditching them, along with countless teas that make promises they don't keep. Why I keep these, I don't know. As a testimony to effort, I guess.

Critics say that the success of alternative approaches is all about the placebo effect. I've read that "placebos are ineffective in the treatment of severe insomnia." Maybe that's why I haven't had more success with these approaches, my insomnia is too severe to be amenable to placebo. But I persist in believing that there's more than the placebo effect to alternative therapies. There's too much that seems right about them: the holistic approach to mind and body, the emphasis on the body's own powers of healing, the attention to the particulars of patients' problems, the concern with chronic conditions. I urge you to try, and I'll go on trying, in my desultory way. (At the top of my list to try next is the Feldenkrais method, a movement and relaxation method that I'm told is effective with insomnia.) We'll see.

I wish mainstream researchers and doctors had more curiosity about the conditions alternative practitioners find everywhere: hypoglycemia, adrenal fatigue, vitamin deficiencies, melatonin or serotonin deficiencies, food allergies. I wish they'd help us sort out the helpful from the hocus-pocus, rather than dismissing it all out of hand. I wish more were known.

Alternative Physicians

What I'd like is a doctor who has an open mind and an imagination, who can move between Western and Eastern, ancient and modern, traditional and alternative approaches. I'm sufficiently my father's daughter to want to see "MD" behind the name of the health practitioner I turn to, but I'd like someone who's willing to use whatever tool or technique works, who knows about nutrition, who takes hormones seriously, who approaches insomnia as though it might have something to do with the body.

There are such doctors, but they are rare. One helped me, not with my sleep but with my thyroid—but since thyroid dysregulation can affect sleep, probably she did help with my sleep. The thyroid regulates metabolism, the rate at which the body converts food into energy. When the thyroid is off, whether it's producing too much or too little thyroid, other things get thrown off, including sleep.

Bear with me here while I tell the story of my thyroid, because thyroid problems, which affect many more women than men, are seriously underdiagnosed, and they're something alternative practitioners are better at picking up than mainstream doctors. In the summer of 1992, I became ill with chills and a high fever, along with a terrible pain in the back of my neck. It would settle in for a few days, then begin to subside, then start up again, and it went on like this for a month. Two doctors diagnosed me as having FUO, which sounded like something from outer space but meant "fever of unknown origin." Finally, a third thought to check for thyroid antibodies, and sure enough, he found antibodies for Hashimoto's, a condition where the immune system attacks the thyroid. I was lucky it was picked up so early; with some people, it goes undiagnosed for years.

For about ten years, I did fine with a synthetic thyroid supplement, but then I began to have symptoms of thyroid deficiency: my skin was very dry, I was putting on weight, and I was cold all the time. Though I'm prone to these conditions more or less all the time, I was also having nosebleeds and hair loss (the ends of my eyebrows were disappearing), and I was unusually sluggish. All are symptoms of thyroid deficiency. But my test numbers were normal, so I could get none of the several doctors I saw to take my complaint seriously. Mainstream doctors test only for thyroid stimulating hormone, or TSH, the signal that the pituitary sends to the thyroid telling it how much of the hormone to make; if your thyroid is making enough TSH, your pituitary will send very little TSH, and

your score will be on the low side, which mine was. Most doctors, seeing numbers in the normal range, proceed no further. Until the 1940s,
says Julia Ross, doctors diagnosed this disorder by symptoms, but now
they look only at the numbers. Ross says she sees a lot of people at her
clinic whose doctors have discounted the possibility of thyroid trouble
because "the numbers are fine." Most doctors don't even feel the gland
to find out if it's swollen, so removed are they from the art of touch—
and the thyroid is easily examined by touch, since it's in the neck, just
above the voice box. Only one of the several doctors I went to about thyroid actually felt it (unfortunately for the point of my story, it was not
the alternative doc).

But alternative doctors are attentive to the symptoms of thyroid deficiency. And they know that TSH is only one of several indicators of
what's going on. Other tests they do are for T4 and T3. T4 is thyroxin,
the less active hormone; this converts to T3, triodothyronine, which is
the more active; but in some people T4 stops converting to T3—which
seems to have happened with me. Since T3 is the more active form of the
hormone, this is critical. The alternative doctor I saw gave me an extract
from pigs' glands which contains not only T3 and T4, but a fuller spec-
trum of T1 and T2. In a month or so, my nosebleeds stopped and I felt
less sluggish; eventually my hair loss diminished and my eyebrows grew
back in. Mainstream docs smile condescendingly when I tell them I'm
taking the porcine supplement, but none of them was able to help me.

I hear stories like this, from a woman whose insomnia came on suddenly: *I am normally a very upbeat, positive person, and I knew I wasn't
depressed. I suspected a change in my hormones. My symptoms felt similar to those I experienced when I had postpartum depression after the birth
of my first son.* But her doctor didn't test for thyroid, discounted her hunch
about hormones, and prescribed antidepressants: *She thought I was way
too young, at forty-five, to be perimenopausal. So I took the antidepressants, but they made me feel even more anxious.* With the help of an
alternative doctor who diagnosed perimenopause and an underfunc-
tioning thyroid, and a nutritionist who advised her about diet and supplements, she found her way to better sleep.

*We need doctors who are willing to work with us, who want to hear the
questions and information we bring in, who are willing to think outside
the box, to take us through whatever is necessary to find the right approach.* So says my friend Roberta. The demand for this kind of doctor is
enormous, write Ralph Snyderman and Andrew Weil: "Most Americans
who consult alternative providers would probably jump at the chance to

consult a physician who is well trained in scientifically based medicine and who is also open-minded and knowledgeable about the body's innate mechanisms of healing, the role of lifestyle factors in influencing health, and the appropriate uses of dietary supplements, herbs, and other forms of treatment"; they would love to find "competent help in navigating the confusing maze of therapeutic options that are available today." Integrative medicine, the name for this approach that combines the best of conventional care with attention to prevention, "insists on patients being active participants in their health care as well as on physicians viewing patients as whole persons—minds . . . spiritual beings . . . physical bodies," write Snyderman and Weil.

Snyderman and Weil describe integrative medicine as "a new movement that is being driven by the desires of consumers." I'd like to say there's a rising tide of such doctors, but in fact, I've found the merest trickle. Alternative medicine requires patience, time, and a commitment to processes that take longer than the quick fix of a drug. The training is time-intensive, and there are not many programs. Even in the San Francisco Bay Area, where you'd expect such practitioners to be thick on the ground, there are not that many, and in some parts of the country, there are none.

Yet this is the direction medicine needs to move if it's going to help people with chronic conditions. We insomniacs need to make our voices part of a rising consumer demand.

CHAPTER 11

Bedding Down with the Beast

I turn and turn, try one pillow, two,
Think of people who have no beds.
Jane Kenyon, "Insomnia at the Solstice"

Try lying on the end of the bed. Then you might drop off.
Mark Twain

Sleep is personal, sleep is intimate, sleep is interwoven into the fabric of our deepest beings. It's not surprising, then, that we have relations to sleep that are as individual and distinctive as we ourselves are.

You must find your own way with insomnia, make your own terms with it, learn what works for you and what does not. Become a close observer of your sleep, which does not mean obsessing about your sleep, but learning your body, how it reacts to foods, drugs, light, time of day. What are your peak times and slump times? How much sleep do you need to do the things you need to do, and how little can you get by with, and for how long? Then cobble together from what you learn a way of life that works. There is no "program" that is right for everybody. There is only what you can find that works.

So I don't have a set of rules, though I do have a few general principles and some things I have found that have helped me and others. I don't use the word *manage* with insomnia, though people like this word. It's a word we find everywhere, a take-charge kind of word: banks tell us to *manage* our accounts, Amazon advises us to *manage* our book orders, a toothpaste ad urges, "*Manage* your smile." I don't want a word like this near my bedroom. Anyhow, manage is what I do all day. When I prepare a class or catch a plane or write a book, I direct my movements in a goal-oriented way. I manage my time, energies, actions. But sleep? Sleep doesn't come under those same principles of control, organization, and efficiency. It's not a take-charge kind of thing. Sleep is not yang, mastering and seizing hold; it is yin, submitting, surrendering. Yang is the mode I try to leave at the bedroom door.

And insomnia? I don't *manage* this beast. I live with it. I live around it. I bed down with it every night, gingerly, cautiously, careful not to provoke it. I do my best to placate it, domesticate it, dull its claws, avoid its fangs, knowing that at any moment it can pounce on me and tear me to bits. But *manage* it? I wouldn't say so.

What I Do

I once knew a woman who was so determined to sleep without drugs that she rearranged her entire life to this end. The last time I saw her, she had quit her job at a biotech company in Silicon Valley and moved home with her mother. She synchronized her habits to the rhythms of dawn and dusk, allowing no bright lights in the house after sunset, engaging in no evening activities that might perk her up; she was in bed by 10 P.M. and up at 6 A.M., without fail. No caffeine, of course, no alcohol or sugar. She spent her days doing meditation, breathing exercises, yoga. No talking on the phone after 6 P.M. Nobody left to talk to, no friends, no guys, no work—no life. But—she told me proudly—no pills.

A claim I cannot make. But I can't let sleep colonize every corner of my life this way, can't yield it my every pleasure and passion. It has to fit into the life I live, leave me room of my own. I sleep to live, not live to sleep.

But I am, as I've said, no model. I'm not good at regularity, not good at saying no to interesting evening activities, not good with rules, though not heedless of them, either. I do constant risk-benefit calculations throughout the day and night: if I drink this, if I eat this, if I don't go home now, if I don't stop working now, it may cut into my sleep—and sometimes I do it anyway. And sometimes it wrecks my sleep, and sometimes it does not. Sometimes the sleep fairy drops by, and sometimes not.

The work I do is bad for sleep, I know. I write, which means I spend vast amounts of time home alone doing close, fussy work. I try to minimize the damage by working in a light room and taking many evenings off, but this doesn't change the fact that writing is close, fussy work that leaves me buzzy with words. (Here's a study someone might do: take a bunch of insomniacs who do close, taxing, indoor work—accountants, computer programmers, lawyers—and send them out into the world to do and see new things, to explore cities, climb the Pyramids, travel, but with the tension of travel somehow removed—I'd volunteer for this one—would their insomnia go away?) The other thing I do is teach, and this generates performance anxiety, but what can I do? It's the way I earn my living, the way I've chosen to earn my living; and I (mostly) love it. You have to work with who you are.

Having said there are no rules, here are a few, if not rules, at least principles that are pretty generally true. The first is—you've heard this so often you've probably stopped listening, but I'll say it anyway—stay away from caffeine. This was a hard lesson for me. I love coffee, I love it so much that it makes me happy just to be in a house where I smell it brewing. I used to make myself a small pot, three scoops of Mocha-Java, ground fine and dripped, to extract the maximum punch. I'd mix it with three-quarters of a cup of warm milk and sip it for the first several hours of the day. I never had any bad effects during the day, but at night I'd wake up with my heart pounding and the feeling of a fist squeezing it tight. Then one morning, a roommate who was a medical student said, "You're crazy to be drinking that stuff with a sleep problem."

"Nonsense," I said, "I've drunk it all my life."

"Yeah, and you've had a sleep problem all your life." I didn't have a really good reply to that. Caffeine, I now know, is a powerful drug. It sets the stress hormones flowing and produces symptoms of hyperarousal that insomniacs don't need more of. Its half-life, the time it takes for half of it to be broken down, is between three and seven hours. This means that if you're on the slow side of metabolizing it, it never leaves your system: if your last cup was at 1 P.M., you still have, at 8 P.M., about half the drug left in your system; at 3 A.M. you have one-quarter of it, at 10 A.M., you have one-eighth of it. If you're a woman in the luteal phase of the cycle, between ovulation and your period, you take about 25 percent longer to eliminate it, and if you're on birth control pills you take about twice the normal time to eliminate it. As you get older and your liver becomes less effective at metabolizing, you take longer still.

So I cold-turkeyed it, and it felt like someone had scooped out my skull and packed it with sawdust—but I was, miraculously, sleeping. I was ecstatic, I thought I'd found the cure—for two weeks or so. Then my old sleep pattern began to reassert itself, and there I was, sleepstarved but with no caffeine to get me through the day. So back I went, this time to half decaf, and that was okay for a while, but then even that got to be too much, and I cut back to all decaf; then, about five years ago, I switched to tea.

So coffee goes on that list of things that make sleep worse but which, when you take them away, don't make sleep all that much better.

I guess that sounds like a logical impossibility, but I think it works this way: if something in the complicated push-pull system of sleep and arousal has you tilted toward wakefulness, like a seesaw that's off-kilter, it takes very little to tilt the system more toward wakefulness, but a lot more to tip it toward sleep. Cutting out caffeine may damp down the arousal but still may not give you the neurological wherewithal you need for good sleep.

These days I drink one or two cups of green tea first thing in the morning (not black tea, which has twice the caffeine of green tea and sets my heart pounding). Most cups of tea contain less caffeine than most cups of coffee, though I suspect there is actually more caffeine in the tea I now drink than there was in the decaf coffee I gave up. But the effect is different: tea has something in it that damps down the stress response, whereas coffee gets the stress hormones flowing. Now when I wake up in the night, I don't feel that fist around my heart. You should know, too, that caffeine hides out in soft drinks and in pain medications. Chocolate has caffeine: never, if you have a sleep problem, drink hot chocolate before going to bed. (*That's* a rule!) These days when I need a pick-me-up before a class, I munch a few pieces of dark chocolate. It's a powerful stimulant.

People have wildly different responses to alcohol: a glass of wine makes Bob sleepy, but it perks me right up, so I've never been remotely tempted to use it for sleep. But many people do use it for sleep; in fact it's the substance most frequently used for insomnia. Alcohol is confusing: it picks you up and it puts you down; it stimulates the stress system and the release of cortisol, but it's also a depressant. Its initial effect is often soporific, though even when it seems to put you out, it gives you shallower sleep and more awakenings, and it breaks down into metabolites that come back to bite you later. It's strong stuff. It affects every organ and system in the body and has a powerful effect on sleep. If a pregnant woman drinks two glasses of wine, you can see the effect in the sleep patterns of the fetus. Even after alcoholics have abstained for months, their sleep continues to be impaired, and sometimes it never returns to normal.

When I read how the body responds to it—"From nature's point of view . . . alcohol is a poison to be eliminated as quickly as possible"—it makes me want to give it up entirely. But I live in a drinking world, and I enjoy social occasions more with it. (As I say, I do constant risk-benefit calculations.) When I drink, as I usually do on social occasions, I try to do it early in the evening, get that quick high, and then switch to fizzy water. If I put some hours between my last glass of wine and sleep, and if I drink no more than two glasses (white, that is, not red), I can get away with it. One glass more, and I wake up with a bad buzz and no chance of getting back to sleep. Usually, that is. Sometimes not.

I guess, in a way that's not helpful for anyone to hear, I'm sort of fatalistic about sleep. *Insomnia has a mind of its own,* as insomniacs often say:

> *It's really a crapshoot—there are nights I come in I'm so exhausted, and I hit the pillow and I'm wide awake. There are other times when I'm not very tired and I read in bed, which you're not supposed to do, and I sleep fine.*

My student Jill told me,

> *I'll have good patches and bad patches, and when I get into a bad patch, I can always find ways to explain it—it must have been this, or that—but "this" or "that" hadn't bothered me at all the week before. You can always find reasons, but I think it's rationalization, not reasons, and why it comes and goes is really mysterious. It makes me feel quite fatalistic.*

Insomniacs describe their insomnia as coming "out of the blue": *I'll be okay for a few days, and then, wham!, it's like somebody slipped caffeine into the calcium pill I take before bed.* And sometimes it doesn't come, just as unexpectedly. I'll never forget the Christmas Eve I drank nearly a bottle of champagne, ate several slices of ham and cake, and slept seven hours straight. "Figure out what you did that night and do it all the time," says my friend Stephanie, the gifted sleeper, who persists in believing that all I need to do is figure out what I'm doing wrong and I'll sleep like her.

"Oh, right." That much champagne is usually a disaster, sugar in the evening is a bad idea, and that much ham can't be good for anyone.

"You must have been relaxed and having a good time."

"I was, but so am I other times."

The sleep fairy came, that's all. Whether we sleep badly or not so badly on a given night seems often to be about some complex, invisible vagary of the inner weather, weather systems that are not on any maps we currently have, that may have to do with what we did the day before, who we saw, what we ate, what we dreamt, the time of month, the time of life, and a whole host of other things about which we know nothing at all. Which does not mean that insomniacs get to throw the rule book out and eat and drink whatever we please. On the contrary, we have to be extra careful because our sleep is so easily wrecked—though following the rules might not do us much good.

For Better or for Worse

"Get plenty of exercise" is a cardinal rule of sleep hygiene. But some studies find that exercise helps and some find that it has no effect. A recent review of many studies attributes these contradictory findings to the different methodologies used: researchers may mean different things by "exercise"; and some studies look at people who are fit, while others look at a more general population. (Few of the studies reviewed looked at women.) Or, it may simply be that exercise helps some people and not others. Anecdotal evidence points this way. I hear, *If I take a two-mile evening walk, I'm set for sleep.* I hear, *Exercise doesn't do a thing for me. I can be out all day, kayaking or skiing, come home, be exhausted, and lie there all night long.* I hear, *The harder I exercise, the worse I sleep.*

Studies suggest that exercise is most likely to help your sleep if you're in good shape. In order to make a difference, it has to be intensive enough to raise core temperature (inside body temperature) two degrees Fahrenheit for about twenty minutes, which happens with twenty to thirty minutes of aerobic exercise: this makes body temperature fall, four to five hours later, to lower than it would be if you hadn't exercised, and may increase deep sleep. Since only people who are in shape can sustain vigorous exercise for twenty minutes or more, they're the ones whose sleep is likely to be improved. (Though if this were the whole story, you'd think a hot bath would do as well.)

Sleep hygiene says we should exercise only early in the day, never close to bedtime. Yet studies don't show that this actually makes a difference. Early in the day? No way. That mellowed-out feeling that comes after a swim does me no good when I have most of a workday still to go. I usually swim from about 6 to 7 P.M., but if there's a pool available I'll swim as late as 1 A.M.; on days I can't swim, I take a two-mile walk up the hill behind my house, and this I also do very late. When I swim a late-night mile (but not when I walk), I'm hit by a wave of sleepiness an hour or two later and drift easily to sleep—though I still wake up two to four hours later; sometimes I can get back to sleep, and sometimes not. Mind you, walking and swimming (the way I do it) are fairly mild forms of exercise, and if you did a really vigorous workout so close to bedtime, you might get the stress hormones flowing and wreck your sleep.

Does exercise help? It helps some people dramatically. I know a woman whose insomnia disappeared when she started biking to work. I do think it's sometimes easier for me, on the days I swim a mile, to get back to sleep without a pill. But the correlation is not so simple, swim a mile and sleep better—yet I know that if I didn't exercise, I'd feel worse, and this would undermine my sleep. So, yes, I think exercise helps.

Here's a principle that's almost a rule, for me, anyway: leave sleep some space. When I plop into bed straight from one of those overscheduled, overcrowded days, with too much to do and too little time to do it, sleep doesn't come, or if it does, it's grudging sleep, ungenerous sleep. When I get into bed so wound up that I can't wait for the next day to come so I can get back to whatever I was doing, the sleep fairy declines to put in an appearance. Coy, she is. Capricious. She needs to feel wanted. Slight her, and she'll slight you. The times when there's too much going on in my life are the times when I most need to make a barrier between the day and bed, and of course, that's when it's hardest. But I must. And I can't allow bedtime to be the first quiet time I've had all day, the first time I'm alone with my thoughts to process the day's events. That way lies disaster.

As for the buffer zone you make between the day and sleep, there are as many kinds of those as there are people. Sometimes I use my late-night walks as a time to decompress. One woman wrote me, *Even stepping outside or onto a balcony to observe the night sky or the night is helpful. Some connection to the outside world.* I know what she means. I used to step outside every night just before bed, when I had a dog, and I did find it pleasant, the smells of the garden, the wind in the trees, the feel of the fog—never enough to put me to sleep, but soothing. Sometimes just tidying up can help, putting away books and papers, doing a few dishes, anything that makes closure to one day and space for the next. Bob plays the piano. That works well for him, rechanneling the neural networks away from the mind-bending work he does, into exertion that's physical but not too strenuous. On the other hand, Bob is a good sleeper and a good pianist, so what works for him might not work for others.

Many people use reading or writing as a way of unwinding. My student Tiffany says, *I can't go to sleep anymore unless I write before I go to bed. Writing quiets the voices, the static of the day. Otherwise I go to bed with voices in my head.* Not me, I don't want anything to do with words or to be anywhere near my computer, even for e-mails—it sets the babbler babbling (though I keep paper and pencil by the bed to jot down anything urgent; but if I keep writing things down, I know I'm not finished with the day). Some people make worry lists, write down every single thing that's bothered them in the course of the day, as the behavioral modification proponents recommend. Not me. When I write about something, I conjure it, bring it alive, and the last thing I want to do is dredge up every troublesome thing. If I've managed to sweep it under the carpet, let it lie. I want to let it go. No more words.

Reading is not my preferred way of unwinding. It's too much like work. No, give me visuals. I crave moving pictures, something that plants new images in my brain and exercises a part of my mind starved by the work I've done all day. When I was a graduate student, I'd watch *The Late Show* and sometimes the *Late Late Show,* and on bad nights, I'd hang in there through *Movies Till Dawn.* (Never in my bedroom.) Back in the days before videos, when we were at the mercy of whatever piece of crap was on the tube, there I'd be at 2 A.M. watching *Night of the Living Dead.* I didn't care, as long as it moved, as long as it wasn't words. And as the night droned on and the ads came thicker, there I'd be, trapped with "Cal Worthington and his dog, Spot." Cal wore a white cowboy hat and moved down the rows of Pontiacs and pickup trucks, slapping their hoods and blatting the price of each. His "dog, Spot" was a tiger on a leash. I'm sure the hours I spent with Cal would add up to months.

If a video or DVD isn't available (and it usually isn't), I'll read the paper. Sometimes I'll flip through one of the zillions of clothes catalogues that arrive in my mail, looking at the pictures. But whatever I'm doing, whether I'm on the couch watching a video or in bed reading or talking to Bob—I do it sitting up. I make sure not to lie down until I'm within minutes of sleep. (This is important, and I've never see it written about.) If I spend any length of time reclining in the evening, it seems to dispel the pressure to sleep, and I'm no longer tired when I try to sleep. If you're built like me, you have to guard, hoard, protect your sleep pressure, what there is of it. If I fall asleep watching a video, even for a few minutes, or if I'm drifting off and awaken just as I'm falling asleep, I don't get back to sleep for hours—all that good sleep pressure built up in the course of the day goes *poof,* up in smoke. I sometimes think coming wide awake after two to four hours may be about having an overly efficient recharge mechanism, not so efficient that it gets me through the day, but efficient enough to perk me up for hours. Not much is known about the way sleep energizes us, though it's known that even a short nap can be reinvigorating. I've found that just getting prone for a few minutes may do the trick: when I need to recharge before a class, it helps if I can lie down, close my eyes, and stretch out, just for a few minutes; it's almost as good as a nap.

Hot baths at night are nice, but tricky. The immediate effect of a hot bath is to energize me—if I'm tired and have to stay up later than I want, preparing for a class, I do it in the bath. But when I've allowed sufficient time after the bath to cool down, I have experienced that drop in temperature that's supposed to happen and, with it, sometimes a wave of sleepiness. And sometimes not.

Warm feet, cool room, this is a rule for me. If my feet are cold, I can't sleep. As experts tell us, the extremities need to be warm for core body temperature to drop. I also need to stop moving around—no more trips to the kitchen, nothing that raises temperature or heart rate. Whether to open the window and risk light and noise, or to keep it quiet and dark, and smother? More risk benefit calculations. When I'm alone I opt for the air, but Bob requires absolute darkness.

Lately we sleep apart more. He used to be such a quiet sleeper, but he's developed a snore. Also I seem to wake him more often—whether it's because his sleep is getting lighter or because I bounce around more, I don't know. There's always a lot of activity on my side of the bed. I'm in and out of bed or changing tapes on my walkman or changing its batteries or knocking a glass of water over on my way to a pill. Then once I know I've awakened him, I lie there not daring to move until I hear him breathe evenly again. It gets fraught. Some people find it soothing to sleep with a person who sleeps well. With us, it works the other way: after a few nights with me, his sleep is as wrecked as mine. It's easier apart, though we both feel the loss. According to the 2005 National Sleep Foundation poll, we're not alone: 20 percent of couples sleep apart on account of a sleep problem.

Sleep Stuff

Anything you can do to feel good about the place you sleep is worth doing—nice sheets, bedspread, décor. I keep my bedroom a clutter-free, work-free zone. For blankets, I use afghans my mother made. They're wonderfully bright, deep reds, purples, blues, and they remind me of her. They're also good because some are light and some are heavy, and I can layer them to make gradations between warm and cool, which I need, since my temperature is all over the place. After a lifetime of sleeping on a make-do mattress, I bought a high-end mattress, and it's one of the best investments I ever made; soft, yet firm, it makes getting into bed a real pleasure. I have an old down pillow so pliable that I can scrunch it down into nearly nothing. I hate those puffed-up monsters they give you in hotels; I stuff a sweater in a pillow case rather than break my neck on them. I've had my pillow forever, and I have no idea where I'll find another—I doubt that anybody makes pillows that can be so scrunched down. It's amazing, the number of things they don't make when it comes to sleep.

Why doesn't somebody begin a line of products for insomniacs? I don't mean those silly things—bath salts, oils, incense, aromatic candles, scented pillows, sachets—you find everywhere these days. Every time you turn around, there's somebody trying to sell you something that promises sleep: a silk jacquard eye mask from the Marquis de Shade; a traveling sleep kit from Chanel, with cashmere socks, a silk eye mask, and silk pillow, that sells for twelve hundred dollars; a mattress for a mere fifty thousand dollars. You can even purchase, in airports, malls, and midtown Manhattan, time in a nap pod, for a nap. No, I mean things that might actually be of use.

Like devices to darken a room. Every insomniac I know remembers that scene in the film *Insomnia* when Al Pacino, crazed by the midnight sun, gets out of bed and, looking haggard as only Pacino can, stares piteously through the thin shade at the glow of the Alaskan night. Then he drags every piece of furniture in the room, piece by piece, over to the window and begins stacking the furniture to block out the light. Most insomniacs have felt that desperate. Window shades, window blinds, miniblinds, even dark curtains just don't do it; sleep masks cling and annoy. In Europe, houses have blackout shutters; you reach out the window, pull them shut, and plunge the room into night. But in this country, we wake with the light, out of some Puritan compulsion to be up and doing. A blogger, European, finds this outrageous:

> With a huge proportion of the population working at night, why do windows have no blinds? . . . There are no built-in black curtains, or roll-down wooden blinds. It is difficult to find such curtains in stores if one wants to install one. What is going on? I have never seen, heard, read about, or experienced another country in the world in which sleep is not sacred and blinds are not an essential part of a house.

He sees this disrespect for sleep as related to Americans' denial that "sleep-need . . . exist[s]."

The world is a glaring, noisy place for the late sleeper or the light sleeper. My friend Roberta plastered tin foil over all her windows and

skylights, blotches of foil splattered throughout her beautiful new con-
dominium. She spent tens of thousands of dollars soundproofing her
windows. A guy I knew in graduate school bricked up his bedroom window in a fit of rage when he found that the double panes he'd installed
failed to muffle the sounds of Seventh Avenue. Bob carries thick black
felt curtains and pushpins when we travel. When we first met, he gave
me, for my birthday, a terrific present: he went to an art supply store and
an upholstery shop and got big pieces of cardboard, a can of black spray
paint, and some black felt. He cut the cardboard exactly to the size of the
bedroom windows, spray painted it black on both sides, and glued the
felt to the edges. He tucked this into my windows, and presto, total
darkness. I no longer wake with the sun. I've had fantasies about patent-
ing this device, whatever you call it, a sort of custom-made inner shut-
ter. I give the idea to you, for our new line of insomnia products.

The paraphernalia I need for sleep are, well, sort of legendary. "Just
take a toothbrush for this one night," said my friend Wendy the good
sleeper, when plans for a trip were getting complicated. Ha! That's like
telling a person with asthma, "Just breathe." When I travel, I pack a suitcase for the things I need and another suitcase for the things my sleep
needs: a white noise machine, a walkman with cassettes of books on
tape, extra batteries, flashlight, nightgown (in case it gets cold), socks for
my feet and a long black sock for my eyes, earplugs, and pills for all
contingencies—aspirin, ibuprofen, antihistamine, Ambien, Ativan or
Restoril, depending on whether I can get to sleep or what shape I'm in
when I wake up after two to four hours. I know it looks absurd, but it's
all useful, every bit of it. The white noise machine makes a lovely blanket like snow, muffling the sounds of dogs, doors, kids, and cars, providing a cocoon that makes it possible to sleep in a London hotel room
or in a small house when there's another human being moving about.
The flashlight enables me to get around in the dark without wrecking my
circadian cycle, such as it is. When you turn on the light, you chase away
whatever melatonin you have in you. Actually, it would be better to have
a flashlight with a red lightbulb, since red doesn't interfere with circadian
rhythms—another thing for our line of products. The long black sock is
to block out the light: I prefer a sock made of cotton or soft wool to any
sleep mask I've ever used: it rests delicately on the lids and the material
breathes better than synthetics. I also pack as many issues of the *New
York Times* as I can fit. If we're traveling by car, I take my pillow and
Bob packs his felt blackout curtains and pushpins; sometimes he even
takes these when we travel by air. I also need a glass of water. And a

banana, if there is one. An alternative doc I saw suggested that I eat before bed, recommending almonds or wheat germ and yogurt. I settled on a banana.

Noise in the Head

So once you've done all you can to make the external environment sleep-friendly, there's the internal environment to negotiate. The externals affect the internals, of course, as when I've worked too late and not made an effective barrier between the day and sleep—this is when I'm most likely to have things racing through my mind.

What sorts of things?

The "pre-sleep cognitive activity" of insomniacs is said to be "negatively toned, . . . more distressing" than that of normal sleepers, "more focused on worry," especially worry about falling asleep. We're said to be preoccupied with the negative effects of not sleeping, to engage in "excessive rumination about sleeplessness." "People with insomnia suffer unpleasant intrusive thoughts and excessive and uncontrollable worry during the pre-sleep period," reports U.C. Berkeley researcher Allison Harvey. Before sleep onset, "patients often describe disturbing *ruminative* thinking of guilt, fear of death, dependency needs, *obsessional* and angry thoughts, overt concern with bodily symptoms," says Eliot Weitzman, formerly director of the sleep center at Montefiore Hospital (my emphasis).

It's difficult to say what goes on in another person's mind—it's hard enough to say what goes on in one's own. But I don't think these descriptions actually fit my thoughts most of the time, and I don't hear many insomniacs describe their "pre-sleep cognition" in such unpleasant terms. My sense here is impressionistic and anecdotal—though I do have an inside track—but I'd say it's a lot more complex and not nearly so negative as these descriptions suggest. What mostly goes on in my head, when I first get into bed, is whatever I've been doing during the day or night, the conversations I've had, the classes I've taught, what's happening tomorrow: I'm like a windup toy that won't wind down. There are times, of course, when something's upsetting me or when I'm anxious about all the things I need to do—then the thoughts may become negatively charged. But more often they're neutral, and the only unpleasant thing about them is that they make too much noise to let me sleep.

I'm talking here about what goes on in my mind when I *first* get into bed, not what happens after I wake up and fail to get back to sleep: *then* it can get bad. There's a big difference between what goes on initially and what goes on later, though I don't see this distinction made in the research. Later is when the anxiety-provoking stuff is most likely to kick in—did I mail that letter of recommendation, did I remember to—and then if I lie there too long, the mind starts its scanning of past and future. I try to count my blessings, go over the good things in my life, but "thoughts leapfrog like evil imps, hell-bent on destruction," as Deborah Bishop and David Levy write. "Every silver lining has a cloud; no slight goes unforgotten." As Ilene says, the demons come out at night. They should not be paid the slightest heed, but it's hard to ignore them, they loom so large. The behavioral modification people are right: get up and do anything rather than let this go on. *Catastrophize* is the word they use; they say we do a lot of it, and that this is why we can't sleep. But this is another of those cart/horse, cause/consequence conundrums: do the dark and dire thoughts cause the insomnia, or do they arise as a result of it?

It seems to me that they're often a consequence. I can't help thinking that researchers *expect* to find insomniacs thinking about unpleasant things—because they believe we are depressed, obsessive, troubled, neurotic—and then, since people see what they believe, they find that we have unpleasant thoughts. As Allison Harvey says, "The tendency towards cognitive interference and worry for the insomnia group . . . is consistent with previous reports characterizing the personality style of the insomniac population as neurotic and obsessively worrisome." Given our "personality style," what else can you expect?

Researchers describe us as obsessive and ruminating. These words turn up often in the literature, used more or less interchangeably—though I don't think they actually mean the same thing. An *obsession* is an anxious, unwanted thought that's recurrent and intrusive. It comes from the Latin verb that means "to besiege" or "to occupy"; the word later took on association with haunting. *Ruminate* means "to chew repeatedly, to chew again what has been chewed slightly and swallowed," and, by extension, "to go over in the mind repeatedly," a term that suggests insomniacs are cud-chewing creatures, ruminants. Cud-chewing, mulling over, may not actually be unpleasant, if you happen to be a ruminant, which I am. That's part of the problem—I often find my thoughts too interesting to let go of, more interesting, certainly, than the blankness I need for sleep.

Obsession, on the other hand, is always unpleasant, at least for me. Everybody's obsessions take a different form, but mine go something like this: *I should have . . . , I shouldn't have . . . , why didn't I . . . , how could I have . . . , how could she have . . . , how dare she . . . , what if I were to . . . ?* This is a fretful state I can get into if something's really gnawing at me, and it's utterly destructive of sleep. "Consciousness then resembles a rat trap whose bars resound with every frenzied scrape of tooth and claw," says poet Walter de la Mare. Do most insomniacs live in this rat cage most of the time? The researchers seem to think we do. I know I don't—if I did, I'd never get to sleep. But I know people who do live there and sleep well: "I live with that gnawing more or less all the time," a friend tells me. "Sleep is the only thing that shuts it *off*. The tide comes in and I'm gone." *That's* sleep pressure!

To hear what insomniacs say about what keeps them awake is to hear of experiences more various and interesting than the researchers describe:

I'll start riffing and not be able to stop.

It's like I'm buzzing or humming or whirring away.

My mind's zinging around like a pinball machine, like billiard balls ricocheting one off the other.

My brain's flying like a trapeze artist from one thing to the next.

There's too much noise in my head, says my student Tiffany. *I can lie there all night long, just thinking about things—not bad things, often they're things I'm looking forward to—but I'll find myself still awake when it's getting light. I keep trying to find my mute button.* I like Tiffany's word *noise* better than *obsession* or *rumination*; it's more inclusive and more neutral.

My student Jill describes her mentation as "thinking":

I start thinking about something at night, and it's just impossible to get my mind to be quiet. I was told to read something really boring at night to put me to sleep. This was when I started reading philosophy.

Reading philosophy didn't lull Jill to sleep—it inspired her to major in philosophy (in addition to English; she was one of the best students I ever had). Insomnia has been called "the philosopher's disease," an affliction of people whose love of thinking makes it particularly difficult to shut down the brain. "Only dolts and drudges sleep," quips Isak Dinesen. "Weary with toil, I haste me to my bed/But then begins a journey in my head," writes Shakespeare in one of his sonnets. It would be nice to think that insomniacs were philosophers and Shakespeares, but I don't buy it. Some of the most high-wired, creative people I know have no trouble shutting off their thoughts, leaving them at the bedroom door, and sleeping peacefully through the night, and my whirring never tosses up anything worthwhile. No, my creativity comes when I'm rested, not when I whir.

I'm not sure what name I'd give to the experience that former poet laureate Billy Collins describes in his poem "Insomnia":

> even though the body is a sack
> of exhaustion
> inert on the bed,
> someone inside me will not
> get off his tricycle,
> will not stop tracing the same
> tight circle
> on the same green threadbare
> carpet . . .
> he keeps on making his furious rounds,
> little peddler in his frenzy.

Is this rumination? Is it obsession? Both these words suggest cognitive activity that's more, well, cognizant than Collins's frenzied circles, which seem to carry on almost independent of him. I don't have a word for it. Nor do I have a word for the tunes that get caught in Allan Berliner's head, that loop teasingly, endlessly, round and round, that he describes (and lets us hear) in his film *Wide Awake*—tunes that become so maddening that he fears listening to certain albums that might start them up.

"Replay" is what I'd call some of my presleep mental activity. When I was reading the plays of Christopher Marlowe for my PhD orals, I had iambic pentameter thundering through my head; as I write this book, the sentences that I've written by day play themselves again by night. *When I was studying Russian, I'd be conjugating Russian verbs all night long,* says my friend Sasha. When I come home from an interesting party, the conversations continue. I'm not thinking about them or *obsessing,* I don't think I'm *ruminating*—they're just humming away, like a washing machine caught in a cycle, churning on and on. If I've spent the evening with an Englishman, I'll hear British accents; if I've spent the evening with Italians, I'll hear Italian accents: *hear,* you understand, not in the sense of a voice speaking to me (I've heard a voice or two, and that's different)—yet the rhythms, the intonations, keep humming away, like those tunes Berliner can't get out of his head.

Occasionally the replay is visual. When I'm at a sleep conference, I'll shut my eyes and the PowerPoint presentations keep on flickering, dots of light bouncing over bar graphs and pie charts in blues, reds, and greens. One night after I'd scrubbed my dog down from an infestation of fleas, I closed my eyes and kept seeing little black dots that were dried flea carcasses, the suds and water running pink from the bloody bites. I'm not ruminating, mulling these things over, they just carry on, independent of thought, independent of *me,* it seems, like a visual or verbal imprint of whatever activity has been most intense during the day. Do other people get these? The replay, the afterglow, makes me wonder if there really is some neural mechanism that's slow to disconnect, some filter that's not screening out, some switch that doesn't flip off. These visuals are not at all like hypnagogia, the hallucinatory images that pop out of nowhere and morph into one another as I descend into sleep. Those release me from the day and lead to sleep; the images I'm describing here are the remains of a day that won't let go.

I don't think "obsessive rumination" begins to describe the things that go on in our heads. Since what goes on in my head can differ from one night to the next, from one time of night to the next, I assume there's an even wider range of experience from one person to the next. Sometimes it's visual or auditory replay, sometimes it's whirring or ricocheting, sometimes it's rumination and sometimes obsession, and sometimes it's things I don't have words for. And sometimes my mind will be quiet and blank, and I'll lie awake anyway: *I can be lying there, not upset about anything, just wide awake. Nothing on my mind, and nothing wrong that I know of. I can lie there till morning, not feeling bad—but when I hear the sound of the garbage truck, then I feel bad.*

It's hard to get the point across that a racing mind is not necessarily about being emotionally upset. One night, some friends were visiting us in the country. We'd stayed up late, talking around the fire, then everyone conked out and had a nice long sea-air-inspired sleep. Everyone but me, that is; I turned off the light and the conversations kept buzzing in my head, and I ended up taking a pill. The next morning, as everyone was talking about how they'd slept, a thing people my age do (or maybe my friends do it more around me), they were all amazed that I'd had trouble going to sleep. "But it was such a pleasant evening, such a nice day," they said, and it was: long walks, conversations by the fire. I was amazed that they were amazed. They'd known me so long, known about my sleep, and they still didn't get it, that I don't need to be emotionally riled up to not sleep.

Then one of my friends, who has a background in neuroscience, began speculating: "Sometimes when there's learning involved, there's a tendency to go over and over it."

"Yes, I can see this happening at a conference," I said, "but not last night. I don't even think I was going over it"—and I tried to explain my idea of the difference between rumination and replay. "Of course a psychologist might say that I'm just too insecure to let go of the day, that I have this neurotic need to hold on."

"Bah," he snorted, "that's psychology for you—make the individual the center and source of everything, refer everything back to intent, conscious or unconscious. Sleep is such a complicated system, so little understood. All you can say with certainty is that in some people, for some reason, things that should go off-line do not. How about having a little humility in face of mechanisms that are so far beyond our understanding, rather than referring the malfunction back to personality, making it all about you, your desire, your will?"

He has a point.

I think the problem has to do with language. I live so much with words, and I don't mean just because I'm reading and writing all day, though that's a part of it, but because I'm a babbler. I babbled in the crib, reciting at night the words I'd learned by day, and I've been babbling ever since. I have conversations with people, imagine their responses, compose e-mails, tell my classes things I forgot to say. I have words running through my head more or less all the time, not just at night, but driving across town, walking in the woods, sitting on the beach, getting into bed; it's as though the words have a life all their own, yammering away. Sometimes I think the only difference between me and those guys on the subway muttering to themselves is that I know how to keep my mouth shut, most of the time. When I tell people about this, I get some pretty weird looks, so maybe not everybody has all this stuff going on—or maybe they just don't tune it in.

Harvard sleep researcher Allan Hobson knows what I mean. "We talk to ourselves all the time," he writes. "We cannot imagine thinking without telling ourselves things; plans for the day, reactions to people, abstract analyses . . . fantasies." Hobson is not, to my knowledge, an insomniac, but novelist Anne Lamott is: "Left to its own devices, my mind spends much of its time having conversations with people who aren't there. I walk along defending myself to people, or exchanging repartee with them, or rationalizing my behavior, or seducing them with gossip, or pretending I'm on their TV talk show or whatever." In her novel *Unless,* Carol Shields describes "the lifelong dialogue that goes on in a person's head, the longest conversation any of us has. O hello, it's me again. And again. The most interesting conversation we'll ever know, and the most circular and repetitive and insane. Please, not that woman again! Doesn't she ever shut up?" No, says Shields, "she" never does shut up, which is why Shields reads novels, so she can escape her "own unrelenting monologue."

Maybe it's louder in some people than in others (loudest in writers?), but I bet it comes with the territory of being human. Man, the speaking animal, the babbling animal. No other creature is like this. Language is what makes us human. Language enables thought, the kind of thought that leads to further thought, that propels us forward to generalization, conceptualization, reflection. It serves us well, in most respects, pushing us to higher-order activities of abstraction and imagination, but then it gets out of control, it won't shut up, to the point that we can be sitting on an idyllic beach, and we go on babbling. The Buddhists call this "the chattering monkey" that scrambles from thought to thought. Lamott compares her inner chattering to a spider monkey tripping on acid: "I wish I could leave it in the fridge when I go out, but it likes to come with me."

Researchers tell us that *mentation,* as they call it, runs through the deepest parts of sleep: sleepers awakened from any stage of sleep report bits and pieces of thought. Maybe if you're not well endowed in terms of sleep pressure, if you don't have that mallet that descends and shuts it off, the noise gets too loud for sleep.

Is this clamor louder in writers than in other people? So many writers are insomniacs—Marcel Proust, Franz Kafka, Mark Twain, Alexandre Dumas, F. Scott Fitzgerald, Jorge Luis Borges, Rudyard Kipling, Victor Hugo, Edgar Allan Poe, Vladimir Nabokov, Charles Dickens, Joyce Carol Oates, Jacqueline Susann, Rick Bragg, Anne Lamott, maybe even Shakespeare—that it's almost an occupational hazard. (For all I know, I came by my insomnia just by hanging around this illustrious lot.) Do people who deal with words all day long sleep worse than people who deal with visuals—do artists have less insomnia than writers? It would be interesting to know.

And how can we get it to shut up?

Getting Quiet

Wherever it comes from, whatever the nature of the noise, you have to get it to quiet down before you can sleep.

The Buddhists use meditation to silence the monkey mind. I have had success with meditation, but not for sleep. I have had no success with the relaxation techniques that many people find effective, such as progressive relaxation, where you focus on tense muscles and try to relax them. When I draw my attention to specific body parts, it only makes me uncomfortably aware of these parts—*Damn, my left knee's hurting again,* and *Is that numbness in my toes?* I could never do breathing exercises, either, not even in yoga—*Breathe!* my instructor would tell me, when I'd freeze into a position. "Observe the breath," writes Dr. Weil. "Focus your attention on your breathing without trying to influence it in any way"—and I lose it right there: tell me to focus on my breathing, and I forget how to breathe. Bob swears that breathing exercises, done right, shut off the babble because, in order to think words, you need to be subvocalizing them, and when you draw breath across the vocal cords, it stops the subvocalizing. (I've come across this idea in sources besides Bob.) I believe in breathing; I recommend it. I just can't get the hang of it.

Some people have success with number games. Dement suggests starting with one hundred and subtracting seventeen, again and again. Not for me—too hard. Others do well with word games. A friend who has an occasional bad night (though is not an insomniac) describes the way she goes through the alphabet, finding words that end in "-ing." *Aching, buzzing, cramming, damming* come to mind. Not for me.

Some people find help in prayer. One woman is soothed by Psalm 4:8: "In peace I will both lie down and sleep; for thou alone. O Lord, makest me dwell in safety." She repeats it silently until sleep comes. She wrote me, *I've used this countless times during the middle of the night—and awakened hours later, thankful that it worked once more! It hasn't worked every time, but has worked more often than not. I've wondered why it's effective. Is it the rhythm and order of the words? Is it the selection of the words themselves, the "dwell in safety" that soothes me?* A friend finds comfort in Psalm 127, "He giveth His beloved sleep." (Hmmm . . . that means, to be without sleep is to be unbeloved? Oh well, whatever works.) She also finds comfort in a poem by Teresa of Avila: *I recite this in the dark watches of the night: Nothing distress you, nothing afright you, everything passes, God will abide. . . . Nothing distress you, cast fear away.* Secular kinds of poetry can also be soothing: *The rhythm can soothe your brain.* I'm reminded of a Renaissance folk remedy, "repeating some well-known rhyme until the monotony produces the desired unconsciousness." Maybe anything helps that tempers that staccato, jazzed-up beat we get into, that brings us back to slower, more regular rhythms, more like our breath and heart.

My friend Cynthia tells me about the Heart Sutra, otherwise known as the Maha Prajnaparamita Hridaya Sutra, which goes like this:

> Avalokitesvara Bodhisattva when practicing deeply the Prajna Paramita
> perceives that all five skadhas are empty
> and is saved from all suffering and distress.
>
> Shariputra, form does not differ from emptiness,
> Emptiness does not differ from form.
> That which is form is emptiness, that which is emptiness form.
> The same is true of feelings, perceptions, impulses, consciousness.
>
> Shariputra, all dharmas are marked with emptiness.
> They do not increase nor decrease. Therefore, in emptiness, no form, no
>   feelings, perceptions, impulses, consciousness.

It goes on for four more verses, a tantalizing combination of the familiar and the unfamiliar, ending "gate gate paragate parasamgate bodhi svaha." Cynthia has spent time in Buddhist monasteries, so the sounds are resonant for her; but it seems like too much effort to me. Anyhow, I don't want anything to do with words.

No, it's visuals I want. When an image drifts by, I try to follow it. Whether it's full-blown hypnagogia or just an odd wacky image like a fragment off a dream, visuals signal sleep. I scan my interior for an image and try to stay with it, ride it to sleep. Visuals are the friends of sleep, and words are the foes. Words keep me caught in my babbling and "managing" self, whereas images are surrender, a sign that sleep is near. Anything that releases me from words into visuals leads to sleep.

If you have any talent for visualization, develop it. I do not, but I'm told it can be a powerful tool. I have tried visualizing the things you're supposed to, a babbling brook, a path through a forest, sunlight dappling the mossy floor, I've tried to dwell lovingly on the details of the scene, as we're told to, but then I go tripping off onto the walk we took last Sunday, or how the redwood tree out back is looking sickly, and the thoughts flood back. Now that I know a little about what goes on in the brain, I can sometimes picture—I know this sounds silly—my thalamus and cortex chattering back and forth. I imagine the two of them buzzing away like unruly students, and I think, "All right, you guys, pipe down," and it's comforting to know it's only me making that ruckus, and I imagine the thalamocortical looping, looping slower, slower, winding down, slower, stiller, and the mind going quiet, allowing sleep to come. "You can rest now," I tell my brain. And give yourself some time to quiet, it doesn't happen all at once, not for some of us. It's like getting into a pool, moving into a different medium, easing yourself in. Maybe for the young and athletic the sudden plunge, but not for me.

And if that doesn't help, here's a visualization technique that often does.

I picture a little man in white overalls, cartoon caricature of a house-painter, baggy pants, cap wedged down around his ears, carrying a bucket of paint. He shuffles out, climbs a few steps up a ladder and paints slowly, deliberately, on a blank white billboard, a big number 100. I follow the movements of his paintbrush with the movements of my eyeballs, tracing the shape of the number through closed lids. When he's done, he turns the page and paints 99. Again, I make my eyes follow his brushstrokes, stubbornly, doggedly, as he paints 98, 97, 96. I make myself pay attention. He's here to help me—I have summoned him, put him to the trouble of coming from a long way. I must concentrate. It is unbelievably boring, so much less interesting than the e-mails I want to compose, the conversations I want to continue. But I know if I don't attend to him, I'll lie there all night chattering away, whereas if I can make myself follow his brushstrokes as he paints 95, 94, 93, then sometimes, miraculously, by the time we get to 80, my breathing slows, and I can feel myself float down, down, to a quieter place, where the babble stops and the images begin.

Now when I go to bed with a racing mind, I summon this little man. He patiently returns, with his ladder and bucket, and sets about his job, painting 100, 99, 98, and so on down. It may also be that the movement of my eyeballs as I trace his brush back and forth is part of the effect, for the same reason that EMDR (the eye movement technique described earlier) has an effect, whatever reason that might be. You're welcome to him, if you can summon him, though he may be mine alone. Maybe we each need our own version of this, a technique that combines concentration and visualization in whatever proportion works for us, whether it's word games, number games, beautiful scenes, or my little man.

After First Sleep . . .

I just assume I'm going to wake up after my "first sleep," as it was once called. That way, I'm not so disappointed or angry when I do. When I used to have expectations about sleeping through the night, I'd get exasperated, and that would make it worse.

To pee or not to pee? That is the question. (Sorry about that dreadful pun—and sorry, too, about these details. It is embarrassing, sleeping in front of strangers, but if I thought that night at the clinic was strange, writing this chapter is stranger.) Okay, so, sometimes it's clear that I need to pee—when I've sat up late the night before, over wine or fizzy water or herb tea, or I've eaten a ton of watermelon, there's no doubt about it. But lots of times it's not so clear, times when I get up to pee and it doesn't amount to much, so to speak. I'm perfectly capable of holding it seven hours when I've had a sleeping pill, so I doubt this is what's waking me up, most of the time. But once I'm awake, I start thinking that I need to, or I ought to, just to get it over with—and then by the time I get back into bed, I'm wide awake. Why can't I just ignore this impulse and turn over and go back to sleep? (If I'm really exhausted, I sometimes can.) *Nocturia*, as it's called, becomes a problem as we age. The bladder, of course, shrinks with age, but something else may be going on. Urine formation normally slows at night, and whatever it is that slows this formation seems to wear out with age. I asked Phyllis Zee, a sleep researcher at Northwestern University, if there was research about this in relation to sleep, and she said there was hardly any. Something I've heard that has worked for some people is "bladder training," which teaches a way to stretch the bladder's capacity. A friend tells me of a method that works for him: he takes a long hot bath just before dinner and it dehydrates him so that he doesn't need to get up during the night. Without his bath, he wakes up after four or five hours; with it, he sleeps eight hours straight. But it has to be before dinner, not after, and the water has to be hot, and he has to stay in it for at least a half hour. The idea of a hot bath before dinner doesn't much appeal to me, so I've never tried it. But it works for him.

I don't know how anybody can turn the clock to the wall, as the behaviorists tell us to. I have to know where I am in the night, to know what stories to tell myself, what techniques to use, what pill to reach for. I find it's actually better to wake up after three hours than four or five, because there's a chance of getting back to sleep; with four or five hours, there's not enough sleep pressure left to put me back under. What matters is not the clock, but that I not clench my mind into anxiety. If the clock has that effect on you, by all means, turn it to the wall, but for me it's more anxiety-producing not to know what time it is.

What matters is that I not let my mind kick in, not start making lists of things I need to do, and above all, not start up with self-recriminations:

I shouldn't have had that second glass of red wine, I shouldn't have had a second bowl of popcorn. . . . Cynthia, who says the Heart Sutra, tells me she tries to "stay in the dream": *When I get up to pee, I try to stay in the dream. If I start to think, I'm lost. A thought to an insomniac is like a drink to an alcoholic. Don't have one.*

There's a thing I sometimes do: I put on hand lotion—I mean, I really rub it in. I keep a bottle of nice-smelling lotion by the bed, and when I'm having a hard time getting back to sleep, I rub it on, slowly, deliberately, grasping one hand with the other, firmly, working it in. Bob says I look like Lady Macbeth trying to wash away my bloody deeds, but I find it comforting. It grounds me. It may be like other techniques I've heard about, such as finger cradling: *Hold your thumb by wrapping your other hand gently around it, hold three to five minutes, then hold the index finger, and so on.* . . . Or a yogic technique, *place the tip of your tongue just above your upper teeth and hold your tongue there.* According to Yoga philosophy, explains Andrew Weil, "this contact closes an energy circuit in the body, preventing dissipation of *prana* [spirit]." Or, *place the palms of both hands on the tummy, makes it nice and warm [and] sort of anchors you in place.* Another version of this might be the eye pillow some people like, *for the soft weight it puts on the eyelids and the sweet smell of herbs. . . . It droops gently over my tired eyes. . . . I feel soothed.* I've tried these things, and I can see how they might help; but I like the lotion. (Also, I have dry hands.)

One study found that babies snugly blanketed (swaddled) sleep longer and wake less often than babies who aren't. There is even a "swaddler/sleep sack" you can buy, "created after the inventor watched her daughter suffer countless sleepless nights because of the involuntary startle reflex, known as Moro Reflex." Maybe grown-ups need swaddling, too. I talked to a woman who told me that wrapping herself tightly in blankets helped her sleep. Maybe anything that makes us feel less free-floating in the universe will help. The startle reflex is thought to disappear at a few months of age, but it doesn't seem to disappear for everyone: many adults recognize that experience of *being startled awake just as I'm drifting off.* (This used to happen to me, but no more.)

On nights when my mind kicks in and the wheels start spinning, and the little man with the paint brush lets me down—I turn to books on tape. Many people get up at this point and read or pay the bills or clean the house. I used to do things like that, but these days, unless I'm ready to give up on sleep, I do not, because once I'm up and doing, I'm up for the duration; also, it's cold and depressing to get up. Sometimes, if it's not too cold,

I turn on the light and read the paper, but I won't get out of bed to do it. Even turning on the light to read is dicey: I'll read, and read, and the sky grows light and I'm still reading. For me, it's best to stay in the dark.

Listening to recorded books is a way of changing the channel without turning on the light. On nights when my mind is revved up, I'll start listening right away, but most nights, I leave it for after first sleep. Having a book on tape to listen to takes the edge off the loneliness of waking in the night, and makes the time less dead and wasted. I tell myself, I'll just see what happens next, in this little world. . . .

I am hopelessly addicted to these things. But it's not so easy to find a tape that's right for sleep. You need just the right kind of story, interesting enough to engage the mind but not so interesting that you need to stay awake to see how it comes out. No page-turners or cliff-hangers, nothing too exciting (*Seabiscuit* got moved out to the car). Nothing with violence or physical awfulness. But it can't be boring, or my mind slips back to my own story. The reader has to have a soothing voice. Women are best, especially British women—their voices are breathier and softer. But they must read at the right pace, not rush through the material. And no shouts or songs or that dumb mood-setting music—it startles me awake; those tapes get moved to the car, or ditched if the music is annoying enough. Novelists who work especially well for me are Jane Austen, Anita Brookner, Penelope Mortimer, Ian McEwan. Memoirs are great because they're not plot-driven: Ivan Doig's *This House of Sky*, a lovely lyrical book about growing up on a sheep ranch in Montana, Nuala O'Faolain's *Are You Somebody?*, Rick Bragg's *All Over But the Shoutin'*, Russell Baker's *Growing Up*, Alexandra Fuller's *Don't Let's Go to the Dogs Tonight*, Bob Smith's *Hamlet's Dresser*. The language is interesting, the characters are engaging, and it doesn't much matter if you fall asleep and miss a scene; you can wind it back and pick it up later. If it's well written, I'm happy to listen to it again. I get to know some of these books quite well, though in a lopsided sort of way: the first part of a tape, I hear over and over; the last part, I may never hear at all. My friend Carol Neely uses recorded books like this, and we've thought about writing blurbs: "This book is great for putting you to sleep." It doesn't sound like a compliment, but it is: it means the book keeps the mind engaged, is sufficiently interesting moment to moment that you're not hanging on to find out what comes next.

Carol listens to biographies, Doris Kearns Goodwin's *Franklin and Eleanor* and David McCullough's *Truman*. She loves them because "they go on forever; they're well written and interesting and you know how it turns out, so there's no suspense." What's great is that there are so many different kinds of readings on tape, mysteries, histories, romances, inspirational, historical. Something for everyone.

Eric Zorn, columnist for the *Chicago Tribune,* uses cassette recordings of talk radio programs. "I find those meditation thingys very distracting—'think of a peaceful beach . . .'—and too much work. Try something that truly takes your mind away, like a big screaming match on immigration or abortion or gun control." He says, "I try not to fall asleep. I try to pay attention to the conversation, follow it carefully, engage in the topic. The next thing I know it's morning and I am rested and refreshed." (This is what the behaviorists mean by *paradoxical intention*.) A respondent to Zorn's blog says, "Nature programs work, too. I have a tape about backyard bird-watching that I've never seen more than five minutes of." One man swears by the Golf Channel.

Not for me: I need a story. I know, I've said words are the enemies of sleep, and here I am listening to all these words. But as long as it's someone else's words, someone else's story, interesting, engaging, but not too exciting, it's okay. Listening to tapes does, of course, create problems, like when I wake up with the wires of the earphones wrapped around my neck, or when I've slept on the wires and they've etched creases down my face—which do not disappear as rapidly as they used to. (If there's nobody with you, you can use a cassette recorder that doesn't need earphones or wires.) And it's a costly habit—I go through about a tape a month, and that's with playing them over and over. I've exhausted entire catalogues. I'm forever scrounging around stores, libraries, yard sales, looking for just the right tape that combines the soothing and the interesting. I'm never happier than when I've just found something wonderful that's really long: Richard Ford's *Independence Day,* Richard Russo's *Empire Falls,* Curtis Sittenfeld's *Prep.* Some are so well performed that they become like a theater in my head. Sometimes the images work their way into my dreams, and I wake not knowing whether the drowning was in the story or in my dream. When I come to the end of one of these long, absorbing novels, I feel bereft, the way I used to feel when I was a kid and finished a novel and was sure I'd never find another I'd like so well; I'd wander around feeling lost until I did. Books have always kept me company, ever since I can remember, but my life as a grown-up leaves me no time to lose myself in them the way I once did. Only insomnia allows this.

Listening may work as well as those punishing routines the behaviorists insist on, where you drag yourself out of bed and stay in another room until you feel sleepy. The study by Ruth Davies that I referred to earlier instructed subjects, when they couldn't fall back asleep after ten minutes, to sit up in bed and read or listen to the radio or watch television—that is, do something that took their minds off their thoughts, though they could stay in bed doing it. Their sleep was significantly improved after four weeks, and was still better a year later, and they hadn't had to regularize or restrict sleep. The crucial thing is to get the mind to stop churning, and anything that can change the channel from your own story onto someone else's may do the trick.

If you love books and don't have time for them in your life, I highly recommend this as a way of getting through insomnia. I've scandalized purists by saying I prefer listening to reading—an English professor, letting down the cause of literature! But I'm not letting it down: in a world where people have so little time for books, listening may save literature. Actually, literature began as a spoken form, with Homer reciting *The Iliad* and *The Odyssey*. Homeric epic, Greek tragedy, Renaissance drama, these were high points of literature, and they were taken in by the ear, not the eye. Most of Shakespeare's original audience did not know how to read—his works were meant for the stage, not the page. Why any author would object to having a novel recorded (as some do), I have no idea: surely it's the prejudice of a print-bound culture to imagine that reading is superior, when hearing is a more direct and immediate way of taking things in (it's certainly been around a lot longer); the sounds and rhythms of words have a far more elemental power and appeal than print on a page. When I want to study a book, learn what's in it, I need to see the words; but for pleasure, let others be bookworms, I'll be a tapeworm.

"There's not a parent who doesn't know the value of a good snoozy story to help lull the little ones to sleep (or make that cranky transition a little easier)," writes a *New York Times* reviewer of children's books. It's a primal pleasure, being read to—it evokes what Anne Lamott calls "the listening child" in us. I'm hooked—and it's a technique I can recommend unequivocally. It can't hurt you, unless you blunder onto a page-turner and lie awake all night to find out who dunnit; then you'll curse me. Otherwise, it's harmless; no side effects.

But there's a technological crisis looming: what to do when there are no more cassettes? All the companies are going over to CDs and iPods, which are useless for dozing to books and not much use even for listening to books, I'm told. Tapes work for sleep because they stop at the end of forty-five minutes, so it's easy to wind your way back to where you were before you fell asleep. But CDs and iPods just keep on going, so you wake up all the way at the end of the book or else lie there worrying about switching it off when you feel yourself getting sleepy. You can't keep track of where you are or manage the controls in the dark, and any aggravation like this wakes you up. Fiddling with the controls of the iPod while driving is, I'm told, worse than aggravating—it's extremely hazardous. Bob has been downloading books from the Web onto CDs and recording the CDs onto cassettes for me to sleep to and for himself to listen to while on the road. But even the equipment to play tapes won't be around much longer. Many listeners, not just insomniacs, are squeezed out by the new technologies.

Please, some entrepreneur, save the book on tape. Or improve the technology of the iPod so that a person listening to a book can listen easily in the dark. People like us are a market, too—and a big one.

Ambivalences

I love to hear about people who have found imaginative ways of getting through their sleepless nights, with yoga or meditation or music or the Internet. One woman tells me she views insomnia as "an opportunity":

> I take to heart a belief that James Hillman expressed in the August 2000 issue of THE SUN. He says insomnia demands a whole new approach, one of looking at those quiet, dark hours as a time to deal with our demons . . . "a chance to meet the other world." I write, study, meditate, read whatever current spiritual guidance book I'm concentrating on.

Another woman, a physician, writes of the years when she was raising children and not getting enough time to herself during the day: *If the only time for myself was 2–4 A.M., I took it. Once I understood that I was waking up because I needed the time, I didn't fight it.* She says that she sometimes sees a patient who does this too: *I do see women and a rare man who can acknowledge that that's the only time they get to read a book or choose what they'll watch on TV.*

One of my favorite stories is told by Lorna Sage in her memoir, *Bad Blood*. When she was ten, she "stopped sleeping, partly from a permanently blocked nose . . . that made it very difficult to breathe." The family doctor "told me that I should consider myself lucky, since I had much more time than people who slept; and he told my mother that she should let me have the light on all night. So he gave me—gave me back—the company of Tarzan . . . and Sherlock Holmes. . . . Remembering his magic words, I'd look out in the dead of night across the countryside, when not another light was burning, and practise feeling pleased with myself." Sage found other advantages too: "Boys and homework were supposed to be incompatible," but since she was insomniac, she had time for both and still came out at the head of her class.

I'm not sure how generalizable her experience is—she was a kid, not a grown-up with grown-up responsibilities, and when she did grow up, she found her way to a fairly freelance existence. She was also exceptionally gifted. I met her once, and she seemed to be one of those Amazing People who moves on an altogether higher plane. But what is generalizable about her experience is that it is always more helpful to see the glass as half full than half empty. This assumes, of course, that you have a glass, that you have something to put in it, and that you have some choice about how to view it—which assumes a lot. If you're working two jobs to put bread on the table, you may not have a lot in that glass or a lot of latitude about how to view it. But if you have any choice, go with the "full." The effect of attitude on sleep has been highly exaggerated, but attitude does make a difference.

If you choose not to get up and do something else, think of it as a choice, not an affliction. Tell yourself how lucky you are *not* to have to get out of bed, how lovely and restful it is to be lying here in the dark, all these nice healing hormones. Feel how good it feels to straighten your back, stretch out long, close your eyes, how lovely the dark; you can rest now, brain, quiet down. "Bear free and patient thoughts," a benediction from Shakespeare's last play, are words I try to remember. Don't lie there cursing your insomnia. Anger has its uses, but not for sleep. And don't let anything I say feed that fire. I've said a lot of dire things in this book (and meant every one), but it's best not to dwell there, if you can help it. Don't go counting up your sleep debt or reckoning the damage done you by your sleepless nights. Nobody knows how the sleep debt works, but it certainly doesn't pile up infinitely or we'd be dropping like flies.

In "The Haunted Mind," Nathaniel Hawthorne describes the time between sleeps as a time of quiet meditation, "an intermediate space, where the business of life does not intrude; where the passing moment lingers, and becomes truly the present": "If you could choose an hour of wakefulness out of the whole night, it would be this." I wish I knew a way to get back to that mellow state our ancestors seem to have enjoyed. I'm sure it helped to have a quieter, less complex life, but it's not like they had nothing to do—and that's what it takes for me, having nothing to do. Then I can glimpse, I can almost imagine enjoying that state between sleeps. But such times are rare, and to tell you the truth, I think I'd rather they be rare. I'm not good at doing nothing.

"I have been one acquainted with the night," writes Robert Frost. As I contemplated the possibility of trying to become "a normal person," I realized how much I'd miss the night, how bereft I'd feel if I never again got to linger in the late-night hours. Night is when the phone doesn't ring, when the boom boxes and the barking dogs (or most of them) quiet down, when the cars go away, when the world is mine. Night is when the light doesn't distract, when the other senses come into play and I can smell the earth and grass and hear the wind in the trees. There is a moment between when the last sounds of night die down and the first sounds of morning start up, a pause when all goes still, even in my urban corner of the world, when I feel suspended, free of time that's so stern a taskmaster during the day. There are nights in the country, when I'm alone with the crickets or the frogs, that I see the beauty of night, and times, on a stretch of summer nights, when I've drifted so free of the world's time that I don't care if I'm still up when the sky turns light, because there's nothing I need to do—nothing but pull down the shades and check out till noon. And I'm not sorry to miss the morning; it seems too brassy, busy, intrusive.

Nighttime is writers' time. Novelist Joyce Carol Oates writes, "When the house is dark and quiet and the entire world turned off for the night, it's a marvelous feeling to be there alone, with a book, or a blank piece of paper. . . . Such moments of solitude redeem all the rushing hours, the daylight confusion of people and duties." Night, she says, "is synonymous with imagination and freedom and solitude—everything you need to be creative—and so I've come to regard my insomnia as something very positive. The night self is a creative self. There is a nocturnal personality, a nocturnal spirit, distinct from that of daylight and available only in solitude." Filmmaker Alan Berliner says this: "The middle of the night is my special haven, the time I do anything I consider really important. . . . I make my films in the silence and solitude of the night . . . the night not only becomes my best friend, but also a source of inspiration." My student Tiffany tells me, *I do my best creative writing at night, between 1 and 4 A.M. Maybe because I'm so tired, it takes away the inhibition. I think in some ways insomnia is my friend—I wouldn't have written the pieces I'm most fond of, without it. I'd have slept through those creative moments.*

Some friend. Fine, if you're up to it, but for creation, I need clarity, I need energy. Late night hours are not my best. Night, I can sometimes call a friend, when there's nothing pressing the next day, but I do not forget those nights I could have howled with rage at being awake, nor the days that followed, bleak, raw, ruined days that would add up to years, days when I needed wits and energy but was stupid as a stump, mornings I'd look in the mirror and think, *This can't go on.* No, insomnia's no friend of mine.

I have no last word, no final pronouncement, on this subject, but I see that even to glimpse the possibility of making peace means I must be feeling better. I wish I could tell you it's meditation that's made the difference, but it's medication, better drugs that enable me to patch together a full night's sleep. It may also be more possible to think such thoughts because I'm on sabbatical as I write this and also because I'm closer to retirement than I've ever been. But I have a jumble of contradictory feelings about that, too. I don't want to stop working, I want to be out there in the world; it's what I've done all my life, it's what I do best. I know I should be better at cultivating my garden, smelling the roses, but that's not who I am.

Also, I know that insomnia is highest among the retired.

But since it is high among the retired, I'll tell this story Ilene told me, about a retired neighbor of hers, recently widowed. "'Poor old Sophie,' I'd think—I'd see her light on at 4:30 in the morning, and I'd think, 'She must be so depressed.' She'd spend her evenings drinking wine, then she'd sleep a few hours, get up, and watch movies. But then I asked her how she was doing, and she said, 'Fine,' she was fine—'When Harry was alive, I always had to go to bed and get up early, on his schedule, and I hated it. Now I get to stay up and see the movies *I* want to see—any time I want to see them.'" Ilene said her assumption that Sophie was unhappy made her realize how easy it is to pathologize a life that deviates from the norm. "I was pathologizing it, but if you can get away from the tyranny of thinking, You have to live like this or be like this, on a regular schedule like the rest of the world, it might be a great help."

I had been telling her what I'd learned about sleep in premodern times and other cultures. I'd been speculating that it might help to know that we of the broken sleep are part of a long and honorable tradition, that people in other times and places have slept in irregular ways. She leapt at this as something that might help her patients: "I think it would help enormously if people didn't have to feel, when they lie awake nights, that they're crazy—these may be natural sleep patterns asserting themselves. So what if they're biologically deficient, compared to some young-healthy-male norm—if the world weren't so rigid, it wouldn't be a problem."

I think she's right. So what if your sleep is odd and eccentric? If you don't have to work nine to five, and if you can patch together enough sleep to get by, why feel you have to hop to the world's tune?

I don't know what to tell you if you have to get the kids off to school or get to an early job. I didn't know what to say to Alan Berliner, whose film *Wide Awake* presents this dilemma, who has a wife and a new baby who inhabit "a different time zone" from his own, a wife who says, "This has to change." But I do know that we all, we insomniacs, have to find a way of making terms with it, find a story we can live with, hang in there and hope that researchers will someday learn why sleep is so difficult for us and come up with therapies that work more effectively, more individually, for us. And meanwhile, do our best to find the consolations, the things that are pleasurable—the quiet, the reading, the loveliness of night—and, perhaps, even, some will find inspiration.

My usual pattern these days is to wake up after two, three, or four hours, take a reading of how likely sleep is to come again, judging by what time it is, what's on my mind, how fast my heart is beating, what I have to do the next day, and whether the first part of sleep has been deep or light (if it's been light, it will only get worse). If there's a chance of getting back to sleep, I'll reach for my walkman and try to ease myself back by listening to a book, and if that doesn't work, I nibble off three to five milligrams of Ambien or take three grams of Xyrem, either of which will give me two to four more hours. When I'm midweek in the middle of a term, I don't usually go through these deliberations; I just reach for a med. When I'm at a conference, I usually take something when I get into bed. I don't like being so dependent on drugs, but I'm resigned to it. It's more realistic than to imagine I can beat myself into a regularity that's no part of me.

Sometimes I think, well, nobody really knows the cumulative effects of these drugs, or the cumulative effects of insomnia, for that matter. Since nobody knows, might as well assume the best, and if it's killing me, the insomnia, the medications I take for it, well, something has to. We none of us get out of this world alive, as a New York cabbie once said to me. You can live with this thing. I have lived with it, not gracefully or as well as I might have lived without it (though that might be a delusion), and who knows for how long I'll live with it. But I get by.

CHAPTER 12

Making Change

What do we have to do to get people to take sleep seriously?
I mean, not just our friends and families, but our bosses, too,
and the people who are looking after our health?

We need a good sleep researcher who might be interested in
all the bits and pieces we know among us, who could help us
put it all together.

There are so many questions that are not being looked at—if
only we had the resources.

Emmanuel Mignot

When my friend Megan spent eight days in a hospital recovering from
major surgery, she couldn't sleep the whole time she was there, not because she was in pain but because it was, as she said, the noisiest place
she'd ever stayed. "The nurses were yakking away all night long, they left
the door wide open, and if I ever managed to get to sleep, someone would
come in and turn on the light, beepers going off, carts rattling by, I
couldn't believe it—how are you supposed to get better, if you can't
sleep?" Nighttime noise levels in patients' rooms get as high as 113 decibels (as loud as a jackhammer); in the intensive care unit, 55 decibels is
usual, about the level of a busy street corner, with spikes up to 80 (a
blender a foot away is 100).

Sleep researchers have been trying to wake up health care professionals to the importance of sleep. They've campaigned to get better hours
for residents, and in 2003, the Accreditation Council for Graduate Medical Education passed a rule limiting residents' hours to an eighty-hour
work week with a maximum of twenty-four hours per shift, ten hours
off between shifts, overnight on-call duty no more than every third night,

one day off per week. But "the new self-imposed rules . . . haven't brought about fundamental change and haven't changed the length of a typical extended shift, which is still four times as long as a normal workday," warns Charles Czeisler, head of the Division of Sleep Medicine at Harvard Medical School. "On this kind of schedule, virtually everyone is impaired." And how do we get doctors to pay attention, when medical textbooks and curricula continue to leave sleep out? "Physicians aren't being trained to recognize sleep disorders," says Czeisler, who notes that in Harvard's four-year curriculum only one semester hour is devoted to sleep medicine. The last time I went for a physical, I noticed that there is still no question about sleep on the routine forms patients fill out.

The National Sleep Foundation has campaigned to get high schools to start later, so that adolescents might actually stay awake for their classes, and it has had some success—in a few school districts. But how to get teenagers to take on fewer jobs, when they're working to buy a car, a cell phone, an iPod, to have and to do all the things that seem so much more urgent than sleep? You may warn parents to take the sleep complaints of their children seriously, caution them that sleep problems may lead to academic problems, drug and alcohol abuse, but will they hear you, when they themselves are so caught up in the frenzy of having and doing it all that they don't take their own sleep seriously?

The National Sleep Foundation has made valiant efforts to raise public consciousness about the hazards of sleepy workers and drowsy drivers, to get transportation departments to adopt more sensible guidelines for truck drivers so that those eighteen-wheelers hurtling down the highway aren't driven by truckers who might as well be drunk. Long-haul drivers sleep on average 4.8 hours, night haulers, 3.8 hours. "The percentage of truck drivers who are exhausted is frightening," says William Dement; "the transportation system is really out to lunch on the danger of this issue."

"It's not true that sleep is on a back burner," Dement told me a friend once said to him. "It's not even on the stove."

There is some urgency to getting it on the stove, in view of the epidemics of diabetes and obesity that are walloping the health care system and the tsunami of aging that's about to hit. More than half of all those who ever lived past seventy are alive today; by 2050, one in five people will be sixty or older. This is a demographic change unprecedented in history. "Aging in place," keeping people healthy and independent enough so they can stay in their own homes and out of nursing homes, will be crucial to society's weathering the coming storm, experts say. Insomnia puts us at greater risk for being placed in nursing homes.

Sleeping well is as key to society's aging well as it is key to an individual's aging well. Policy makers would do well to pay it some attention.

Let's think in this chapter about what we might do—and my "we" includes insomniacs, physicians, researchers—to get sleep and sleep disorders on the stove.

On a Personal Level

We insomniacs need first to be clear in our own minds that insomnia is not something we're bringing on ourselves—unless, of course, we are bringing it on ourselves, by eating, drinking, stressing ourselves more than our systems can take, in which case we need to change what we're doing, insofar as we can. Once we've modified our behavior to the best of our abilities, we need to ditch the idea that insomnia is something that's happening to us because we're weak-willed or morally deficient. We need to come out of the closet and own up to this problem, communicate with friends, family, co-workers, colleagues, doctors that this is a serious condition, debilitating, depressing, dangerous, that even though we may look okay to them, we may *not* be okay. We are dragging an invisible weight up an invisible hill, and if it looks like we're letting down our side as a worker, a spouse, a parent, well, there's this weight, there's this hill. People don't want to hear about our problems—they have problems of their own—so it's tricky. We need to find a way of saying, "Look, this is real, even if you can't see it, and no, it's not going to go away if we take a hot bath or quit worrying," while not being in their face, not sounding like we're asking for special dispensation.

The workplace is a daily challenge when you can't count on sleep. Since insomnia is not seen as a disability—sleep is not, as we saw, defined as one of the "major life activities" protected by the Americans with Disabilities Act—we need to appeal to employers, fellow workers, and colleagues for their understanding and cooperation, to be allowed to do our work on our own time. Changes are occurring in the workplace that make it easier for employers to accommodate employees with irregular needs. Information technology allows people to work at home; schedules staggered to relieve traffic congestion allow people to get to work at a later hour. But changes are also occurring that make for less flexibility: as workers become more disposable, bosses have less incentive to accommodate them. It's the workers who are expected to accommodate, and quickly, too, or be left in the dust.

Also going against us are the age-old prejudices against anyone who sleeps late or asks for unconventional arrangements around sleep. Night people are viewed—as we saw earlier—as lazy, undisciplined, unpunctual, or as having an attitude problem. "It's the early bird that gets the promotions, the pat on the backs . . . because he'll always be in the office at 7 A.M. Whereas the guy who stays late doesn't get the same recognition," says a night person interviewed in *Birds of a Different Feather,* Carolyn Schur's study of night owls and early birds. People who work late shifts or work at home find themselves out of the loop and up against a glass ceiling that keeps them from getting ahead. Such arrangements may also increase their sense of isolation, and no insomniac needs more of that.

Night people have been speaking out against this bias, though, until recently, mainly in a humorous vein. Schur, in the summer of 2006, called a conference of night owls, the first international "Parliament of Owls," in Saskatoon, Saskatchewan. On the Web I click into a "Nocturnal Society," a nightworkers.com, and a "Nightowl Network." I come across a thirty-one-page "Late Sleeper's Bill of Rights" with entries like "From this moment henceforth, 'morning' shall commence at 10 AM . . ."; "H/she who sleeps late, sleeps last." But in January 2007, night owls in Denmark began a serious push for change. They formed the "B-Society," which argues that the model of starting work early harks back to an agricultural era that's outmoded in today's industrialized world, and that companies can attract more skilled professionals and increase productivity by providing conditions amenable to night people. Companies can become "B-certified" by showing that they're willing to accommodate the needs of late risers. By March 2007, the B-Society had three thousand members and was attracting the support of trade unions, politicians, and policy-makers interested in making a more flexible workplace.

It's about time. Some night owls absolutely cannot adjust to early-bird schedules, and their efforts to do so may turn them into full-blown insomniacs, as we've seen. Here's a study for somebody to do: take a bunch of insomniacs and let us self-regulate, find the schedules that work for us, then surround us with people who adjust to *our* rhythms, who hold meetings and arrange deadlines around *our* needs. Would we sleep better, feel better, and be all around better "adjusted"? You bet. Those who make the rules are always going to be the better adjusted.

But since the world is not likely to rearrange itself to our liking or even to provide us with the equivalent of wheelchair ramps or larger bathroom stalls, our best hope is to find a line of work that allows us to stay as clear as possible of the world's rules, and try not to leave this to luck.

This is something bad sleepers and night people should give serious thought to when choosing a line of work, assuming that they have a choice, so they don't end up in jobs where sleep is a lifelong torment.

At one of the sleep conferences I attended, I had just heard a talk about the difficulties shift workers have, adjusting to night work, when the woman sitting next to me turned and said, "They never tell the whole truth about this, because they look only at the day workers who've been screwed up by night shifts—what about the night people who get screwed up by morning hours?" She told me she'd been miserable as a respiratory therapist working the day shift. "I didn't feel like I could function until noon; I felt dangerous in the ICU. Then I went to a later shift and I was fine. My favorite is working 2 to 2." She said, "When I counsel high school students, I tell them, 'Follow your body rhythms; don't try to fight them. When you're choosing your career, think about your normal rhythms, because otherwise, you are going to be very unhappy. Find a position that fits your body.'"

Excellent idea, to advise young people that their sleep tendencies and circadian rhythms are as much a part of their "aptitude" as a gift for mathematics or athletics, that if they sleep badly or late, they should probably not set their hearts on becoming surgeons or anything else that requires them to be in top form at the crack of dawn. (Surgeons should probably also not be doing 7 A.M. surgeries on people like me, whose peak times are so obviously much later, but that's another issue.) Get students to become aware of their sleep patterns. I have begun to do this, a little; as a faculty advisor, I often talk with students about their futures. I now bring sleep into the conversation.

Some natural self-selection takes place anyway. Troubled sleepers and late sleepers tend to gravitate toward certain kinds of work—the arts, entertainment, shift work, freelance work that allows them to get jobs done on their own time. How about sleep lab technician? Sleep research? Sleep researchers tell me how difficult it is to stay awake all night and study sleep; it doesn't sound all that hard to me. "Academia is a good place," says late-riser Bella DePaulo, a professor of psychology at the University of California, Santa Barbara: "If you're doing 80 hours of work, what does it matter what 80 hours you work?" *Night time is geek time. Geek time is my time,* said a student I interviewed. *At first I had a hard time accepting I was insomniac and tried to sleep; now I actually enjoy my insomnia—I design Websites, write programs, that kind of thing.* Computer work is a haven for the diurnally challenged. Says Matt, an insomniac professor of computer science, *When I was in graduate school, the only time we could get access to the computers was when everyone else was asleep. Since I was a teenager, being in computer science has always really helped because I've been able to set my own hours.*

But, he tells me, *I am terrified of when my kid starts school.*

Matt and his early-bird wife worked well together, sharing the parenting responsibilities for their son while he was a preschooler, but soon, when he needs to be at school at the crack of dawn, it won't be so easy. And there's the rub: insomniacs are forever bumping up against the world's rules. Even I, with a maximally flexible teaching schedule, run afoul of early bird rules all the time: morning appointments, planes to catch, committee assignments. I can schedule my classes for afternoons and evenings, but when it comes to committees, I'm at a loss. An 8 A.M. meeting means I get three hours' sleep (and that's with a pill), and I'm good for nothing all that day and the next day too. I can't just tell people, "I'll feel like hell," because they have problems of their own, but I can try to make the case that, if I do something that undermines my sleep so radically on a regular basis (committees at my college meet once a week), it will impair my functioning in the job I was hired to do, which is to teach. If people knew more about sleep disorders, knew that chronic sleep loss can be seriously incapacitating, I might get somewhere with this argument, but right now it gets taken about as seriously as my suggestion that we schedule meetings after my last class, at 10 P.M. We need researchers to get these messages out, and we ourselves need to get these messages out, so that when we ask an employer that we be allowed to do the work on our own time, we have some leverage.

I am, for the millionth time, struck by how little tolerance there is on this issue, by how self-righteous early risers are, as though sleeping late were a mark of degeneracy (and where were they at 1 A.M., when I was grading papers?). Lighten up, I want to say: there are differences. Obviously, some things have to happen early in the day: the mail must go out, trains have to run, but much of the inflexibility is just hidebound conventionality. "Or jealousy," said Ilene, who admitted that she was intolerant of her ex's sleeping in, partly because she was jealous that she had to go to work while he got to sleep, even though she knew he had problems sleeping. But then, as we've seen, attitudes toward sleep do not always bring out the best in people. A friend who's a philosopher, Elizabeth Minnich, sees this intolerance as a "virtue challenge": "It's where we find deviations from prescribed norms linked with virtue that we get these unsympathetic judgments. There's something virtuous about sleeping less, getting up early, having your sleep under control. People are uncomfortable about virtue challenges in a way they're not about a case of hives, say."

We need to encourage people to think more imaginatively about sleep. A way to begin might be simply to talk about sleep, introduce it into conversations, break the silence that has until recently surrounded it. When I began researching this book, I went around asking everyone I met about their sleep. Initially, I'd bring it up because I was in search of fellow insomniacs and their stories, but then I found myself just sort of generally becoming interested in the relations people have to sleep, the ways they fit it into their lives, the attitudes they have toward it, the rituals they have around it. At first, I met with awkwardness and nervous laughter, but over time, maybe because sleep has been getting more press lately or because I got better at introducing it into the conversation, I found it was a marvelous way of bringing people out. When people see that you're really interested, they become interested, too, and they open up—and there you are with this total stranger, in her bedroom, as it were, plunged into the most intimate details of her life, learning about her childhood, her relationships, and it is fascinating, not in a voyeuristic way, but as a way of getting to know who a person is. Then, too, there's the excitement of seeing a light-bulb click on when a person makes a connection, as in, "I think I was jealous" or "I never realized, that's what I was doing." I began these conversations as a researcher, but I see now that they're not going to end with this book, that it's become a kind of crusade to get people to think about this third of their lives that they take so for granted that they scarcely know it exists, let alone that it can be so problematic for some people.

"I didn't know there were people like you. My head hits the pillow and I'm out"—I hear this often. Well, now they know.

We can carry on our own personal campaigns even if we don't have a public forum, simply by talking about sleep, making clear that it's not a ridiculous or a trivial thing to talk about or a concern only to the old or ill. We can all do our bit to bring this subject to light.

State of the Science, June 2005

Before I say more about what we all might do, I want to describe the NIH State-of-the-Science Conference, "Manifestations and Management of Chronic Insomnia in Adults," because it shows where we are and how far we have to go. This was a conference unlike any I'd ever been to. It was all about insomnia, unlike the annual sleep meetings, which are only incidentally about insomnia, and it was intense, with many of the major researchers gathered together in one small auditorium for three days. (The annual conferences have more than five thousand people in attendance—this had a few hundred.)

The last NIH conference on insomnia had been in 1983, and this was a long-awaited event. What comes out of NIH consensus conferences has lasting consequences: if change is going to happen, this is where it occurs. This turned out not to be a "consensus" conference, since there wasn't enough basis for consensus—it was called a "State-of-the-Science" conference instead—but the report it produced will have consequences nonetheless. A panel appointed from areas related to sleep—psychology, psychiatry, neuroscience, epidemiology, statistics, geriatric medicine, nursing, community medicine—was charged with writing the report. The panel was given a list of questions to address—about the etiology, diagnosis, prevalence, consequences, and public health burden of insomnia; the efficacy and safety of available treatments; directions for future research. It was then to bring the report back to the audience, on the third day, rewrite it in light of discussion, and post it on the Web. This is now "the state of the science" on insomnia.

And change did occur. The NIH insomnia conference twenty-two years earlier had defined insomnia as "primarily a symptom of other underlying disorders" and recommended treating the underlying disorder as the first line of treatment. That view demoted insomnia to secondary status, stripping it of an existence of its own, with effects that we've seen. But the 2005 final report does not use the term *secondary*; it refers to insomnia as a *comorbid* condition, meaning a condition existing simultaneously with, but usually independently of, other medical conditions, such as depression and anxiety. Comorbid conditions often accompany insomnia, there may be considerable overlap among them, but this *doesn't tell you which causes which*. As Daniel Buysse says, "This sounds like a small matter of wording, but it's a huge step, from thinking of insomnia as a symptom to seeing it as comorbid." It's a momentous shift: now insomnia can be viewed as a "stand-alone disorder" and not simply the effect of some other cause. This means that it's now a legitimate object of research in its own right.

But it will take a while for this new understanding to filter into popular consciousness. As Thomas Roth says, "It's almost second nature to assume that insomnia is secondary to something." "You'd be surprised at how many treating insomnia are unwilling to see it as anything other than a symptom of depression," says a speaker at the 2005 sleep conference. A U.K. researcher wrote in 2005, "Many insomnia specialists, particularly in the EU, would argue that the condition of primary insomnia might not exist at all." Still, it's a beginning.

But what kind of a stand-alone disorder? Once you let go of the notion that insomnia is secondary to and caused by depression, anxiety, or some other primary disorder, you're left with the question: What *is* it caused by? It may be caused by lots of things, as we've seen, but an important suggestion was made by two NIH presentations that addressed possible neurophysiological etiologies: Clifford Saper talked about the sleep switch, and Gary Richardson talked about other physiological models. On the third day, when the panel brought its report to the audience for feedback, I was surprised to see, under the section about "important future directions for insomnia-related research," no mention of a need to investigate neurophysiological etiologies. The report called for studies of "genetic etiology" and "family history, along with a systematic search for specific genes," but where was the neurobiology or neuroendocrinology of insomnia? That whole *physiological* side of *psychophysiological* insomnia was missing again. These two papers had taken forty minutes out of the eleven hours of presentations, not as much as this line of inquiry warranted, but their arguments were compelling enough to have made it into the final recommendations. I read the report over several times, thinking, surely I've missed something—but no.

I waited for someone in the audience to notice this omission and point it out. I kept waiting for someone to say something, but the discussion went on, and on, and—nothing. Please, I kept thinking, somebody say it, so I don't have to get up in front of this group again. (I'd spoken before, and I hated it, a television camera on me, a microphone I couldn't get to work, or was it my voice that I couldn't get to work, my heart pounding, palms sweating, knowing that everyone in the room is wondering, Who *is* that woman?) But the session was coming to an end, so I hauled myself over to a mike and said, "In view of the excellent presentations of Dr. Saper and . . . [I blanked on the other guy's name] on possible neurophysiological etiologies, shouldn't there be some mention of research into the neurobiology of insomnia?" So this sentence got added: "The neural mechanisms underlying chronic insomnia are poorly understood." I wasn't saying anything original: I was only reiterating what the *National Sleep Disorders Research Plan* said in 2003, that research into the pathophysiology, the neurobiology, of the disorder is urgently needed. But nobody else said it.

Then came the press conference, on the last hour of the last day, an entire hour reserved for questions from the media. I'd been caught up in the rallying cry for more research, for "a substantial public and private research effort" that would include the development of new research tools and longitudinal studies (studies that follow subjects forward through time are sorely lacking in insomnia research)—though I was drawn up short by a crack overheard during a break: "Just where do they think the money for all this research is coming from?" I was expecting to see television cameras roll in, lights flash, reporters elbowing each other out of the way in their eagerness to ask questions (well, maybe not quite), but when the hour for the press conference finally came, only ten or so representatives of the press showed up, most from journals I'd never heard of. If Lauran Neergaard of the Associated Press hadn't been there, the event would have had even less visibility than it did; as is, it was nearly invisible. So few questions were asked that the press conference ended with twenty-five minutes to spare—which was poignant, since time had been in such short supply during the previous two days that speakers had had to rush at high speed through their presentations.

To the media, the NIH conference on insomnia was a nonevent. Some celebrity gets strung out on Ambien and they're all over it, but when the real issues are on the table, they're nowhere in the room.

Also puzzling to me was the press release issued by the conference: "Many of the medications widely used to manage chronic insomnia have not yet been rigorously evaluated for long-term use. . . . The panel was concerned that many of the drugs now used to treat insomnia, such as antidepressants and antihistamines, have not been approved for this indication," that "their efficacy in treating chronic insomnia has not been proven." This is what got picked up and reported, when the conference was reported at all. "Insomnia Sufferers Need Better Care, Experts Say," announced a headline in the *American Journal of Health-System Pharmacists News,* explaining that there is "misplaced faith" in antidepressants and over-the-counter remedies, when "what works" is "currently marketed benzodiazepine hypnotics and benzodiazepine-receptor agonists."

This was puzzling. Many people do fine on those older drugs and prefer to stay on a low dose of trazodone or doxepin than to hazard the benzodiazepines and nonbenzodiazepines. Anyhow, this was hardly the main point of the conference. The point I heard emphasized again and again was that chronic insomnia, a condition from which untold millions suffer and about which very little is known, is a condition that needs a great deal more research. If I had written the press release, I'd have said, "Until we know more about insomnia, we won't be able to develop better treatments." I'd have quoted Daniel Buysse: "Quite simply, we still do not know what insomnia really is, in the sense of what causes it, but we need to know this in order to develop rational treatments." I'd have quoted Marcia Angell: "You first have to understand the nature of the disease you want to treat, what has gone wrong in the body to cause it. That understanding needs to be fairly detailed, usually at the molecular level, if there is to be any hope of finding a drug that will safely and effectively interfere with the chain of events responsible for the disease." That kind of understanding needs basic research, the slow, gradual, brick-by-brick building of knowledge about how the sleep system works and what can go wrong with it. I'd have made a point none of the conference speakers did, that this will take more than the $3.8 million a year that the NIH spends on basic research on insomnia at the present time.

"Fundamental advances are the result of tiny increments in knowledge," writes David Gershon in *The Second Brain*. "Little steps add up, but they are not by themselves spectacular, and even the people who are taking the little steps may not know where they lead." But basic research has had a hard time of it lately. The tendency, as Gershon says, is to fund the applied, the practical, which is always easier to justify because it has a known purpose. "The money always goes to the quick fixes," as Peter Hauri told me. This is why so many researchers are drawn to apnea, and why most insomnia research goes to treatments and therapies, rather than the search for a cause.

Finally, as of June 2005, insomnia exists. Now the NIH needs to act like it believes it.

Getting Organized

When I was a graduate student, I'd sit by my window on the tenth floor of an Upper West Side apartment and gaze out at a building across the way, where, on a floor as high as mine, I'd see a lone light, night after night. "The lonely beacon of the insomniac," as Aminatta Forner calls it, describing, as she moves through the empty streets of London, "the sight of the solitary light in an otherwise dark row of terraced houses." I used to wonder who that person was, whether he or she saw my light and was wondering about me too.

Now we have the Internet, forums like Sleepnet.com and Talkabout
sleep.com, chat rooms, message boards, blogs, and newsgroups to put us
in contact with one another, allowing us ways of sharing our experiences, offering support, advice, and information about doctors, drugs,
online pharmacies, insurance. *I thought I was the only person in the
world who was suffering this bad, I thought it was only me,* I read on
the forums. *Now I know that somebody's listening who cares.* But we
could use the Internet to do much more. *Wouldn't it be great if we could
organize the way other diseases have,* says my friend Roberta, *have a
central organization that would speak for our interests, ride herd on
Congress to make sure there was research money, check in with researchers to find out what they're doing, make a newsletter or a journal?
Other disease groups have done this. Why not us?*

"Would it help draw attention to the problem if insomniacs got together and became activists?" I asked Peter Hauri.

"*Yes,*" came the response, unhesitating, emphatic. "That has happened
in other areas. But insomnia patients have never been that well organized."

"Why is that?" I asked.

"They don't want everybody else to know they have insomnia; also,
they still lead productive lives, they have no time. Mainly, I think, they
don't want to expose themselves." I would bet also that it's because
we've been talked out of recognizing insomnia as the sort of problem
anything can be done about. Insomnia was only in 2005 recognized as a
condition in its own right. We've been told it's a symptom of some other
problem, that it's within our individual power to control—which intensifies our self-blame for having it and leaves us all the more alone. It's difficult to peel down through these layers of confusion and see insomnia
as a problem in its own right that needs more research and a different
kind of research.

It's not easy to make a movement when it's all you can do to get
through the day, and when the stigma attached to your condition makes
you want to hide it rather than publicize it. But others have done it,
women a lot sicker than we are (most health advocacy has been women's
work). Women in the 1960s broke through "barriers of secrecy and
shame," as Barbara Ehrenreich terms it, to make a movement that revolutionized health care.

From small beginnings: "A group of us in the late 1960s, about 25
strong, began to meet weekly in our kitchens and living rooms. As we
talked about what had happened to us during pregnancy, in labor, in our
gynecologists' offices, in our bedrooms, the first thing we learned was

that we were not alone" and that "we knew as much about ourselves as our doctors did—in fact, often we knew more." Women those days had the energy of the 1960s behind them, the momentum and optimism of the women's movement. "Pro-choice rallies united us," recalls Jane Pincus, one of the original eleven who incorporated, in 1972, as the Boston Women's Health Book Collective. The following year, they published *Our Bodies, Ourselves,* a compendium of information about women's bodies, a book translated into a dozen languages and reissued in a half dozen editions. Though none of the founders had degrees in health, they learned that they could read the scientific literature, and they remained firm in their insistence that "we, as women, are the best experts on ourselves."

"We discovered that every one of us had a 'doctor story,' that we had all experienced feelings of frustration and anger . . . toward those doctors who were condescending, paternalistic, judgmental, and uninformative," write the founders of that collective. In 1969, Barbara Seaman published an exposé of the birth control pill, *The Doctor's Case against the Pill,* that linked the pill with strokes, heart disease, diabetes, depression. Her book led to the 1970 congressional hearings on the safety of the pill that got package inserts for oral contraceptives. This exposé and others galvanized a grassroots movement that swelled in numbers, until "by 1975, nearly 2,000 [women's self-help medical projects] were scattered across the U.S.," recounts Cynthia Pearson of the National Women's Health Network.

In the 1980s, as women woke up to the fact that one in nine gets breast cancer (today it is one in eight), they began speaking out. They found one another in cancer support groups, they read about one another in newspaper or magazine articles, they began meeting in living rooms. In cities throughout the country, groups mushroomed into existence, then those groups formed alliances. These women didn't start out as activists—they were homemakers, nurses, social workers, lawyers, real estate agents, artists, mothers, grandmothers—but they soon became activists. They heard the AIDS slogan SILENCE = DEATH and saw the AIDS activists getting what they wanted. They began marching, lobbying, making noise, converging in Washington in May 1991, to form the National Breast Cancer Coalition, an organization that soon included several million members. That spring they flooded Congress with 650,000 letters. The coalition succeeded in getting Congress to allocate $406 million to breast cancer research, nearly tripling the budget from the year before. They gained access to advisory boards that set research priorities and policies—they got "a seat at the table."

"When I think of the beginnings of the women's health movement, I think, above all, of the stories women told," recalls Barbara Ehrenreich. That was where it all began, women talking, telling their stories. They told their stories to support groups they joined or formed, to congressional subcommittees, to the media. Some wrote journalistic exposés, some wrote personal narratives of illness, disability, and survival, publishing books about breast cancer, AIDS, chronic fatigue syndrome, Parkinson's disease. However they chose to tell their stories, breaking the silence was the first step toward collective action, and the first step toward changing public consciousness.

The women's health movement is a stunning example of grassroots activism that has brought about widespread changes at local and federal levels. In 1990, the NIH established the Office of Research on Women's Health for the purposes of addressing "inequities in women's health research and to ensure that women are included in clinical studies." For the first time ever, a woman was made director of the NIH, Dr. Bernadine Healy. In 1991, Healy launched the Women's Health Initiative, a massive fifteen-year study involving 160,000 postmenopausal women, looking at questions about hormone replacement therapy and the effect of diet and exercise on coronary heart disease, breast cancer, and colon cancer. By 1997, about a third of hospitals in the United States had some kind of women's health center. Patient advocacy groups have proliferated, and though many of them have lost touch with their grassroots beginnings, they ensure that people who are faced with ADD, aging, AIDS, Alzheimer's, anxiety, autism (we're not even out of the A's yet) have a place to turn.

Insomniacs could learn from the women's health movement. We could also learn from the people who made the Restless Legs Syndrome Foundation and Narcolepsy Network. They too have told their stories: in *Sleep Thief: Restless Legs Syndrome,* Virginia Wilson makes me feel what it's like to have legs that "have minds of their own," legs that feel so jumpy and crawly that they push her to pace the room the whole night through. She describes the cataclysmic effects RLS has on people's lives, lets us hear the sufferers speak for themselves: *I was a legal secretary for 32 years and now I can hardly get my dishes done;* and *I was a police officer. . . . I was forced to retire. . . . It cost me my 28-year marriage. . . . Even my dog can't sleep with me.* In *Narcolepsy: A Funny Disorder That's No Laughing Matter,* Marguerite Jones Utley makes me feel what it's like to be so drowsy that you fall asleep every time you ride in a car, to lack the energy to do the things you want to do, to experience terrifying dreams while you're awake. I hadn't fully taken it in that, since emotions trigger these attacks, people with narcolepsy become fearful even of laughing or playing with their kids, and consign themselves to a drab affectless zone.

People with RLS and narcolepsy have lots of "doctor stories," stories of physicians who dispense useless advice about diet and lifestyle, prescribe drugs that do more harm than good, and/or blame the sufferers, implying that the problem is something they're bringing on themselves. Utley recounts, "I was told I was depressed, I was fed handfuls of antidepressants and sedatives—imagine, sedating someone with narcolepsy!" Narcolepsy used to take around twenty-five years to diagnosis, which left plenty of time for misdiagnoses, and it is often, to this day, attributed to laziness and stupidity. Over time, as lawyer and patient advocate Bob Cloud says, people with narcolepsy may "start to believe that they are lazy, unmotivated, irresponsible."

The advocacy groups these people formed show what a few determined people can accomplish. In 1990, Oron F. Hawley of Escondido, California, who was then over ninety, began exchanging letters with eight fellow sufferers of RLS, all of them quite elderly. They shared information on medications and therapies and ways of coping. Virginia Wilson, one of these original nine, volunteered to do a newsletter, *The Night Walkers*. As letters poured in, she realized that many millions were struggling with this problem—an estimated 6 to 15 percent of the population. She then began collecting information. She made up a questionnaire about medical history and family background and required anyone wishing to join an RLS support group to complete the questionnaire. RLS had not been thought to come on in childhood, but the survey indicated that almost 20 percent of the hundred respondents could recall the onset of symptoms before the age of ten. She sent the data to Dr. Arthur Walters, who used them in a study of RLS that confirmed that, sure enough, RLS occurs in children. The group opened a bank account in 1993 with a gift of one thousand dollars and established a medical advisory board selected by Dr. Walters. The first International Symposium on Restless Legs Syndrome was held in 1994. Today the RLS Foundation has 120,000 members and representatives who work with NIH.

The Narcolepsy Network similarly emerged from small beginnings, from the vision of thirteen women who came together from self-help groups in 1984. It now has over twelve hundred members, and, as one of them told me, "now NIH comes to us for ideas." As a result of its work publicizing this disease, "in the last twenty years, the average time from onset of symptoms to diagnosis has dropped from twenty-five years to nine"—a major accomplishment! Members of the Narcolepsy Network also made a big difference by testifying to Congress against pressure to restrict GHB to a schedule I classification; if it had been so restricted, we would not have Xyrem today.

Support groups are crucial. They're the only place sufferers can find "someone else in the world who really understands what you go through and how you feel," writes Utley of narcolepsy. "Join an RLS support group," urges Wilson. "If one is not available, form one." The RLS foundation has ways of encouraging people to do this: a quarterly newsletter for support group facilitators, a facilitator Listserv, and an online discussion forum that keeps facilitators in touch with one another. In 2003 there were more than eighty RLS support groups in the United States and three in Canada.

Insomniacs also have lots of complaints about doctors:

> *The doctor I saw was condescending and pompous. He told me he would test me for sleep disorders, and if none were found, he would refer me to a psychologist to help me learn better ways to sleep. It seems he hadn't bothered to notice that I am a psychologist and I could have done that for myself.*

From a "U.K. insomniac," I hear,

> *I am not at all anti–traditional medicine, but the closed minds, ignorance, and above all, the writing off of middle-aged women as "neurotic"—especially if you are highly educated and practising in a profession—fills me with frustration and despair.*

Insomniacs make their most damning statement about doctors simply by staying away from them. "The great majority of patients with frequent insomnia are not speaking to their doctors about this problem," reported Nalaka Gooneratne, director of a sleep disorders clinic at the University of Pennsylvania Medical School, to the NIH conference in June 2005. "When we ask why, many said they were uncertain whether a doctor would really help them, would take it seriously, would have anything to treat it. Very few felt their doctors could help them."

People with narcolepsy and RLS can point to scientific breakthroughs that show the neurobiological basis of their problems. On account of postmortem studies that turned up hypocretin deficiency in the brains of narcoleptics and the insufficiency of the iron transport receptor in the brains of patients with RLS, they can now tell their doctors and friends and families that what they have is a neurological disorder, not a psychological problem. As a matter of fact, the RLS Foundation, which has worked with the Brain Bank at Harvard since 2000, played a major role in the studies that revealed the iron deficiency, by providing the brain tissue to be studied. They were quite literally the brains behind the project. The foundation has 720 more people lined up to donate their brains.

But insomniacs have nothing like these breakthroughs to point to, no way of arguing that their problem has a neurobiological basis, so it continues to be described as psychological and behavioral, a condition the sufferers are bringing on themselves. "We [doctors] believe people about other things," says a physician friend, "but even the sleep docs don't believe patients about insomnia, when they say it's ruining their lives." He compares insomnia to chronic pain, which is also a problem for which you have to take the patient's word:

> Doctors used to be this bad about pain—if you went in and said, "I hurt" and they couldn't see anything, you used to have a harder time being taken seriously. Docs have got better about this, because more is known about pain—now you can point to neurological pathways. But you can't point to anything with chronic insomnia. It's barely begun to be recognized as a distinct entity. It still doesn't have legitimacy. I suspect in time they'll come around, but it's going to take awhile.

This has made it difficult for us to organize, difficult for us to see that we have a problem worth organizing for, or that we ourselves are worth organizing for, which may be why we never have.

But we need to organize. We could learn from the way the Narcolepsy Network and the RLS Foundation have established lines of communication among patients and researchers and medical professionals, see how they've organized support groups, launched studies and conferences, lobbied legislators, published newsletters, got the word out—and they got this going before the Internet. We could learn from the National Organization for Rare Disorders, a group that's raised consciousness about rare disorders that nobody had ever heard of: sickle-cell anemia, Tay-Sachs disease, cystic fibrosis, and multiple sclerosis. This group has created a Rare Disease Database and a Patient Services Department, administers yearly research grants to young researchers, and is a presence on Capitol Hill, thanks to its tireless president, Abbey Meyers.

We need an organization that is by us, of us, and for us, not organized by the doctors and not run by the drug companies. We need to make our own way, free of entangling alliances with anyone who has their own agenda, whether medical or corporate. Above all, we need to be careful of corporate influences. One of the ways drug companies do their marketing is through patient advocacy groups, supporting them, infiltrating them, taking them over, even establishing groups of their own. Patient groups are useful to drug companies because they're considered unbiased, but there's a big difference between "Astroturf" groups, as they're called, and genuine grassroots groups. I'm told advocacy groups can't get far without pharmaceutical industry support—about two-thirds of patient advocacy groups accept such support—and I'm assured there are ways of accepting it without compromising goals. But it's a fine line to tread.

If we organize an insomnia advocacy group—*when* we organize—we must not allow it to be turned into a group for the promotion of sleeping pills, as there will be pressure to do. Daniel Kripke told me, "Put this in your book, IN BIG LETTERS: some billionaire who has a relative with terrible trouble sleeping, or terrible trouble himself, should endow a private foundation. There should be patient advocacy groups for insomnia—but they'll need to stay independent of the pharmaceutical companies!"

Patients and Physicians

Patients have become, thanks to the patient advocacy movements, a lot less patient these days, less ready to believe that "doctor knows best." The old paternalistic, authoritarian model has given way to a more activist view of the patient's role that allows us a say in our treatment. The Internet has given us access to information that once belonged exclusively to physicians, breaking the monopoly over medical knowledge that doctors once held. We can now find, within seconds, up-to-the minute information about treatments, conditions, drugs. "It's a massive revolution," says Dr. Rita Charon of the Columbia University College of Physicians and Surgeons. "It altogether shifts what goes on when a patient comes in with pages of downloaded stuff and half the time the doctor looking at it has never seen it before."

There's a lot of nonsense on the Web, of course, people making easy promises and selling magical cures, and many doctors resent the precious time it takes to explain to the patient why a drug or treatment picked up off the Internet might not be the best idea. But doctors who attend to the information their patients bring in find that it "can sometimes do more good than harm." One physician says, "I've had a bunch of people say, 'I've been chasing down my symptoms and this is what I think it is and my doctor hasn't paid attention to me.' About 50% of the time when I see patients like that, they're correct." Patients, for their part, need to know that they must bring in studies and articles from refereed journals if they're going to get their physician's attention—not "I heard somewhere" or "I read in a chat room." Anecdote has its uses, but it won't get you far with a physician.

Why don't they listen? is a lament I hear from insomniacs again and again. Face it, the seven-minute shuffle we get from most doctors won't make much headway with a problem like chronic insomnia, even if the doctor is the best listener in the world. The way health care is structured today, doctors don't have time to listen. "You can't sit and talk and really get an entire history," says an internist who sees five thousand patients a year, interviewed for the *New York Times*. "So you do what you were taught as a resident: do more tests, don't spend more time with patients, getting to know them."

So in asking doctors to pay attention to what we say, we're asking them to go against the considerable pressures on them to practice speed medicine. But I'll urge it anyway: Doctors, please hear us out, find out what we know. "Patients are goldmines of information to a doctor who's willing to listen," writes Sidney Walker, in *A Dose of Sanity*. We are, after all, the ones who are most motivated to find out what's wrong. To us, we're the main event; to you, we're just one more patient. Be open to the possibility that we might know something you do not, might have come across something that you've missed. Don't tell us we're stressed out or depressed if we insist that we are not, and don't shunt us to "psychiatry" unless we look like we really need it. If we say we think our problem might be hormones, hear us out. If we describe symptoms of hypothyroidism, consider the symptoms and not just the test numbers. Don't tell us we're getting all the sleep we need if we say we're not. Please don't trivialize or dismiss us just because you see so many people who have problems that are worse.

I, like most insomniacs, have many "doctor stories." But I'll say, too, that the doctors who turn up at the sleep conferences are a pretty impressive bunch, judging from the concern I hear in their voices, the perceptiveness of their questions. Maybe these are just the interested ones, the ones who want to learn about sleep, I don't know, but I love their questions: "Something I've noticed is . . ." "Might there be a relation between . . . ?" "Might there be a point in trying . . . ?" Their comments are often more original and informative than the talks themselves. But they go by too quickly: "Wait a minute, stay with that thought, answer that question—how does that tally with what we've just heard?" I want to say. When a physician has something interesting to say, some hunch or intuition, some success with a therapy, there's no place to go with it. There's no panel at the conferences, no forum or venue where speculation or anecdote has a say.

An observant physician may well turn up something that's ahead of the guidelines or the literature. History offers a long line of physician-observers and experimenters who have made breakthrough discoveries. William Withering, in the eighteenth century, noticed that a woman had improved her "dropsy"—swelling in the lower limbs—by drinking an herb tea, and set out to discover what was in that tea. He identified foxglove, *Digitalis purpurea,* which became the basis of the digitalis used today for congestive heart failure. Edward Jenner, also in the eighteenth century, paid attention to the lore that people who'd had cowpox were protected against smallpox, and his experimentation lead to vaccinations for smallpox. We might not want docs to go around injecting us with cowpox and the like, but look at Warren Warwick, the doctor Atul Gawande wrote about in the *New Yorker,* whose cystic fibrosis clinic outperforms all others, who does "whatever he can" to keep his patients' lungs open, experimenting, inventing. "Good doctors," writes Gawande, "are supposed to follow research findings rather than their own intuition or ad-hoc experimentation," but Warwick credits his own intuitions and observations and "is almost contemptuous of established findings. National clinical guidelines for care are, he says, 'a record of the past, and little more—they should have an expiration date.'" That can be said of official guidelines for insomnia, in my opinion. Why hasn't insomnia fired the imagination of a doctor like Warwick? Maybe it has, and we just haven't heard.

Where would we hear? No place I know of. Why not have a session at the sleep meetings where doctors can take their ideas? Find out what they know?

Research

If I've convinced anyone of anything, I hope it has been to credit the subjective experience of those who live with this condition, to hear what we have to say. Every way we turn, sleep is turning out to be larger than our conceptions of it, more complex than our categories, descriptions, measurements. One way to cast a wider net might be to invite "others" into the discussion, to allow the patients, the subjects, the sufferers a role in the research process—and if what we say collides with existing theoretical models, rethink the models.

Advocacy groups have shown doctors and researchers that people who live with afflictions have something to teach, that nonscientists can play a role, not only in fund-raising and lobbying, but in working with scientists to help direct research efforts. Researchers would find in insomniacs a huge pool of untapped resources, would see that there are many of us ready to donate our time, energies, talents, our hearts, minds, money—and yes, our brains, once we've finished with them.

Listening to patients' concerns, learning how they weigh risks and benefits, for example, might "better define which research questions should be studied," writes Jody Heymann of Harvard Medical School. "Research would change in a number of ways if we spent more time listening to patients while we were designing studies, . . . talking with the people we hope our research will help. . . . If patients' concerns were addressed, there would be more research on the side effects of treatments," she suggests. "Patients with chronic conditions often know that they will be living with a particular disease and its symptoms, treatment, and side effects for the rest of their lives. They need information about . . . long-term consequences." David Healy, the Welsh psychopharmacologist and outspoken critic of the overuse of SSRIs, has found that "certain personality types—as established by questionnaire—seemed to do better than others on [SSRIs]," writes Jerome Burne in *The New Statesman*. "Teasing out these differences," says Burne, "could make prescribing a far less hit-and miss affair than it is at present. . . . Making patients partners in the trials, rather than just clinical fodder, could restore a genuine spirit of scientific inquiry."

One thing researchers would learn, listening to us, is that we're not all alike—as the older researchers well knew. In 1972, Ismet Karacan made what seems like a stunningly simple observation: "There are different kinds of insomniacs." The insomniacs he looked at "were all alike in that they reported sleep problems, but they were different from one another in the type of sleep disturbance revealed by EEG recordings. . . . A very important future research area will be the assessment of various psychological, biochemical, physiological and EEG measures from insomniacs, with the aim of delineating the sub-types of insomnia," he said, adding that the classification system to come out of this delineation of types should "be based on the developmental history of the disorder, the psychological characteristics of the patients, the biochemical responses characteristic of patients," and the patients' responses to various treatments. Such differences, he argued, "need to be understood before we can develop effective treatments," since each type "probably requires a tailor-made treatment."

This has not been the direction research has taken, as we've seen. "Variability has been largely overlooked on sleep research," concludes a 2005 review by University of Pennsylvania sleep researchers. "Individual variabilities in sleep and wakefulness remain understudied scientifically" and are rarely taken into account, in theories or practices. "One often-neglected issue in this area is the extreme heterogeneity of insomniacs," writes Peter Hauri. "I used to believe," Hauri told me, that "insomniacs are all one group. Now I get incredibly interested in how wide the variety is from one to another, when I talk on an individual level and try to find what their life situation is." Hauri describes himself as a "splitter": "There are 'lumpers' and 'splitters' in the world. The lumpers emphasize the communality in all insomniacs[,] . . . the splitters emphasize the differences among us. If you really get to know each insomniac, you will see that each has a little different cause for his poor sleep. So, tracing these differences might make you more able to help the insomniac."

Hauri was onto an important distinction with his work on childhood-onset insomnia, as we saw in chapter 5. If that subset of childhood-onset insomniacs had been more thoroughly studied, it would have made the point that only *some* people's insomnia is precipitated by a stressful event or events, whereas others have had theirs "just always"—and this latter category is where you'd look for a genetic component. But childhood-onset insomnia is not studied anymore. It was not even mentioned at the NIH conference.

Another distinction is, of course, that many of us are women. "Sleep researchers need to make greater efforts to understand the effects of sex on human sleep and its pathophysiologic implications," writes Fred Turek in 2006. "Animal models are needed to elucidate the molecular, cellular, and physiologic mechanisms by which the sex-related neuroendocrine environment influences the sleep-wake cycle." There are many basic questions that nobody's asking, as far as I can tell. Do women have more sleep-maintenance insomnia, difficulty staying asleep, than men do? Can we distinguish between women whose insomnia is hormonally driven and those whose insomnia is not? What is it about me that gave me such a strong reaction to pregnancy hormones that I slept blissfully through so stressful a time?—and please, somebody, put it in a pill, or maybe tweak the progesterone I take as part of my HRT so it has that effect. Is my supersensitivity to my own hormones a sign of a stress system on permanent alert? (*Is* my stress system on permanent alert? I don't even know. I've been unable to inspire enough curiosity from a physician or researcher to help me figure it out.) Might a hyperactivated stress system be related to those "exquisite sensitivities" to drugs, caffeine, sugar that Hauri found in some insomniacs? There are tests that can tell us about what our stress systems are up to—why not use them as a means of differentiating among insomniacs? Studies of insomniacs' hormonal profiles, the few that have been done, suggest that ours are different from normal sleepers', higher in cortisol and lower in melatonin. But what about our other hormones—thyroid, prolactin, estrogen, progesterone, growth hormone—what do they look like? And might such differences be made the basis of intervention?

What first needs doing, as Karacan argued in 1972, is to make distinctions, break insomnia down into various types, then zero in on the causes of those differences. Insomniacs could help with this process. That grassroots epidemiology that Wilson and her group did is inspiring: a patient devises and administers a questionnaire that turns up information, which then becomes the basis of a research study. Why couldn't we devise a questionnaire that asks basic questions about hormonal and metabolic issues, family histories, childhood stresses and traumas, head injuries, the work we do and how it affects our sleep, what we eat, digestive problems and peculiarities, and what we think is the source of our problem? Cast as wide a net as possible, as Alice Stewart, the first lady of epidemiology, advised. If she were alive, she'd help us—but surely we can find someone who's savvy about statistics, who knows about designing epidemiological studies, to help us devise a questionnaire. See what kinds of things turn up.

When the genetic basis to delayed phase syndrome was discovered, an important subset of insomniacs came to light, people who would not be insomniac if they were allowed to sleep according to their own clocks. Identifying the genes associated with insomnia will be, as the NIH conference report stated, one of the main challenges of future research. The depression study I described in chapter 6, which followed subjects through time and found an association between two short versions of the 5-HTT gene and vulnerability to stress, might be a way to approach insomnia. But a longitudinal study of this sort, which follows subjects forward through the years, takes years. Meanwhile, a model more within the realm of immediate possibility might be a study of chronic fatigue syndrome done by researchers at the Centers for Disease Control, published in April 2006. Chronic fatigue syndrome, first recognized in the 1980s, has had a hard time being recognized as "real," since there are no objective markers. The afflicted are overwhelmed by fatigue, problems of memory and concentration, muscle aches and pains; often there is a slightly elevated temperature, enlarged glands, faintness, nausea, emotional volatility—and insomnia. Tests reveal "nothing wrong," and sufferers, mainly women in their forties, fifties, or sixties, are said to be hypochondriacs, hysterics, malingerers. Activists have formed an international network of support groups, advocacy groups, Websites, and chat rooms, and have had considerable success getting this condition taken seriously; but women still get told they have the "yuppie flu."

A Centers for Disease Control study took 227 people with chronic fatigue syndrome into a hospital and did intensive evaluations, looking for factors that might be in any way related to the illness. They measured their sleep; looked at their "psychiatric status," cognitive functioning, memory, and concentration; and took urine and blood tests that yielded information about subjects' neuroendocrinal systems and levels of inflammatory markers. "We've brought together a whole bunch of different types of data," says lead researcher Suzanne Vernon, "genetics, gene activity, clinical information, physiological markers, ways to describe how the person is feeling—and wrapped that all together to try to generate a molecular profile." The researchers found that subjects' stress systems were in a hyperaroused state, and discovered variations in genes that mediate the ability to respond to stress that might account for this state. William Reeves, a researcher on the project, says this provides "an underlying biologic basis," if not "a single simple marker" for the disease. The study is a major step toward getting chronic fatigue syndrome validated.

Why not take a group of insomniacs who are from families of insomniacs and have the same kind of insomnia—isolate a subset—and do this kind of analysis of them? Find out what's going on with their neuroendocrine systems, take measures of their gene expression, generate this kind of detailed molecular profile—and try to find the genes associated with the disorder? While we're at it, why not study the good sleepers— I mean the *really* good sleepers who retain their gift for sleep throughout life, whose gift runs in the family—find out about their genetic profiles?

I'm intrigued by the autoimmune connections I keep finding, the high incidence of insomnia in people who have chronic fatigue syndrome, fibromyalgia, thyroid problems—conditions that affect many more women than men. Of course, anything that causes pain or discomfort may disrupt sleep, but given the close involvement of sleep with the immune system, might there be something subtler going on? Some sleep disorders seem actually to have come about as a result of an autoimmune response. Researchers think the damage to the hypocretin center in narcoleptics' brains is caused by an autoimmune reaction. Studies suggest that the hypothalamic damage found by Baron Von Economo in the autopsies he did on patients who died from sleeping sickness may also have been due to autoimmune damage. What if there's been this kind of damage with some insomniacs?

And the eyes. Insomniacs are always complaining about their eyes— sore eyes, tearing eyes, itching eyes, twitching eyelids, eyes so red that they draw comment from friends. There are mornings I think I'll be okay, but then I look in the mirror and see that red glow, those deep dark bags, and I know I'll nosedive in a few hours: the eyes are a sure sign. What is it about sleep loss that makes such dramatic effects? And what is it about sleep that restores the eyes? I find one study that describes a connection between sleep problems and problems of vision, that suggests visual impairment may prevent the light from reaching the circadian clock and thereby dysregulate the circadian rhythms. But what if some visual impairments are the *effect* rather than the cause of sleep disturbance? And those dark, wavy effects at the edge of my visual field, and the dead green spot I see on days after I've taken a benzo-type drug—but, interestingly, *not* after I take Xyrem—what's that about? And the skin: what is it about sleep loss that turns me gray? Is this question so obvious that nobody's addressing it, or is it so complex that nobody's addressing it?

Researchers now understand why the hormonal havoc wrought by sleep starvation makes us hungry. "There has been an avalanche of studies in this area," says Mignot. "It's moving very rapidly." But there is not much work on "the plumbing," as David Dinges says, on the enteric nervous system, that system located in the sheaths of tissue lining the esophagus, stomach, small intestine, and colon. This extraordinarily complex, self-contained network contains more nerve cells than the spinal cord; it can act independently of the brain, learn, remember, and produce "gut feelings." It contains every type of neurotransmitter and neuromodulator found in the brain, including those most crucial to sleep—GABA, histamine, norepinephrine, and dopamine. Gershon calls it "the second brain" because it produces 95 percent of the body's serotonin and is a rich source of natural benzodiazepines. It produces four hundred times as much melatonin as the brain's pineal gland, though the production is influenced not by light but by food, especially foods containing tryptophan.

Its workings are closely coordinated with sleep. During sleep, the brain in the gut produces ninety minutes of slow muscle contractions followed by short periods of rapid muscle movements, cycles that correspond to the cycles of deep sleep and REM. When the brain is in deep sleep, the gut quiets down (there is "decreased small intestinal motility"), whereas REM has "immediate stimulatory effects on colonic motility" like those that occur with arousals and waking. When you disrupt the rhythmical movement of the peristaltic action of the intestines, you disrupt REM patterns; when you disrupt REM, you disrupt peristaltic action—and along with this, regular bowel activity. Am I the only one who's noticed that when you stop sleeping you just sort of plug up, and when you sleep, you unplug? (Or am I the only one indelicate enough to mention it?)

The gut and the brain send messages back and forth, via the vagus nerve, and the gut sends more messages than the brain. "The information content of the messages sent by the bowel to the brain is not entirely known," says Gershon. Might some guts be saying, "Wake up, wake up"? I've long had this feeling, a gut feeling, that the tension that grips me when I wake up after three hours emanates from my gut—there's this sense, hard to describe, not hunger, not indigestion, not pain, not anything I can name, just this unease, not a knot, exactly, not so localized as a knot, but a sort of tension, as if the whole area's awake. Of course, any stomach upset may disturb sleep. An estimated 26 to 55 percent of people with irritable bowel syndrome have sleep disturbances (again, the wonder to me is that *anyone* with this condition could sleep through it). They also seem to have more REM than other people do, which points to that mysterious interaction between gut and brain. I wonder about subtler irritations that may go undetected. Gastroesophageal reflux may not give obvious heartburn symptoms, yet may still cause frequent awakenings. One insomniac discovered that she had a subclinical gastric irritation, a sort of pre-ulcer condition, in a part of the stomach where you don't feel pain; she started taking Tagamet and her insomnia went away. I come across several people who sense that their sleep problems started with giardia or parasites. Might there be other kinds of subclinical irritations, unknown disorders of the enteric nervous system, that affect our sleep?

I go to conference after conference and find nothing about the relation of insomnia to the most fundamental of questions, how what we eat affects the way we sleep—in spite of recent discoveries about the connections between the appetite and sleep-regulating centers in the brain and the powerful effect sleep deprivation has on hunger. And I wonder about those conditions alternative practitioners find everywhere, food allergies, hypoglycemia, adrenal fatigue: do they affect sleep? The indifference of doctors and researchers to alternative approaches is also an indifference to chronic conditions that can't be fixed. It amounts to an indifference to the well-being of women and the elderly as well, since these are the people who disproportionately suffer from such conditions.

When I run these questions by researchers, they nod and say, Yes, that sounds interesting. But they also say that, in the current climate, funding is so tight that they're just trying to hang on to their current projects. "All NIH is suffering from the prioritizing of war over life," as UCLA sleep researcher Michael Irwin told me: "There's a no-growth budget, but research costs haven't stopped growing—they go up while the budget remains flat, so these are real cuts. As funding becomes more competitive, the grants go to the easy. The innovative approaches that are really pushing the envelope—they're the ones that languish." Science is under assault, and we're seeing the effects. "The U.S. is losing its dominance in the sciences," reports the *New York Times*. Fewer students are choosing science careers. The percentage of patents being granted in the United States is declining relative to other countries.

It is poignant to see sleep research so exciting, so on the verge of breakthroughs, as the ground is being cut out from under it. As the understanding of sleep deepens, as the stream is fed and enriched by neuroscience, molecular biology, genetics, the funding shrinks and important projects are shut down. And with these cuts goes hope for the research that might bring truly safe and effective treatments for insomnia. Researchers need to have a clearer sense of what's gone wrong with our sleep systems before they can come up with medications to set it right.

In the spring of 2005, Emmanuel Mignot, who did breakthrough work leading to the discovery of hypocretin's role in narcolepsy, announced to the Narcolepsy Network that his program had been cut. "We are sorry to announce that after 18 years of operation and many discoveries, our Program Project grant on narcolepsy, funded generously over the years by the NIH's National Institute of Neurological Diseases and Stroke, will not be renewed after June 1st 2005." Dr. S. Nichino, who discovered the hypocretin deficiency in the cerebrospinal fluid of humans with narcolepsy, will "not have any federal funding left to work on narcolepsy." Mignot told me that this calls a halt, for the time being, to the search for the human narcolepsy gene. "We will also be unable to provide service and information as we have to patients in the past."

At this time more than ever, researchers need us. We need to put pressure, make noise, make it clear that we're here and we're not going to go away.

Miles to Go

"There is so much more to know," Dement told a Stanford audience in February 2005, "but if you knew how hard it was to get this far, you'd be amazed at how much we do know." Dement said to me, "I used to think, if I die before I know why we sleep, I'm going to die unhappy. But sleep continues to elude us, and now I'm more resigned." At the 2003 conference in Chicago, the fiftieth anniversary of the discovery of REM, pioneer sleep researcher Michel Jouvet, one of the most distinguished figures of the field, addressed a football-stadium-size ballroom full of people, saying, "We have not been able to solve this great mystery, so I give this to you young people, one of the greatest of all mysteries—of sleep. This last mystery, this last frontier, what is the meaning of this journey we go on every night? I leave it to you."

Change is in the air. In 2005, sleep medicine was recognized as an independent specialty by the American Board of Medical Specialties, which represents validation at the highest level. With this new recognition as a medical field, only MDs (not PhDs) may be certified as "sleep diplomates," that is, sleep doctors. The shift toward a biomedical model may turn out to be good for insomnia, but I hope it doesn't make second-class citizens of PhDs; some of the best insomnia research has come from PhDs. I hope it doesn't tilt the field further toward pulmonary medicine. And I hope the specialty isn't flooded by doctors looking for "nonemergency" fields. This has been the trend in medicine: those specialties that offer "controllable lifestyles," where you don't have to be on call and can keep regular hours, are attracting the most doctors. Dermatology is suddenly hot, with a 40 percent increase in students going into it in the past five years, "compared with a 40% drop in those interested in family practice," reports the *New York Times*.

Sleep medicine may look easy, but it's anything but easy. It's a challenge and an adventure that holds rewards more than economic, an opportunity for discovery, for making a difference in people's lives—if, that is, it doesn't fall into the rote and formulaic, the perfunctory prescribing of a medication or the rehearsal of old rules. Anybody can do it poorly; the challenge is to do it well. Done well, it can give people back their lives—an expression I hear from both patients and physicians—for the gift of sleep is the gift of life. To treat chronic insomnia, just common, ordinary, garden variety insomnia, to give it the art, skill, patience, perseverance, and imagination it requires, is not for the faint of heart.

At the 2005 annual sleep conference in Denver, a week or so after the NIH conference, I ran into Michael Bonnet at a poster session. He'd had to leave the NIH conference before the press conference I found so dispiriting, and he asked me how it had gone.

"Hardly anybody came," I told him. "I guess what's so important to us doesn't matter much to the world."

He sighed, shook his head. "But I'm hopeful," he said. "Look around"—and he gestured at the crowds swarming the poster boards, tripping over each other to read about the new studies—"It's a vital field. It's a great field to go into—there are so few sleep specialists in relation to the number of people who have sleep disorders. And there's no lack of researchers. Besides," he went on, "we're capturing the interest of the best neurophysiological researchers—we've got them to write grants on insomnia. Some of the best in the field are becoming interested in insomnia, Clifford Saper, Bob McCarly, Dennis McGinney. That's what we need, the neurophysiological model, to get beyond this idea that insomniacs are crazy, to get the NIH to think of it as a neurophysiological problem. There's tremendous money in it—it could lead to better drugs. Researchers ought to be interested."

I looked around, took in the scene, all these people milling around, men and women of all sizes, shapes, colors, a multitude of accents, languages, passions, tremendous energy.

"Now," he said "what we need is for the insomniacs themselves to stand up and say, 'There are a lot of us, send resources our way.' Exert some force, make your presence known. Tell the world that you're here, that this area needs resources."

He's right, I think. If these forces can converge—insomniacs, scientists, the NIH—who knows what we might do?

Notes

See www.SleepStarved.org for a fuller version of these notes, as well as citations for researchers' comments that are taken from conference talks or interviews.

CHAPTER 1. INSOMNIA

1   **Look on the Web**   Occasionally, when I've come across the same thoughts or feelings expressed again and again, I've made composites or pastiches of voices. I do this for purposes of clarity, concision, and effect.

2   *someone opened a tap*   "Gray Matters: Sleep and the Brain," Vancouver Public Radio International, www.dana.org/books/radiotv/gm, accessed January 2003.

2   **Says Romanian writer**   E. M. Cioran, interview, ed. Jason Weiss, *Writing at Risk: Interviews in Paris with Uncommon Writers* (University of Iowa Press, 1991), pp. 4–5.

2   **risk factor for suicide**   Taylor et al.

2   **risk factor for alcoholism**   Stoller.

2   **Ancient Egyptian hieroglyphs**   Goldberg and Kaufman, p. 3.

3   **They include anointing**   Wright, pp. 188–91.

3   **Surveys indicate**   These are the figures agreed upon by most researchers. The 2002 National Sleep Foundation Sleep in America Poll (www.kintera .org/atf/cf/%7BF6BF2668-A1B4-4FE8-8D1A-A5D39340D9CB%7D/ 2002SleepInAmericaPoll.pdf) gives a higher figure, with over a third (35 percent) reporting they experienced at least one of four insomnia symptoms (difficulty falling asleep, waking a lot, waking up too early, and waking feeling unrefreshed) every night or nearly every night in the previous year, and over half (58 percent) reporting at least one of these symptoms at least a few nights a week.

3   **Among the poor, the female, and the elderly**   Foley et al.

3   **Sleep researchers estimate**   Hajak.

3   "Insomniacs are seen as neurotics"   Coleman, p. 135.

3   *I'm not an insomniac, I just can't sleep*   David Goding, "Eyes Wide
         Open," *Sydney Herald Sunday Magazine* (July 7, 2002): 40–44; His-
         lop and Arber, "Understanding Women's Sleep."

4   "underground ailment"   Diamond.

4   Sleep has little part   R.C. Rosen et al., "Physician Education in Sleep
         and Sleep Disorders: A National Survey of U.S. Medical Schools," *Sleep*
         16 (1993): 249–54.

5   A myth that's been called into question   Bliwise.

5   When 501 physicians   Daniel Everitt et al., "Clinical Decision-Making
         in the Evaluation and Treatment of Insomnia," *American Journal of
         Medicine* 89 (1990): 357–62.

5   "the patient with a chronic complaint"   Orr et al.

6   "You're probably not 'getting enough'"   "Every physician to whom I
         spoke," writes Phyllis Rosenteur, "said he had no insomniacs among
         his happily married patients. 'A satisfactory sex act,' one said, 'is safer
         and surer than a sleeping pill.' Another distinguished doctor sent me off
         with what he called a fool-proof formula: 'Frustration keeps one
         awake; satisfaction sends one to sleep.'" Rosenteur, p. 111.

7   *People cannot hear that*   Baddiel, p. 120. Baddiel's routine is described
         in "Diary of an Insomniac," by "an anonymous coward" (self-desig-
         nated), www.room23.org/2252.html, accessed March 2003.

7   "Insomniacs may be naturally short sleepers"   Mark Chambers,
         "Alert Insomniacs: Are They Really Sleep Deprived?" *Clinical Psy-
         chology Review* 13 (1993): 649–66.

8   "Worries by such insomniacs"   Horne, "Dimensions to Sleepiness,"
         p. 174.

8   "Although [insomniacs] may report"   Horne, *Why We Sleep*, p. 208.

9   "We do not know the real causes"   Buysse, "Rational Pharmacother-
         apy"; Daniel Buysse, "Response to Dr. Jacobs," *Sleep* 27, 2 (2004):
         348–49.

9   "We do not know . . . the nature"   Richardson and Roth, "Future
         Directions."

9   There is little agreement   Walsh, "Insights."

9   far from consensus   "There wasn't enough evidence for consensus."
         Karl Hunt, "Report on 2005 NIH Conference" (19th Annual Meeting
         of the APSS, Denver, June 2005).

9   NIH . . . spent . . . less than $20 million   This is according to the
         NIH's figures. "Computer Retrieval of Information on Scientific
         Projects, Hit List," National Institutes of Health, http://crisp.cit.nih
         .gov/crisp/crisp_lib.query, accessed December 2006. "If one evaluates
         the overall progress in sleep disorder research, it is both surprising and
         disappointing that research on various aspects of insomnia has lagged
         behind." Kiley.

9   **Sanofi-Aventis spent *$123 million* . . . advertising Ambien**   Saul, "To Sleep, Perchance to Eat."

10   **no comparable explanation for why we sleep**   Siegel, "Why We Sleep."

10   **"The mystery of sleep function"**   Hobson, *Sleep,* p. 189.

10   **"It's a fabulous field to work in"**   Quotes for which citations are not provided are from interviews conducted between 2002 and 2006, from conversations or e-mails, or from presentations at the meetings. Citations are provided in the fuller version of notes at Sleepstarved.org.

11   **"the meeting place for mind and body"**   Horne, *Sleepfaring,* p. 258.

11   **people have to begin somewhere**   The "fundamental Western division between mind and body" is something "our society, for all its sophisticated caveats, still endorses," says Luhrmann, p. 8.

11   **Nearly everyone who comes at insomnia**   When I began researching this project, I was struck by the fact that nearly everything published about insomnia was in the psychology library at Berkeley, in journals like the *Journal of Abnormal Psychology, Archives of General Psychiatry,* and *Journal of Clinical Psychopathology*—and *Sleep,* the premiere journal of the field, is there, too. The items on my list required only an occasional run to the "bio-sci" library.

11   **"the unfortunate consequence of discouraging research"**   Drummond and his colleagues checked out the eighty-four grants "identified by the key word 'insomnia'" funded by the National Institutes of Health and found that "only five of these (as of 2002) address issues related to how disease severity is associated with neurological and/or neuroendocrine abnormalities in humans." Drummond et al.

11   **there's enormous variability**   "If we could see a person's chromosomes as clearly as we can see her face, we would perceive in those long, spiral molecules the same degree of individuality." Braun, p. 104.

11   **"Some people have better/stronger"**   Michael Bonnet, interview by author, May 31, 2002.

11   **many of which are now known to be genetic**   Susan Redline, "Heritability of Sleep and Sleep Disorders," in *Encyclopedia of Sleep and Dreaming,* ed. Mary Carskadon (Macmillan, 1993), pp. 277–79; D.E. Kolker and Fred Turek, "The Search for Circadian Clock and Sleep Genes," *Journal of Psychopharmacology* 13, 4, suppl. 1 (1999): S5–9.

13   **"Though we want to be neutral"**   Atul Gawande, "The Pain Perplex," in *Complications* (Holt, 2002), p. 118.

14   *controlled substances*   These are drugs or chemicals whose manufacture, sale, and distribution come under the authority of state or federal law, specifically, the Controlled Substances Act of 1970 (21 U.S.C. 811), www.usdoj.gov/dea/pubs/abuse/1-csa.htm, accessed April 2007.

15   **"one of the few disorders where the diagnosis"**   Horne, *Why We Sleep,* p. 208.

17   **I find us quoted three times**   By Frankel in 1976; Gaillard in 1978, "Chronic Primary Insomnia"; and Carey et al. in 2005, discussed below.

17   **I find no such books on insomnia**   The few first-person narratives I find, by Rosenteur, Rubenstein, and Armour, tend to self-parody. (Armour, best known for his book *It All Started with Columbus,* happened, weirdly enough, to teach in the same small English department where I've taught since 1974.) I also find Hayes's *Sleep Demons: An Insomniac's Memoir,* but this is primarily a memoir (as its title indicates), a coming-of-age story by a man who happens to have insomnia. John Wiedman writes as an insomniac, but his is a self-help book focused on managing insomnia. Goldberg and Kaufman, whose interest in insomnia is motivated by their insomnia, write the most interesting of these books.

17   **"Insomnia is a subject"**   Laura Miller, "Just Do It," Booknotes, *New York Times Book Review,* January 11, 2004.

18   **"the throes of life"**   Coren, p. 157.

18   **In the 2005 study I referred to earlier**   Carey et al.

19   **Anecdote is not highly regarded**   Dylan Evans, p. 21.

20   **"Chronic anxiety neurotics"**   Richard Coleman et al., "Sleep-Wake Disorders Based on a Polysomnographic Diagnosis: A National Co-operative Study," *Journal of the American Medical Association* 247, 7 (February 19, 1982): 999–1003.

21   **"It may not be news"**   Dement and Vaughan, p. 410.

21   *One night a month*   Jennifer Hunter, "The Facts of Night," June 2004, *North Shore Magazine,* www.northshoremag.com/cgi-bin/ns-article?articlewhat=articles/12-01-the_facts_of_night.dat.

22   **Stewart advised her research team**   Greene, pp. 216, 219.

23   **"sleep complaints are twice as prevalent in women"**   *National Sleep Disorders Research Plan,* sec. 4, "Sleep, Sex Differences, and Women's Health," 2003, National Heart, Lung, and Blood Institute, www.nhlbi.nih.gov/health/prof/sleep/res_plan/section4/section4a.html, accessed April 2007.

23   **it is certainly a women's issue**   When a recent survey asked a random sample of one thousand adults ages twenty-five to seventy-four, "What is the most important factor in your happiness?" 51 percent of women said sleep (only 14 percent said sex, as opposed to 34 percent of men who said sex, and 26 percent who said sleep!). "What America Hungers For," www.usaweekend.com/05_issues/051002/051002food_poll.html, accessed October 2, 2005.

CHAPTER 2. SLEEPSTARVED

26   **sleep deprivation is a time-honored form of coercion**   Adam Hochschild, "What's in a Word?" Op-Ed, *New York Times,* May 23, 2004.

27   **"Sleep-deprived people"**   Martin, pp. 63–64; Horne, *Why We Sleep,* p. 55.

29   "the most powerful predictor of school failure"   D. Blum et al., "Re-
        lation between Chronic Insomnia and School Failure in Preadoles-
        cents," *Sleep Research* 19, 1 (1990), abstract, cited in Stoller.

29   Researchers think it might . . . be linked to the attention deficiency disor-
        ders   R.E. Dahl, "The Impact of Inadequate Sleep on Children's Daytime
        Cognition Function," *Seminars in Pediatric Neurology* 3, 1 (1996): 44–50.

30   Americans with Disabilities Act   Linton, p. 32n2.

33   insomniacs have a hard time getting jobs   Stoller; Damien Leger et al.,
        "Medical and Socio-Professional Impact of Insomnia," *Sleep* 25,
        6 (2002): 625–29.

33   *I can't believe I'm fucking awake*   Through a Glass Darkly, darkglass
        .org/blog8/23/0.

33   Sleep deprivation makes people indifferent and listless   M. Engel-
        Friedman et al. found that "effortful behavior is negatively affected by
        sleep loss." "The Impact of Naturally Occurring Sleep Loss on Effort,
        Mood, and Sleepiness," in *Proceedings of the 17th Annual Meeting of
        the Associated Professional Sleep Societies* (Associated Professional
        Sleep Societies, 2003), abstract 046.I, p. 186.

33   "It's not working"   Coren, pp. 67–69.

34   "Chronic insomniacs don't reach the top"   L.J. Johnson and C.L. Spin-
        weber, "Good and Poor Sleepers Differ in Navy Performance," *Mili-
        tary Medicine* 148 (1983): 727–31.

34   Lord Roseberry, prime minister   Quoted in Goldberg and Kaufman,
        p. 34.

35   Sleep loss increases pain sensitivity   Charles Morin et al., "Self-
        Reported Sleep and Mood Disturbance in Chronic Pain Patients," *Clin-
        ical Journal of Pain* 14 (1998): 311–14.

35   If you deprive young, healthy adults   Gail Davis, "Improved Sleep
        May Reduce Arthritis Pain," *Holistic Nursing Practice* (May–June
        2003): 128–35. If you force young women to awake every hour of the
        night for seven nights, subjects report more aches and pains the next
        day and have heightened pain perception. M.T. Smith et al., "The Ef-
        fects of Sleep Deprivation on Pain Inhibition and Spontaneous Pain in
        Women," *Sleep* 30, 4 (2007): 35–52.

35   if you give arthritis sufferers sleep medication   James Walsh et al., "Ef-
        fects of Triazolam on Sleep, Daytime Sleepiness, and Morning Stiffness
        in Patients with Rheumatoid Arthritis," *Journal of Rheumatology* 23,
        2 (1996): 245–52.

35   Subjects were less able to secrete *insulin*   Spiegel et al., "Impact of
        Sleep Debt."

36   "stronger predictor" of "nursing home"   Charles Pollack et al., "Sleep
        Problems in the Community Elderly as Predictors of Death and Nursing
        Home Placement: Its Significance for Hospital Practice," *Journal of
        Community Health* 15, 2 (April 1990): 123–35.

36   "most important predictor"   Dement and Vaughan, p. 262.

36   **A study that looked at healthy elders**   Mary Dew et al., "Healthy Older Adults' Sleep Predicts All-Cause Mortality at 4 to 19 Years of Follow-Up," *Psychosomatic Medicine* 65 (2003): 63–73.

36   **Insomniacs have two to three times**   Stoller.

36   **more than twice the rate of auto accidents**   Hauri and Linde, pp. 3, 4.

36   **annual cost of insomnia**   Stoller estimates both direct and indirect costs as coming to around $100 billion.

36   **"People with chronic insomnia are distressed"**   Meir Kryger, "Burden of Chronic Insomnia on Society" (paper presented to the "National Institutes of Health State-of-the-Science Conference on Manifestations and Management of Chronic Insomnia in Adults," June 2005, 13–15). Also, D. Katz and C. McHorney, "The Relationship between Insomnia and Health-Related Quality of Life in Patients with Chronic Illness," *Journal of Family Practice* 51 (2002): 229–35; Drake et al.; Leger et al.

37   **"astonishing anachronism"**   Chip Brown, "Stubborn Scientist," quotes Thomas Roth saying: "as though we'd flown to Mars. . . ."

38   **Doctor Samuel Johnson**   Quoted in Ekirch, "Sleep We Have Lost."

38   **As for the social sciences**   Taylor.

38   **many medical textbooks, leave sleep out**   Orr et al.

38   **"the most moronic fraternity"**   Vladimir Nabokov, *Speak, Memory: An Autobiography Revisited* (1947; reprint, Vintage, 1967), pp. 108–9.

38   **"something to be gotten over"**   Edward Said, *Out of Place: A Memoir* (Vintage, 1999), pp. 294–95.

38   **"Sleep puts even the strongest"**   Coe, p. 177.

39   **"the indifferent judge between the high and low"**   Sir Philip Sidney, *Astrophel and Stella*, sonnet 39, *The Norton Anthology of English Literature*, ed. M.H. Abrams et al. (Norton, 1968), p. 474.

39   **"Sleep is something we share"**   Marcus Aurelius, *The Meditations*, trans. Maxwell Staniforth (Penguin, 1964), bk. 8, p. 123.

39   **sleep, unlike death, is a realm**   Hamlet, in act III, scene I, describes death as "The undiscover'd country, from whose bourn / No traveller returns."

39   **"The individual who lives out his allotted"**   Rosenteur, p. 7.

39   **Even in classical Greek and Roman times**   Coren, p. 278.

40   **More than 80 percent of Americans believe**   According to a survey quoted by Dement and Vaughan, p. 121.

40   **"Guys like General Electric's Jeffrey Immelt"**   Wells.

40   **"In the corporate world"**   Groopman.

40   **One-fifth of the workforce does shift work**   R.G. Bursey, "A Cardiovascular Study of Shift Workers with Respect to Coronary Artery Disease Risk Factor Prevalence," *Occupational Medicine* 40 (1990): 65–67.

40   **Home Depots, Wal-Marts**   Groopman.

40   A new principle of "incessance"   Melbin, pp. 3, 8.

40   In 1910, people slept an average of nine hours a night   Wilse Webb
        and J.R. Agnew, "Are We Chronically Sleep Deprived?" *Bulletin of the
        Psychonomic Society* 6 (1975): 47–48; Webb, "Twenty-Four-Hour
        Sleep Cycling," in *Sleep: Physiology and Pathology; A Symposium,* ed.
        Anthony Kales (Lippincott, 1969); Coren, p. 3.

40   the second-most traded   Silvia Franceschi, "Coffee and Myocardial
        Infarction: Review of Epidemiological Evidence," in *Caffeine, Coffee,
        and Health,* ed. Silvio Garattini (Raven Press, 1993), p. 208.

40   Starbucks . . . a household word   Nicole Nolan, "Starbucked!" *In
        These Times,* November 11, 1996, pp. 14–17.

40   "Energy drinks are a $3.7 billion industry"   Michael Mason, "The
        Energy-Drink Buzz Is Unmistakable. The Health Impact Is Unknown,"
        New York Times, December 12, 2006.

40   The wake-up drug Provigil   Graham Lawton, "Get Ready for 24-
        Hour Living," NewScientist.com, February 18, 2006, www.newscientist
        .com/article/mg18925391.300; O'Connor.

40   "You would think that the tangible"   Vaughn McCall, quoted in
        Jennifer Wilson.

41   residents to work 100 to 120 hours per week   S.R. Daugherty et al.,
        "Learning, Satisfaction, and Mistreatment during Medical Internship:
        A National Survey of Working Conditions," *Journal of the American
        Medical Association* 279 (1998): 1194–99. A 2001 study by Owens
        et al. found that medical residents at a major teaching hospital average
        3.7 hours of sleep the nights they're on call.

41   "I have heard doctors say"   Coren, pp. 203–6.

41   1999 report from the Institute of Medicine   Cited in Owens et al.

41   As recently as 1977 . . . Ray Meddis   His comment provoked an in-
        somniac to write him, "Sir, you are a bloody idiot." Meddis, p. 104.

41   Rechtschaffen . . . subjected rats to total sleep deprivation   Rechtschaf-
        fen et al., "Physiological Correlates."

41   Later work suggested   Carol Everson, "Clinical Manifestations of
        Prolonged Sleep Deprivation," in *Sleep Science: Integrating Basic Re-
        search and Clinical Practice,* ed. W.J. Schwartz (Basel, 1997), p. 52.

41   Lugaresi could do nothing   Elio Lugaresi et al., "Fatal Familial In-
        somnia and Dysautonomia with Selective Degeneration of Thalamic
        Nuclei," *New England Journal of Medicine* 315 (1986): 997–1003.

42   Institute of Medicine issued a report   *Sleep Disorders and Sleep De-
        privation.*

42   *Power Sleep*   Maas et al.

43   *frontal cortex . . . most affected*   Harrison et al.; Horne, *Sleepfaring,*
        pp. 74–75.

43   where humans are thought to "form their sense of who they are"
        Braun, p. 191.

43   **Creative thinking . . . takes a beating**   Horne, "Sleep Loss and 'Divergent' Thinking Ability."

43   **We dream in every stage of sleep**   Rechtschaffen et al., "Interrelatedness of Mental Activity during Sleep," *Archives of General Psychiatry* 9 (December 1963): 26–37.

44   **there is *rebound***   Jouvet, pp. 8, 152, 160.

44   **insomniacs tend to remember lots of dreams**   Schredl.

45   **babies dream**   Dement and Vaughan, p. 106.

45   **late-term fetuses seem to dream**   H.P. Roffwarg et al., "Ontogenetic Development of the Human Sleep-Dream Cycle," *Science* 152 (1966): 604–19.

45   **The species whose young are born the most helpless**   Jerome Siegel, "Why We Sleep." Siegel does not, however, believe that REM is associated with learning.

45   **the role of REM in learning**   Hobson, *Sleep,* p. 50; A. Karni et al., "No Dreams, No Memory: The Effect of REM Sleep Deprivation on Learning a New Perceptual Skill," *Society for Neuroscience Abstracts* 18 (1992): 387.

45   **people who take antidepressants that wipe out REM**   Lavie, pp. 140–45.

45   **when researchers wake people out of REM**   Stickgold, "Why We Dream," p. 581.

46   ***Procedural memory . . . declarative memory***   Researchers differentiate not only between different kinds of memories but between different steps in acquiring memories, which they call encoding, consolidating, reconsolidating, and enhancing. They are finding that sleep is involved in all, and that all stages of sleep are involved. See Walker and Stickgold; Empson, pp. 167–68; C. Smith, "Sleep States and Memory Processes," *Behavioral Brain Research* 69 (1995): 137–45.

46   **different kinds of memory are dependent on different kinds of sleep**   Walker and Stickgold; Empson, p. 167–68; C. Smith; W. Phihal and Jan Born, "Effects of Early and Late Nocturnal Sleep on Priming and Spatial Memory," *Psychophysiology* 36 (1999): 571–82.

46   **animals or humans are taught a new task**   Ulrich Wagner et al., "Sleep Inspires Insight," *Nature* 427 (January 22, 2004): 304–5.

46   **Memory is related to *plasticity***   Walker and Stickgold; also, T.T. Dang-vu et al., "A Role for Sleep in Brain Plasticity," *Pediatric Rehabilitation* 9 (April 2006): 98–118.

47   **"We are taking in so much information"**   Stickgold, on *To the Best of Our Knowledge,* "Sweet Dreams, Sleepless Nights," interviewed by Jim Fleming, Public Radio International, www.wpr.org/book.

47   **"off-line memory reprocessing"**   Stickgold et al.

47   **to lay down new tracks**   "Brain cells, after collecting new information in the form of biochemical changes during the wake cycle, need some downtime to fix those changes," says Harvard neuroscientist Clifford

Saper; quoted in William Cromie, "Waking Up to How We Sleep and Dream," *Harvard University Gazette,* November 17, 2005, news.harvard .edu/gazette. For a fascinating account of what goes on in the brain to make this happen, see M. Massimini et al., "Breakdown of Cortical Effective Connectivity during Sleep," *Science* 309 (2005): 2228–32. "Sleep is the price we pay for plasticity," explains Giulio Tononi, a researcher on the study. Quoted by Beth Azar, "Wild Findings on Animal Sleep," *Monitor on Psychology* 37, 1 (January 2006), American Psychological Association Online, www.apa.org/monitor/jan06/wild.html.

47   **we need also to retain memories**   Hobson, *Sleep,* pp. 199–200.

47   **Subjects who've been taught . . . Alpine Racer II**   Stickgold, "Why We Dream," p. 584.

47   **"review and recombine memories"**   Stickgold quoted in "'Study Not Sleep' Is Exam Boost," BBC News, November 2, 2001, www.news.bc.co .uk/1/hi/health/1634019.stm.

47   **"arguably among the most sophisticated human"**   Stickgold, "Sleep-Dependent Memory."

47   **compromises our ability**   Durmer and Dinges.

47–48   **nurse who . . . "didn't make the connection"**   Kryger quoted in Jennifer Ozols, "Time for Bed," *Newsweek,* March 3, 2005, www.msnbc .msn.com/id/7077587/site/newsweek.

CHAPTER 3. BLAME THE VICTIM

49   **"When all else fails, invoke a psychoneurosis"**   Gershon, p. 177.

50   **"If you were chained"**   Gershon quoted in Harriet Brown, "The Other Brain, the One with Butterflies, Also Deals with Woes," *New York Times,* August 23, 2005.

50   **"When I was a medical student"**   Gershon, telephone interview by author, April 11, 2003.

50   **irritable bowel syndrome may also originate in the gut**   Gershon, p. 121.

50   **"Migraine, we used to believe"**   Silberstein quoted in Kamen, p. 88.

50   **Obsessive-compulsive disorder was described by a Freudian**   Shorter, p. 270.

50   **obsessive-compulsive disorder is a "neurobiological illness"**   Quoted by Amy S. Wilensky, *Passing for Normal: A Memoir of Compulsion* (Broadway Books, 1999), p. 210.

50   **"schizophrenogenic mother"**   This was the notorious phrase of Freida Fromm-Reichmann, a refugee German analyst. Quoted in Shorter, p. 177.

51   **"We would have all these erudite conversations"**   McGlashan quoted in Benedict Carey, "A Career That Has Mirrored Psychiatry's Twisting Path," *New York Times,* May 23, 2006.

51   **the heritability of schizophrenia**   Ridley, p. 106.

51   **"We used to believe"**   Then, once "the relevant hormone, neurotransmitter, or genetic abnormality . . . is discovered," says Robert Sapolsky,
"the psychogenic disease is magically transformed into an organic
problem—'oh, it wasn't your personality after all.'" *Zebras,* p. 271.
Stuttering may be added to this list. In the past, stuttering has been explained in terms of "sexual fixations, emotional disorders, nervousness,
and persistence into adult life of infantile nursing activities," reports
Andrew Pollack, "To Fight Stuttering, Doctors Take a Close Look at the
Brain," *New York Times,* September 1, 2006. But "brain imaging studies have shown that the brains of people who stammer behave differently from those of people who don't when it comes to processing
speech."

51   **In the nineteenth century, the condition was attributed**   Seiji Nishino
and Emmanuel Mignot, "Pharmacological Aspects of Human and
Canine Narcolepsy," *Progress in Neurobiology* 52 (1997): 27–78.

51   **"I was sent for psychotherapy"**   Utley, pp. 13–14.

52   **discovery . . . of a mutated gene**   L. Lin et al., "The Sleep Disorder Canine Narcolepsy Is Caused by a Mutation in the Hypocretin (Orexin)
Receptor 2 Gene," *Cell* 98 (August 6, 1999): 365–76.

52   **Within weeks of Mignot's study**   R. M. Chemelli et al., "Narcolepsy
in Orexin Knockout Mice: Molecular Genetics of Sleep Regulation,"
Cell 98 (August 20, 1999): 437–51.

52   **Yanagisawa . . . investigating . . . role in feeding behavior**   T. Sakurai
et al., "Orexins and Orexin Receptors: A Family of Hypothalamic Neu-
ropeptides and G Protein-Coupled Receptors That Regulate Feeding
Behavior," *Cell* 92 (1998): 573–85.

52   **"We didn't aim at, or expect"**   Yanagisawa quoted in Jack McClintock, "Let Sleeping Dogs Arise," *Discover,* February 2000, www
.discovermagazine.com/2000/feb/featdogs.

52   **Mignot's group made the leap to humans**   S. Nishino et al., "Hypocretin (Orexin) Deficiency in Human Narcolepsy," *Lancet* 355 (2000):
39–40.

52   **postmortem examinations of narcoleptics' brains**   C. Peyron et al., "A
Mutation in a Case of Early Onset Narcolepsy and a Generalized Ab-
sence of Hypocretin Peptides in Human Narcoleptic Brains," *Nature
Medicine* 6 (2000): 991–97.

52–53   **"We think that there's something that specifically kills"**   Jerome Siegel
also believes the problem is autoimmune damage. "Narcolepsy."

53   **Hypocretin . . . a mastermind**   Mignot, "Commentary on the Neurobiology."

53   **"We were taught"**   Mahowald quoted in Chip Brown, "Man Who
Mistook His Wife."

53   *Restless legs syndrome* **. . . afflicts 6 to 15 percent**   Barbara Phillips et
al., "Epidemiology of Restless Legs Symptoms in Adults," *Archives of
Internal Medicine* 160 (July 24, 2000): 2137–41.

53   sufferers are . . . "judged as psychotic"   Virginia Wilson, p. 104.

53   they're making up "imaginary ills"   Ibid., p. 45.

53   or concealing some deep, dark deed   Ibid., p. 99.

53   "The missing iron may cause certain neural signals to misfire"   Restless Legs Foundation, "Restless Legs Foundation Annual Report" (RLS Foundation, 2003), p. 3.

54   "Freudian psychology and its offshoots"   Dement, "Personal History."

54   "Today this would never pass"   Dement and Vaughan, pp. 35–36.

54   "The disturbance of sleep is a neurotic symptom"   Ernst Simmel, "Symposium on Neurotic Disturbances of Sleep," *International Journal of Psycho-Analysis* 23, 2 (1942): 65.

54   "Like alcoholism or homosexuality"   F. S. Caprio, "Bisexual Conflicts and Insomnia," *Journal of Clinical Psychopathology* (October 1949): 376–79.

54   "schizoneurosis, with anxiety-hysteric"   Valentine Ujhely, "Oedipal Jealousy and Passive Dependency States in Insomnia," *Journal of Clinical Psychopathology* 11, 2 (1950): 65–69.

54   "the struggle between her id"   Otto Fenichel, *The Psychoanalytic Theory of Neurosis* (Norton, 1945), p. 63.

54   "Here we have a veritable catalogue"   Jacob Conn, "Psychogenesis and Psychotherapy of Insomnia," *Journal of Psychopathology* 11, 2 (1950): 85–91.

55   "do[ing] something crazy"   Conn.

55   "There is always a reason"   Leonard Gilman, "Insomnia in Relation to Guilt, Fear, and Masochistic Intent," *Journal of Clinical Psychopathology* 11, 2 (1950): 63–64.

55   "Psychotherapists have ample case material"   Caprio.

55   "psychopathological basis . . . was obvious"   F. R. Riesenman, "Anxiety and Tensions in the Pathogenesis of Sleep Disturbances," *Journal of Clinical Psychopathology* 11, 2 (1950): 82–84.

56   Depression, . . . "a despairing cry for love"   Walter Bonime, "The Psychodynamics of Neurotic Depression," *Journal of American Academy of Psychoanalysis* 4 (1976): 1073–78. This definition was generally accepted by psychoanalysts.

56   It became difficult to believe in the value of a long Freudian analysis   Not that the entire profession all at once jettisoned all of Freud. There's much that remains, and much good that remains, of the Freudian approach. That we may be in thrall to parts of ourselves that we're not aware of, that we may, by working back and working through, loosen the hold of the past and the compulsions that bind us—these assumptions inform the practices of psychotherapists I admire. But Freudians left an unfortunate legacy regarding insomnia.

56   "nearly all of Freud's central concepts"   Hobson and Leonard, p. 62.

56   "Physiological factors are seldom the primary cause"   Kales and Kales, p. 80.

56   "The majority of chronic insomniacs"   Anthony Kales et al., "Bio-psychobehavioral Correlates of Insomnia, III: Polygraphic Findings of Sleep Difficulty and Their Relationship to Psychopathology," *Internal Journal of Neuroscience* 23 (1984): 43–56.

56   Insomniacs feel "inadequate, insecure" . . . "entitlement"   Kales and Kales, p. 46.

56   Insomniacs "tend to be obsessional"'   Ibid., pp. 170–71.

56   "manage stress ineffectively . . . high levels of psychopathology"   Ibid., p. 119. They have "maladaptive coping mechanisms," say the Kaleses (p. 112).

56   "possibly schizoid"   Ibid., p. 102.

56   "The well-established importance of psychiatric factors"   Alexandros Vgontzas et al., "Usefulness of Polysomnographic Studies in the Differential Diagnosis of Insomnia," *International Journal of Neuroscience* 82 (1995): 47–60.

57   Throughout the twentieth century   Robert Coursey, "Personality Measures and Evoked Responses in Chronic Insomniacs," *Journal of Abnormal Psychology* 84, 3 (1975): 239–49; Larry Beutler et al., "Psychological Variables in the Diagnosis of Insomnia," in *Sleep Disorders: Diagnosis and Treatment,* ed. Robert Williams and Ismet Karacan (Wiley, 1978), pp. 69–70; Damien Leger, "Public Health and Insomnia: Economic Impact," *Sleep* 23 (2000): S69–76.

57   "tense, complaining, histrionic"   Quentin Regenstein quoted in Goldberg and Kaufman, p. 142.

57   Insomniacs have an "internalizing or obsessive personality style"   Dorsey and Bootzin.

57   "Good sleepers appear busier"   Marchini et al.

57   Insomniacs score high   Thomas Roth et al., "The Nature of Insomnia: A Descriptive Summary of a Sleep Clinic Population," *Comprehensive Psychiatry* 17, 1 (1976): 217–20.

57   according to some studies (though not all)   Dorsey.

57   Critics point out   Paul, pp. 45–73. Paul notes that the MMPI was revised in 1989, with an expanded base of twenty-six hundred persons of more varied social backgrounds, but that it retained its basic assumptions—and 84 percent of its original items.

57   said to be "emotionally seclusive"   Marchini et al.

57   a "distressed, pessimistic, worried group"   E. Shevy Healey et al., "Onset of Insomnia: Role of Life-Stress Events," *Psychosomatic Medicine* 43, 5 (1981): 439–51.

57   "greater difficulty in interpersonal relationships"   Kales and Kales, pp. 96–97, 113.

57   tendency to deny . . . "considering sleeplessness"   Ibid., pp. 163.

57   they have a "strong resistance"   Ibid., pp. 217-18.

57   Even when they deny that they're depressed   Ibid., p. 124.

58   "stress-related psychophysiological problems"   Ibid., p. 120.

58   Here's the language   *Diagnostic and Statistical Manual,* p. 599.

60   In medicalese, a *symptom* is   Billiard and Bentley.

60   *sign* or objective indication   *Signs, symptoms, syndromes,* and *diseases* are defined by Buysse, "Diagnosis and Classification of Insomnia Disorders," in *Insomnia: Principles and Management,* ed. Martin Szuba et al. (Cambridge University Press, 2003), pp. 4-5.

60   *Complaint,* in the language of medical professionals   Roehrs and Roth, p. 414.

60   In 2004, insomnia was promoted from symptom to syndrome   "A syndrome is a set of symptoms (subjective complaints from the patient) and signs (objective, physician-assessed indicators) that occur together and characterize a particular abnormality or form an identifiable pattern." *Stedman's Medical Dictionary* (Lippincott, 2004).

60   Insomnia can't be termed a disease   "A disorder generally only graduates from its status as a syndrome [to disease] when its underlying pathological causes or 'etiologies' . . . are uncovered," writes Howard Kushner in *A Cursing Brain? The Histories of Tourette Syndrome* (Harvard University Press, 1999), p. 4.

60   What does it matter   It matters in terms of the distribution of resources that we have "a reasonably clear idea, first what a disease is, and second, which diseases are most worth the investment of time and money." Jackie Leach Scully, "What Is a Disease? Disease, Disability, and Their Definitions," *European Molecular Biology Organization* 5, 7 (2004): 650-53.

60   "The naming of diseases"   Shenk, pp. 183, 78-79, 74.

61   And researchers know it   Jack Edinger, "Classifying Insomnia in a Clinically Useful Way," *Journal of Clinical Psychiatry* 65, suppl. 8 (2004): 36-43.

61   "The inability to accurately define"   Kiley.

62   Health plans give less compensation   Nina Schuyler, "Out of the Shadows," *In These Times,* February 8, 1998.

62   It is deeply engrained in the American psyche   Solomon, pp. 361-62.

62   "Patients who present themselves to doctors"   Gershon, p. xiv.

62   "There is little sympathy for"   Ibid., pp. 309-10.

63   "appear insistent and tiresome"   Eduard Estivill, "Behaviour of Insomniacs and Implication for Their Management," *Sleep Medicine Reviews* 6, suppl. 1 (2002): 53-56.

63   "Poor sleepers . . . weak and negative personalities"   Meddis, p. 110.

63   Women's problems are more likely than men's   Council on Ethical and Judicial Affairs, American Medical Association, "Gender Disparities in

Clinical Decision Making," *Journal of the American Medical Association* 266, 4 (1991): 559–62. This report cites studies.

63   **Hauri recounts approaching a psychiatrist**   Hauri and Linde, p. ix.

64   **"It is clear"**   Luce and Segal, p. 85.

64   **their "own worst enemies"**   Colligan, p. 33.

64   **"Some people really produce"**   Hartman, quoted in Goldberg and Kaufman, p. 243.

64   **"There are people who exploit their insomnia"**   Luce and Segal, p. 68.

64   **"Those are persons for whom"**   Segal, quoted in Hauri and Linde, p. 86.

64   **"Insomniacs are usually highly invested in"**   Kales and Kales, p. 44.

64   **"At work they typically function"**   Ibid., p. 44.

64   **"avoid family . . . interactions" . . . "may even demand"**   Ibid., p. 167.

64   **The Kaleses' idea of *secondary gains***   "Because of their preoccupation with their symptoms and investment in the secondary gain they receive, these patients are difficult to treat." Ibid., p. 48.

64   **"difficult to give up their sleep disorder"**   Lavie, p. 171.

65   **Harvard study gave doctors the case histories**   Herbert Hendin, *Suicide in America* (Norton, 1995), 216; cited in Solomon, p. 247.

65   **But some of the nuttiest people**   I find two researchers who acknowledge that "many people with severe psychiatric disorders sleep well, and a large proportion of patients with insomnia do not have psychiatric disorders." Arthur Spielman and Paul Glovinsky, "The Varied Nature of Insomnia," in *Case Studies in Insomnia,* ed. Peter Hauri (Plenum, 1991), p. 3. I find two researchers who say, "Though evidence of increased neuroticism, anxiety, and worry have been found in insomniacs, there are no doubt many persons experiencing these problems who do not have difficulty sleeping." Freedman and Sattler. But researchers do not make much of this point that seems so important to me.

68   **"sensation avoiders"**   Hauri and Fisher describe insomniacs as "more aversive to change and challenge," as "seek[ing] routine tasks for both jobs and hobbies."

69   **Charles Morin, examining the beliefs**   "Dysfunctional Beliefs and Attitudes about Sleep among Older Adults with and without Insomnia Complaints," *Psychology and Aging* 3, 3 (1993): 463–67, my emphasis.

71   **I do not have that natural pressure**   Stepanski et al. suggest that insomniacs may have "a diminished homeostatic response to sleep loss" that "may represent a neurophysiologic abnormality."

71   **"about 70% of persons suffering from chronic pain"**   Davis.

72   **"every time the sleeper was 'shot'"**   Hobson, *Sleep,* p. 98. But the story of a thirty-seven-year-old man who slept through being shot—literally—tops it all. Michael Lusher awoke nearly four hours after a small-caliber bullet struck him in the head, to notice blood oozing from his head. That's sleep pressure for you! "Man Sleeps through Gunshot

to the Head," SFGate.com, May 21, 2007, www.sfgate.com/cgi-bin/
article.cgi?f=/n/a/2007/05/21/national/a130837D64.DTL.

72 **many of the personality traits** Hauri and Fisher.

73 **You could make them depressed** Ford and Kamerow; Perlis et al.,
"Self-Reported Sleep Disturbance as a Prodromal Symptom in Recurrent
Depression," *Journal of Affective Disorders* 42, 2–3 (1997): 209–12; and
many other studies.

73 **In fact, in a study of eighty-six patients** D. Morawetz, "Depression
and Insomnia: Which Comes First?" *Australian Journal of Counseling
Psychology* 3, 1 (2001): 19–24.

73 **A 1946 paper** Fred Turek describes this paper in "The Prevailing Culture of Sleepiness," *Sleep* 28, 7 (2005): 798–99.

73 **"The causal web"** Rechtschaffen, "Laboratory Studies," p. 168.

74 **"the psychogenic bucket"** Sapolsky, p. 271.

76 **"The status of night people"** Colligan, pp. 154–55.

76 **"Early to bed, early to rise"** St. John and Williams.

76 **"Until about one hundred years ago"** Alvarez, p. 6.

76 **"Murderers and thieves"** Ekirch, *At Day's Close*, p. 8.

77 **"Good people love the day"** Quoted in Verdon, p. 66.

77 **"When it was said of any man"** Ekirch, *At Day's Close*, pp. 31–32.

78 **"The best pillow is a clear conscience"** L. E. Wexberg, "Insomnia as
Related to Anxiety and Ambition," *Journal of Clinical Psychopathology* (October 1949): 373–75.

CHAPTER 4. SLEEPLESS IN SEATTLE

79 **guy looking for his wallet** Peter Hauri, interview by author, May 16,
2003.

79 **in 1960 . . . Rechtschaffen "called"** Hauri and Linde, p. 5.

82 **a lunchtime event** Margaret Moline, "Sleep across the Life Cycle"
(paper presented to the 16th Annual Meeting of the APSS, Seattle, June
10, 2002).

82 **Seventy-five percent of sleep research** 2003. *National Sleep Disorders
Research Plan.*

83 **menopause is a biological . . . event** Sherwin; Landis and Moe.

84 **study . . . catches my attention** Tarja Porkka-Heiskanen et al.,
"Orexin A and B Levels in the Hypothalamus of Female Rats: The Effects
of the Estrous Cycle and Age," *European Journal of Endocrinology*
150, 5 (2004): 737–42.

85 **Where have I heard this before?** Dr. B. Karpman, "Paraphiliac Preoccupations and Guilt in the Etiology of Insomnia," *Journal of Clinical Psychopathology* (April 1950): 75–78.

86   **physicians don't take time**   P.M. Nicassio et al., "Insomnia: Non-pharmacological Management by Private Physicians," *South Medical Journal* 78 (1985): 556–60.

89   **drug companies paid over 60 percent**   Angell, *Truth,* p. 139.

89   **going to a used car salesman**   D.R. Waud, "Pharmaceutical Promotions," *New England Journal of Medicine* 327 (1992): 351–53.

89   **researchers with financial ties**   Cohen, p. 133.

90   **exposé after exposé**   Books by Abramson, Angell, Avorn, Cohen, Critser, Kassirer, and Moynihan and Cassels came out in 2004–05.

91   **he himself had written about this**   Mendelson, "Do Studies of Sedative/Hypnotics Suggest the Nature of Chronic Insomnia?"

91   **"the dark side"**   Kripke's book, *The Dark Side of Sleeping Pills,* is available on the Web. Also, see Kripke, "Chronic Hypnotic Use: Deadly Risks, Doubtful Benefit," *Sleep Medicine Reviews* 4, 1 (2000): 5–20.

98   **"surprising how little is known"**   Ernest Hartmann, in Goldberg and Kaufman, p. 249.

99   **"To be a working scientist"**   Luhrmann, p. 165.

99   **"a feeling for the organism"**   This is the title of Evelyn Fox Keller's biography, *A Feeling for the Organism: The Life and Work of Barbara McClintock* (Freeman, 1983).

105   **"I have spent twenty-seven years of my life sleep-depriving people"**   Dinges's remarks, unless otherwise indicated, are taken from "Manifestations of Sleepiness" (paper presented to the 16th Annual Meeting of the APSS, Seattle, June 10, 2002); "Sleepiness and Performance" (paper presented to the 18th Annual Meeting of the APSS, Philadelphia, June 8, 2004); "What Is Sleep Debt?" (paper presented to the European Sleep Research Society 17th Congress, Prague, October 7, 2004).

105   **"There is some cognitive price"**   Durmer and Dinges.

105   **"Sleepiness is relentless"**   Dinges and Nancy Kribbs, "Performing while Sleepy," in *Sleep, Sleepiness, and Performance,* ed. Timothy Monk (John Wiley and Sons, 1991), p. 121.

105   **"Some people are resilient"**   Van Dongen et al., "Systematic Interindividual Differences."

106   **"something in the genes"**   As it is turning out to be: A.U. Viola et al., "PER3 Polymorphism Predicts Sleep Structure and Waking Performance," *Current Biology* 17 (April 2007): 613–18.

106   **landmark study discussed earlier**   Spiegel et al., "Impact of Sleep Debt."

107   **They then looked at people who restrict their sleep voluntarily**   B. Mander et al., "Short Sleep: A Risk Factor for Insulin Resistance and Obesity," *Sleep* 24 (2001): A74.

107   **80 percent increase in Americans with diabetes**   N.R. Kleinfield, "Diabetes and Its Awful Toll Quietly Emerge as a Crisis," *New York Times,* January 9, 2006.

107   **One in three children**   "The Royal Route to Obesity," *Sleepmatters* (NSF), 5, 4 (Fall 2003): 3.

107   **both as related to the reduction of hours that we sleep**   C. Meisinger et al., "Sleep Disturbance as a Predictor of Type 2 Diabetes Mellitus in Men and Women from the General Population," *Diabetologia* 48 (2005): 235–41. There are also studies that find associations between sleep duration and body mass index. See James Gangwisch et al., "Inadequate Sleep as a Risk Factor for Obesity: Analyses of the NHANES I," *Sleep* 28, 10 (2005): 1289–96, among others.

107   **"the royal route to obesity"**   "The Royal Route to Obesity," *Sleepmatters* (NSF), 5, 4 (Fall 2003): 3.

107   **Insulin resistance moves us down this route**   McEwen and Lasley, p. 201.

107   **reduced levels of growth hormone push us along**   Eve Van Cauter et al., "Interrelations between Sleep and the Somatotropic Axis," *Sleep* 21, 6 (1998): 553–63.

107   **18 percent decrease in leptin levels**   Spiegel et al., "Leptin Levels Are Dependent on Sleep Duration."

108   **"The body is screaming famine"**   Eve Van Cauter, "Sleep Loss: A Role in the Epidemic of Obesity" (paper presented to the Annual Meeting of the APSS, Chicago, June 7, 2003). Several of Van Cauter's remarks are taken from this talk.

108   **"if animals are in a situation"**   Karine Spiegel, "Sleep Loss and Metabolism" (paper presented to the European Sleep Research Society 17th Congress, Prague, October 6, 2004). "We are the only species that voluntarily elects to go without sleep," say Dinges et al.

108   **28 percent increase in levels of ghrelin**   Spiegel et al., "Leptin Levels Are Dependent on Sleep Duration."

108   **"like Rollerblading uphill"**   Van Cauter, quoted in Steve Fishman, "Are You Sleeping?" *Bazaar* (April 2001).

108   **less than half the immune response**   Karine Spiegel et al., "Effect of Sleep Deprivation on Response to Immunization," *Journal of the American Medical Association* 288, 12 (September 5, 2002): 1471–72.

108   **One study found that those who got a good night's sleep**   Tanja Lange et al., "Sleep Enhances the Human Antibody Response to Hepatitis A Vaccination," *Psychosomatic Medicine* 65 (2003): 831–35.

108   **Even modest sleep loss . . . reduction of NK cell activity**   Irwin et al., "Partial Sleep Deprivation." Irwin et al. found that after only one night of being awake from 11 P.M. to 3 A.M., subjects had significantly higher levels of tumor necrosis factor and interleukin 6. "Sleep Deprivation."

108   **Sleep loss . . . raises levels of *cytokines***   Alexandros Vgontzas et al., "Circadian Interleukin-6 Secretion and Quantity and Depth of Sleep," *Journal of Clinical Endocrinology and Metabolism* 84, 8 (1999): 2603–7; Vgontzas and Chrousos, "Sleep," 2002.

109 **Inflammatory markers may also account for the pain** M. Haack et al., "Sleep Restriction Increases Il-6 Levels and Pain-Related Symptoms in Healthy Volunteers," in *Proceedings of the 18th Annual Meeting of the Associated Professional Sleep Societies* (Associated Professional Sleep Societies, 2004), 137; T. Akerstedt and P.M. Nilsson, "Sleep as Restitution: An Introduction," *Journal of Internal Medicine* 254 (2003): 6–12.

109 **Inflammatory markers . . . associated with heart attack** B. Lindahl et al., "Markers of Myocardial Damage and Inflammation in Relation to Long-Term Mortality in Unstable Coronary Artery Disease," *New England Journal of Medicine* 343, 16 (2000): 1139–47; and other studies.

109 **poor sleep . . . and . . . cardiovascular risk** N.T. Ayaset et al., "A Prospective Study of Sleep Duration and Coronary Heart Disease in Women," *Archives of Internal Medicine* 163 (2003): 205–9. Skai Schwartz et al. suggest that "the insomnia–coronary heart disease association may be comparable" to the classic risk factors for heart attack, smoking and diet. "Insomnia and Heart Disease: A Review of Epidemiologic Studies," *Journal of Psychosomatic Research* 47, 4 (1999): 313–33.

109 **sleep deprivation activates the inflammatory response** H.K. Meier-Ewert et al., "Effects of Sleep Loss on C-Reactive Protein, an Inflammatory Marker of Cardiovascular Risk," *Journal of the American College of Cardiology* 43, 4 (2004): 678–83. This may also explain the recently discovered link between lack of sleep and the progression of periodontal disease. M. Kibayashi et al., "Longitudinal Study of the Association between Smoking as a Periodontitis Risk and Salivary Biomarkers Related to Periodontitis," *Journal of Periodontology* 78, 5 (May 2007): 859–67.

110 **"the body's own best state of defense"** Hobson, *Sleep,* p. xiv.

111 **the field "is growing so fast"** Dinges quoted in Chip Brown, "Man Who Mistook His Wife."

CHAPTER 5. THE BRAIN OF AN INSOMNIAC

112 **"Insomnia may not be in their head"** Buysse, "New Visions for Insomnia" (paper presented to the 18th Annual Meeting of the APSS, Philadelphia, June 8, 2004).

112 **"spent . . . over 200 hours staring at the eyes"** Dement, "Knocking on Kleitman's Door."

113 **More was learned . . . Decade of the Brain** Damasio, "How the Brain."

113 **"It's dark in there"** Quoted in Margaret Atwood, *Negotiating with the Dead: A Writer on Writing* (Cambridge University Press, 2002), xxiv. "We're at the same stage in brain research that biology was in the 19th century," says Vilanur Ramachandran, director of the Center for Brain and Cognition at the University of California, San Diego. "We know almost nothing about the mind." Quoted by Lawrence Osborne, "Savant for a Day," *New York Times Magazine* (June 22, 2003).

114   **"Whether one is awake or asleep"**   Hauri, "Primary Insomnia," p. 636.

114   **"complex push-pull system"**   Hobson, *Sleep,* p. 11.

114   *homeostatic*   Homeostasis refers to the organism's need to maintain this steady internal state—*homeo* means "same" and *stasis* means "balance."

114   **"biggest mistake the evolutionary process ever made"**   Rechtschaffen, "The Control of Sleep," in *Human Behavior and Its Control,* ed. W. A. Hunt (Shenkman, 1971), 75–92.

114   **works best "under relatively narrow conditions"**   Rechtschaffen, "Function of Sleep. "

115   **"Mice are so much easier to study"**   Feinberg, interview by author, U.C. Davis, April 24, 2002.

116   **Jouvet . . . performed a series of elegant operations**   Jouvet, pp. 84, 149.

116   **A study headed by Larry Sanford found**   Larry Sanford et al., "Influence of Contextual Fear on Sleep in Mice: A Strain Comparison," *Sleep* 26, 5 (2003): 527–40.

116   **their sleep has many features of ours**   Paul Shaw et al., "Correlates of Sleep and Waking in *Drosophila melanogaster,*" *Science* 287, 5459 (March 10, 2000): 1834–37.

116   **These flies don't "complain a lot"**   "Animal Models: Drosophila" (paper presented to "A Primer of Sleep Research," Sleep Research Society, February 11, 2006, La Jolla, Calif., on C. Cirelli et al., "Reduced Sleep in *Drosophila* Shaker Mutants," *Nature* 434 [2005]: 1087–92).

117   **"they cannot learn"**   Daniel Bushey et al., "Drosophila Hyperkinetic Mutants Have Reduced Sleep and Impaired Memory," *Journal of Neuroscience* 27, 20 (May 16, 2007): 5384–93. This study identified a gene that controls the flow of potassium into cells—which is very important, since this is essential to deep sleep. "Without potassium channels, you don't get slow waves, the oscillations shown by groups of neurons across the brain that are the hallmark of deep sleep," says Chiara Cirelli, senior author of this study. "Scientists Identify Second Sleep Gene," University of Wisconsin, Madison, May 22, 2007, www.newswise.com/p/articles/view/530254/.

117   **"a state of most intense stupor"**   Morris Rickman, "Von Economo Encephalitis," *Archives of Neurology* 58 (2001): 1696–98; Lavie, pp. 152–53.

118   **"It looks as if this cluster"**   Saper, quoted in O'Connor.

118   **published these groundbreaking findings**   Saper et al., "Sleep Switch"; Saper and Scammell.

118   **"You can actually correlate sleep loss"**   Saper's remarks are from
"Discovering the Neurobiological Pathways of Sleep and Wakefulness"
(paper presented to the 19th Annual Meeting of the APSS, Denver, June
20, 2005), and "Neurobiology of Insomnia" (paper presented to the
NIH Conference, Bethesda, Md., June 13, 2005).

118   **"sends outputs to"**   Saper et al., "Hypothalamic Regulation."

118   **wake-promoting signals ascending from the brainstem**   Buysse et al.;
Siegel, "Brain Mechanisms." I'm focusing on nonREM in this chapter
because it seems to be most crucial to falling asleep and staying asleep.

118   **neurons that generate the wake-up neurotransmitters histamine and
hypocretin**   Other neurotransmitter systems that play a role in arousal
are acetylcholine, norepinephrine, serotonin, and glutamate.

119   **The *thalamus* is key**   Mircea Steriade et al., "Thalamocortical Oscillations in the Sleeping and Aroused Brain," *Science* 262 (1993): 676–85.

119   **these neurons must cease their rapid firing**   Buysse et al.

119   **"in either a clearly waking or sleeping state"**   Saper et al., "Sleep Switch."

120   **"as if a chemical factor builds up"**   Siegel, "Brain Mechanisms."

120   **what the key substance is**   Amy Blanchard and Bashir Chaudhary,
"Medications and Their Effects on Sleep and Wakefulness," in *Sleep
Medicine,* ed. Teofilo Lee-Chiong Jr., et al. (Elsevier, 2002), p. 570.

120   ***adenosine***   T. W. Dunwiddie and S. A. Masino, "The Role and Regulation of Adenosine in the Central Nervous System," *Annual Review of
Neuroscience* 24 (2001): 31–55.

120   **"at certain levels of adenosine"**   McCarley quoted in William Cromie,
"Awakening to How We Sleep," *Harvard University Gazette,* March 5,
1998.

120   **no one sleep substance**   Antonio Culebras, "Normal Sleep," in *Sleep
Medicine,* ed. Teofilo Lee-Chiong et al. (Hanley & Belfus, 2003), p. 2.

120   **multiple substances . . . interact complexly**   *Cascades* is a term often
used. See James Kreuger and Ferenc Obal Jr., "Sleep Regulatory Substances," in *Sleep Science: Integrating Basic Research and Clinical
Practice,* ed. W. J. Schwartz (Basel, 1997), pp. 178, 182–83.

121   **If you lesion this nucleus**   N. Ibuka and H. Kawamura, "Loss of Circadian Rhythm in Sleep-Wakefulness Cycle in the Rat by Suprachias-
matic Nucleus Lesions," *Brain Research* 96 (1975): 76–81.

121   **"weak thalamic gating"**   Wei Wang et al., "Mismatch Negativity and
Personality Trait in Chronic Primary Insomniacs," *Functional Neurology*
16 (2001): 3–10. A. Besset et al., "Homeostatic Process and Sleep Spin-
dles in Patients with Sleep-Maintenance Insomnia: Effect of Partial
(21h) Sleep Deprivation," *Electroencephalography and Clinical Neurophysiology* 107 (1998): 122–32.

121   **excessive hypocretin or overly active hypocretin**   Tamas Horvath
and Xiao-Bing Gao, "Input Organization and Plasticity of Hypocretin Neurons: Possible Clues to Obesity's Association with Insomnia,"

Cell Metabolism 1, 4 (April 2005): 279–86; David Prober et al., "Hypocretin/Orexin Overexpression Induces an Insomnia-Like Phenotype in Zebrafish," *Journal of Neuroscience* 26, 51 (2006): 13, 400–10.

121   **"Parents have long observed"**   Hobson, *Sleep*, p. 83.

121   **"in such a complex 'push-pull' system"**   Hauri, "Primary Insomnia," p. 636.

121   **"Just as there are various levels of intelligence"**   Hauri, "Insomnia Manual."

122   **end of a continuum . . . some "yet to be identified"**   Hauri, "Primary Insomnia," p. 636.

122   *I am an insomniac and have been all my life*   "Diary of an Insomniac," www.room23.org/2252.html.

122   **"Primary Insomnia typically begins"**   *Diagnostic and Statistical Manual*, p. 601.

122   **two Stanford researchers**   Christian Guilleminault and T.F. Anders, "Sleep Disorders in Children," *Advances in Pediatrics* 22 (1976): 151–75.

124   **These findings were confirmed**   Hauri, "Cluster Analysis of Insomnia."

125   **one looked at two patients**   Regenstein and Reich.

125   **The abstract**   Gaillard et al.

125   **Hauri's observation of a "relative absence of"**   Hauri and Olmstead, "Childhood-Onset Insomnia."

125   **The final investigation**   Philip and Guilleminault.

125   **nobody's really looking**   "Work on a possible early predisposition to insomnia is still in its infancy," write Drake et al.

126   **which I'm sure they often are**   Richard Ferber's book *Solve Your Child's Sleep Problems,* which teaches parents limit-setting techniques, is widely praised; many parents have had success with this behavioral approach.

126   **Idiopathic insomnia is defined**   *International Classification of Sleep Disorders*, p. 12.

129   **Babies have irregular sleep patterns**   Dement and Vaughan, pp. 111–12.

130   **"Relatively mild psychological stressors"**   "Insomnia Manual"; Hauri and Fisher.

130   **"It seems almost impossible"**   "Primary Insomnia," p. 637.

131   **In *Sleep Demons***   Hayes, p. 3.

131   **The DSM-IV acknowledges that**   *Diagnostic and Statistical Manual*, p. 602.

131   **A 2000 study**   Bastien and Morin.

131   **A study done a few years later**   Dauvilliers et al.

132   **moving fast**   Stephanie Maret and Mehdi Tafti, "Genetics of Narcolepsy and Other Major Sleep Disorders," *Swiss Medical Weekly* 135

(2005): 662–65. Genetically engineering strains of rodents, producing knockout mice and genetically modified lines, is the means of many of these studies.

132   **Narcolepsy . . . may run in families**   Siegel, "Narcolepsy."

132   **Fatal familial insomnia**   Peretz Lavie, "Genetics Wakes Up for Human Sleep," *Sleep Medicine Reviews* 9 (2005): 87–89.

132   **"If you have two parents who sleepwalk"**   Clete Kushida, talk at Stanford University, February 5, 2005. Also, H. Bakin, "Sleep Walking in Twins," *Lancet* 2 (1970): 446–47; C. Hublin et al., "Prevalence and Genetics of Sleep Walking: A Population-Based Twin Study," *Neurology* 48 (1997): 177–81; C. Hublin, "Sleeptalking in Twins: Epidemiology and Psychiatric Comorbidity," *Behavior Genetics* 28, 4 (1998): 289–98.

132   **Between a third and a half of all cases of restless legs syndrome**   Anup Desai et al., "Genetic Influences in Self-Reported Symptoms of Obstructive Sleep Apnea and Restless Legs: A Twin Study," *Twin Research* 7, 6 (2004): 589–95.

132   **researchers refer to them as *traits***   Franken et al.

132   **The first recordings of twins' EEGs**   W. W. Zung and W. P. Wilson, "Sleep and Dream Patterns in Twins: Markov Analysis of a Genetic Trait," *Recent Advances in Biological Psychiatry* 9 (1966): 119–30, cited in Mehdi Tafti and Paul Franken, "Functional Genomics of Sleep and Circadian Rhythm," *Journal of Applied Physiology* 92 (2002): 1339–47.

132   **Large-scale studies of twins**   Markku Partinen et al., "Genetic and Environmental Determination of Human Sleep," *Sleep* 6, 3 (1983): 179–85.

133   **all adult twins enrolled in the Australian Twin Registry**   Andrew Heath et al., "Evidence for Genetic Influences on Sleep Disturbance and Sleep Pattern in Twins," *Sleep* 13, 4 (1990): 318–35.

133   **Belgian researcher**   Paul Linkowski et al., "Genetic Determinants of EEG Sleep."

133   **Linkowski estimates that the heritability of deep sleep**   Linkowski et al., "EEG Sleep Patterns in Man," 73; Linkowski.

133   **Family studies have found**   Kenneth Kendler and Carol Prescott, "Caffeine Intake, Tolerance, and Withdrawal in Women: A Population-Based Twin Study," *American Journal of Psychiatry* 156, 2 (1999): 223–28.

133   **A team of researchers in Zurich**   J. V. Retey et al., "A Functional Genetic Variation of Adenosine Deaminase Affects the Duration and Intensity of Deep Sleep in Humans," *Publication of the National Academy of Sciences* 43 (October 25, 2005): 15676–81.

133   **"It seems that when this enzyme is inhibited"**   Hans-Peter Landolt, quoted in Sarah Taber, "A Passport to Never-Never Land," *World Almanac E-Newsletter*, 5, 12 (December 2005), www.worldalmanac.com/dyk/dyk.htm.

133   "About ten percent of people have inherited"   Landolt quoted in Kate Ravilious, "Can't Sleep? Blame Your Parents," *The Guardian,* October 11, 2005.

134   "For certain sleep disorders such as insomnia"   Landolt quoted in Taber, "A Passport to Never-Never Land."

134   genes related to the processing of other sleep substances   Such as GHRH, which regulates the pituitary release of GH, and somatostatin, which may be similarly implicated in the amount and intensity of deep sleep. Franken et al.

134   A 2002 study that found a mutation   Andreas Buhr et al., "Functional Characterization of the New Human GABA(A) Receptor Mutation Beta-3 (R192H)," *Human Genetics* 111 (2002): 154–60.

134   "we abandoned this project"   Erwin Sigel, e-mail, August 27, 2006.

134   A 1998 study by Mignot and other   Daniel Katzenberg et al., "A Clock Polymorphism Associated with Human Diurnal Preference," *Sleep* 21, 6 (1998): 569–76.

134   A team of researchers looked at three generations   Christopher Jones et al., "Familial Advanced Sleep-Phase Syndrome," *Nature Medicine* 5, 9 (1999): 1062–65; K.L. Toh et al., "An hPer2 Phosphorylation Site Mutation in Familial Advanced Sleep Phase Syndrome," *Science* 291, 5506 (2000): 1040–43.

134   The study is "convincing evidence"   David White quoted by Kathryn Senior, "Family with 'Early to Bed, Early to Rise' Gene Mutation Discovered," *Lancet* 354 (September 4, 1999).

134   it could be that the gene functioning is affected   Louis Ptacek, interview by author, December 21, 2006.

134   British researchers   Simon Archer et al., "A Length Polymorphism in the Circadian Clock Gene per3 Is Linked to Delayed Sleep Phase Syndrome and Extreme Diurnal Preference," *Sleep* 26, 4 (2003): 413–15.

134-35   "shorter variant of the gene"   Simon Archer, press release, University of Surrey, June 16, 2003.

135   A twin study found that "if one identical twin"   Martin, p. 279; K. Belicki and D. Belicki, "Predisposition for Nightmares," *Journal of Clinical Psychology* 42 (1986): 714; C. Hublin et al., "Nightmares," *American Journal of Medical Genetics* 8 (1999): 329.

135   Jouvet tells an intriguing story   Jouvet, pp. 18–19.

135   One of the most fascinating interviews I had   Michael Young, interview by author, May 4, 2005.

135   "If the overall shape of human sleep-wake behavior"   Michael Young and Steve Kay, "Time Zones: A Comparative Genetics of Circadian Clocks," *Nature Reviews* 2 (September 2001): 702–15. See also Scott Rivkees, "Time to Wake-Up to the Individual Variation in Sleep Needs," *Journal of Clinical Endocrinology and Metabolism* 188, 1

(2003): 24–25: "These observations underlie why it is difficult to change sleep patterns, if we are fighting inherent physiology."

136   "like changing your height or eye color"   Mahowald quoted in St. John and Williams.

136   "a false dichotomy"   Ridley, pp. 101.

137   "The field of sleep disorders medicine lags behind"   Nofzinger, "Advancing the Neurobiology"; "Neuroimaging and Sleep Medicine."

137   "Sleep is a moving target"   Many of Nofzinger's remarks are taken from "Regional Cerebral Glucose Metabolism during Sleep in Humans" (paper presented to the 16th Annual Meeting of the APSS, Seattle, June 12, 2002), and "Neuroimaging Studies and Sleep" (paper presented to the 17th Annual Meeting of the APSS, Chicago, June 4, 2003). Also, "What Can Neuroimaging."

138   Decreased activity in the frontal cortex   Horne, "Dimensions to Sleepiness"; Horne, "Human Sleep, Sleep Loss, and Behaviour."

138   hold off assigning causality   Nofzinger, "Advancing the Neurobiology."

138   "still pretty gross"   There are other kinds of scans that have promise: PET and SPECT tracers that attach specifically to cells that regulate certain neurotransmitters and thereby reveal the density of those neurotransmitters in various area of the brain. But these are not being used for sleep at the present time.

138   When I asked Allan Rechtschaffen   Rechtschaffen, telephone interview by author, May 20, 2002.

139   "National, NIH-supported brain tissue banks"   National Sleep Disorders Research Plan, sec. 3, "Portmortem Brain Analysis in Sleep Disorders Patients," National Center on Sleep Disorders Research, 2003, National Heart, Lung, and Blood Institute, www.nhlbi.nih.gov/health/prof/sleep/res_plan/section4/section4a.html, accessed April 2007.

CHAPTER 6. SLEEP, STRESS, AND STAGES OF LIFE

141   "It's stress related, you're such a busy person"   Quoted in Carey et al.

142   whether their temperature might be higher   Deborah Sewitch, "Slow Wave Sleep Deficiency Insomnia: A Problem in Thermo-Downregulation at Sleep Onset," Psychophysiology 24, 2 (1987): 200–15.

142   everybody who comes after Monroe   "Unresolved and internalized psychological conflicts lead to emotional arousal and in turn to physiologic activation before and during sleep," say Kales and Kales, pp. 119, 45, 73, 80, 121; D. Schneider-Helmert, "Clinical and Conceptual Aspects of Sleep and Emotional Stress," in Sleep 1980: 5th European Congress of Sleep Research (Karger, 1980), 107–13.

142   "poor sleep . . . a physiological . . . event"   Bonnet and Arand, "Review Article."

143   hyperarousal is a twenty-four-hour problem   "24-Hour Metabolic Rate."

143   "physiological factors are equally"   Bonnet, "Update on Insomnia: Focus on *Physiology* and Treatment" (paper presented to the 18th Annual Meeting of the APSS, Philadelphia, June 6, 2004).

143   After a week of "caffeine-degraded sleep"   Bonnet and Arand, "Caffeine Use."

143   "more pathological [MMPI] personality profiles"   Bonnet and Rosa.

143   Insomnia . . . has been "treated behaviorally"   Bonnet and Arand, "Consequences."

143   I interviewed Bonnet   May 31, 2002. Bonnet quotes are from this interview unless otherwise indicated.

144   The symptoms of hyperarousal that he and other researchers are finding   "Increased heart rate, body temperature, metabolic rate, and secretion of [stress hormones] corticosteroids and adrenaline are all indicators of increased sympathetic nervous system activity." Bonnet and Arand, "Heart Rate Variability."

144   *vagal brake*   McEwen and Lasley, pp. 74, 82.

144   "Old individuals of all sorts"   Sapolsky, p. 203.

144   "Insomniacs have . . . increased"   Bonnet and Arand, "Review Article."

144   When Alexandros Vgontzas   Vgontzas et al., "Chronic Insomnia," 1998.

145   Some insomniacs have stress systems that are as activated   M. W. Johns et al., "Relationship between Sleep Habits, Adrenocortical Activity, and Personality," *Psychosomatic Medicine* 33 (1971): 499–508.

145   If you make insomniacs exercise   Hauri, "Effects of Evening Activity on Early Night's Sleep," *Psychophysiology* 4, 3 (1968): 266–77.

145   If you tell a group of insomniacs   T. K. McClure et al., "Sustained Endocrine and Sleep Responses to Psychological Stressor in Primary Insomnia," in *Proceedings of the 18th Annual Meeting of the Associated Professional Sleep Societies* (Associated Professional Sleep Societies, 2004), abstract 636, p. 283.

145   "Whether the increased arousal"   Stepanski, "Etiology of Insomnia."

146   We lose it in the natural course of aging   Sapolsky, p. 203.

146   women faster than men   Seeman and Robbins.

146   "neurobiological scar"   Ralf-Michael Frieboes et al., "Nocturnal Hormone Secretion and the Sleep EEG in Patients Several Months after Traumatic Brain Injury," *Journal of Neuropsychiatry and Clinical Neurosciences* 11 (1999): 354–60.

146   Early abuse or neglect   Erica Weiss et al., "Childhood Sexual Abuse as a Risk Factor for Depression in Women: Psychosocial and Neurobiological Correlates," *American Journal of Psychiatry* 156, 6 (1999): 816–28.

146   **Studies of women who've experienced**   Christine Heim et al., "Pituitary-
Adrenal and Autonomic Responses to Stress in Women after Sexual
and Physical Abuse in Childhood," *Journal of the American Medical
Association* 284, 5 (2000): 592–97.

146   **Such changes are found in rats who've experienced maternal neglect**
Noha Sadek and Charles Nemeroff, "Update on the Neurobiology
of Depression," August 24, 2000, www.medscape.com/Medscape/
psychiatry/treatmentupdate/2000/tu03/public/toc-tu03.html, valid for
CME until August 24, 2001.

146   **rats exposed to prenatal stress**   C. Henry et al., "Prenatal Stress Increases the Hypothalamic-Pituitary-Adrenal Axis Response in Young
and Adult Rats," *Journal of Neuroendocrinology* 6 (1994): 341–45.

146   **surprisingly few studies**   Alice Gregory et al., "Family Conflict in
Childhood: A Predictor of Later Insomnia," *Sleep* 29, 8 (2006):
1063–67, found that family conflict at age seven to fifteen years predicted insomnia at eighteen years. But looking at three hundred pairs
of eight-year-old twins, Gregory et al. found (that same year) "little evidence of a substantial association between childhood anxiety and
sleep problems" and a "moderate" "correlation between total sleep-
problem score and depression," a correlation that was "mainly explained by genes." "Associations between Sleep Problems, Anxiety,
and Depression in Twins at 8 Years of Age," *Pediatrics* 118, 3 (2006):
1124–32.

147   **20 to 30 percent suffer long-term effects**   Xiangdong Tang et al., "Rat
Strain Differences in Freezing and Sleep Alterations Associated with
Contextual Fear," *Sleep* 28, 10 (2005): 1235–44.

147   **what makes the difference?**   For a fascinating account, see Avi
Sadeh, "Stress, Trauma, and Sleep in Children," *Child and Adolescent Psychiatric Clinics of North America* 5, 3 (1996): 685–700.
Sadeh surveyed a wide range of studies of children's responses to
stress and found some studies that "have documented improved or
deeper sleep" following experiences such as terrorist activities or attack by ballistic missiles. He suggests that an issue "that has escaped
thorough investigation is the issue of individual . . . differences."
These "have rarely been the focus of a sleep-related study" (as we'll
see in chapter 12).

147   **"different individuals respond differently"**   Rubinow et al.

147   **Some strains of mice and rats**   Larry Sanford et al., "Influence of Contextual Fear on Sleep in Mice: A Strain Comparison," *Sleep* 26, 5 (2003):
527–40.

147   **The genetic determinants for such differences**   McEwen and Lasley,
p. 128.

147   **847 New Zealanders**   Caspi et al.

148   **"a higher set point that could be genetic or induced"**   Bonnet and
Arand, "24-Hour Metabolic Rate"; "Review Article."

148   **patterns of cortisol release . . . are more similar**   Paul Linkowski et al., "Twin Study of the 24-h Cortisol Profile: Evidence for Genetic Control of the Human Circadian Clock," *American Journal of Physiology* 264 (1993): E173–81.

148   **"insomnia might be a heritable trait"**   C. Bastien and Michael Bonnet, "Do Increases in Beta EEG Activity Uniquely Reflect Insomnia? A Commentary on 'Beta EEG Activity and Insomnia,' by Michael Perlis et al.," *Sleep Medicine Reviews* 5, 5 (2001): 377–79.

148   **"The set point of the HPA axis is genetically determined"**   O. Van Reeth et al., "Interactions between Stress and Sleep: From Basic Research to Clinical Situations," *Sleep Medicine Reviews* 4, 2 (2000): 201–19.

148   **We are dealing . . . with a powerful stressor**   Bruce McEwen, "Sleep Deprivation as a Neurobiologic and Physiologic Stressor: Allostasis and Allostatic Load," *Metabolism: Clinical and Experimental* 55, suppl. 2 (2006): S20–S23.

148   **When sleep is disturbed**   Van Cauter et al., "Modulation of Neuroendocrine Release by Sleep and Circadian Rhythmicity," in *Advances in Neuroendocrine Regulation of Reproduction*, ed. S. Yen and W. Vale (Plenum, 1990), pp. 113–22; Van Cauter and Spiegel.

149   **But after a sleep-deprived night**   Leproult et al.

149   **it impairs its resiliency**   P. Meerlo, "Sleep Restriction Alters the Hypothalamic-Pituitary-Adrenal Response to Stress," *Journal of Neuroendocrinology* 5 (2003): 397–402.

149   **Spiegel and her colleagues found**   Spiegel et al., "Impact of Sleep Debt on Metabolic and Endocrine Function."

149   **"a feed-forward cascade of negative effects"**   Leproult et al.

149   **"These observations challenge"**   Van Cauter and Spiegel.

149   **"It is possible," says Van Cauter**   Van Cauter, p. 271.

149   **This is a vicious circle**   Andrea Rodenbeck et al., "Interactions between Evening and Nocturnal Cortisol Secretion and Sleep Parameters in Patients with Severe Chronic Primary Insomnia," *Neuroscience Letters* 324 (2002): 159–63.

149   **elevated levels of cortisol damage . . . *hippocampus***   The hippocampus is "one of the important negative feedback sites in the brain for controlling glucocorticoid secretion," say McEwen and Lasley (p. 108). "Truly prolonged exposure to stress or glucocorticoids can actually kill hippocampal neurons," as Sapolsky found (pp. 191–92). Sapolsky describes a "feedforward cascade": glucocorticoids "hasten the death of hippocampal neurons. . . . The tendency of glucocorticoids to damage the hippocampus increases the oversecretion of glucocorticoids, which in turn leads to more hippocampal damage, more glucocorticoids, spiraling downward" (p. 313).

150   **Insomniacs may have trouble sleeping**   Rodenbeck and Hajak.

150   **In *Sleep Demons***   Hayes, p. 3.

150   **a student who's had raging insomnia**   Other *corticosteroids,* as
they're called, include cortisone, ACTH (adrenocorticotropic hormone), prednisolone, triamcinolone, dexamethasone, and methyl-
prednisolene.

152   **In the year 2000, Americans put in the equivalent**   Porter Anderson,
"Study: U.S. Employees Put in Most Hours," CNN.com, August 31,
2001, www.archives.cnn.com/2001/Career/trends/08/30/ilo.study/. This
article refers to a report by the United Nations International Labor Organization, "Key Indicators at the Labor Market, 2001–2002." See
also Stephanie Rosenbloom, "Please Don't Make Me Go on Vacation,"
New York Times, August 10, 2006.

152   *burnout*   A study from the National Institute of Psychosocial Factors
and Health, Stockholm, found that burnout is associated with disturbed sleep. Marie Soderstrom et al., "Sleep and Sleepiness in Young
Individuals with High Burnout Scores," *Sleep* 27, 7 (2004). Social
workers, teachers, nurses, therapists, physicians, dentists—those who
most need to care—seem particularly prone to it. A. Weber and
A. Jaekel-Reinhard, "Burnout Syndrome: A Disease of Modern Societies?" *Occupational Medicine* 50 (2000): 512–17.

152   **"a state of vital exhaustion"**   World Health Organization, *International Classification of Diseases,* 10th rev. (ICD-10) (World Health
Organization, 1992).

153   **53 percent of American workers**   John Schwartz, "Always on the Job,
Employees Pay with Health," *New York Times,* September 5, 2004.

153   **The conditions of today's work world**   Bob Herbert, "An Economy
That Turns American Values Upside Down," *New York Times,* September 6, 2003.

153   **Twenty percent of American workers saw their jobs disappear**
Sounds incredible, but this is from "Policy Statements Adopted by the
Governing Council of the American Public Health Association," No-
vember 15, 2000, "Public Health Impacts of Job Stress," *Association
News,* sec. 200018, p. 502, www.ajph.org/cgi/reprint/91/3/502.

153   **"The hire-and-fire culture"**   Anne-Marie Mureau, "Workplace Stress:
A Collective Bargaining Issue," Economic and Social Department, International Metalworkers' Federation, www.ilo.org/public/english/dialogue/
actrav/publ/126/mureau.pdf.

153   **"It used to be"**   Worker quoted in NIOSH Working Group, Steven
Sauter et al., "Stress . . . at Work," National Institute for Occupational
Safety and Health, www.cdc.gov/niosh/stresswk.html.

153   **"We will need to reskill ourselves"**   Burke quoted in Gleick, p. 81.

153   **We can also expect**   More than 19 million people spend an hour and
a half or more on the road to and from work. "Audio Publishing Industry Continues to Grow," Audio Publishers Association, September
12, 2006, www.audiopub.org/i4a/pages/Index.cfm?pageID=3617.

153   **As Barbara Ehrenreich learned**   *Nickel and Dimed,* p. 220.

153   **Seventy percent of American women with children under eighteen**   Jon Cohen and Gary Langer, "Working Moms Make It Work," *ABC News,* May 8, 2005, based on an ABC News/Washington Post poll conducted by telephone among a random national sample of 1,007 adults.

153   **"The reality of mid-life women's sleep"**   Hislop and Arber, "Sleepers Wake!"

154   **I find the term *electronic leash***   Philipson, p. 4.

154   **"The people who are under someone's thumb"**   McEwen quoted in Anahad O'Conner, "Cracking under the Pressure? It's Just the Opposite, for Some," *New York Times,* September 10, 2004.

154   **"You're all nerved up"**   Shipler, p. 228.

154   **The few studies I find of ethnicity and sleep**   Carl Stepnowsky Jr. et al., "Effect of Ethnicity on Sleep: Complexities for Epidemiologic Research," *Sleep* 26, 3 (2003): 329–32; Judi Profant et al., "Are There Ethnic Differences in Sleep Architecture?" *American Journal of Human Biology* 14 (2002): 321–26; Jean-Louis Girardin et al., "Sleep Duration, Illumination, and Activity Patterns in a Population Sample: Effects of Gender and Ethnicity," *Biological Psychiatry* 47 (2000): 921–27.

154   **In New Zealand**   Sarah-Jane Paine et al., "Who Reports Insomnia? Relationships with Age, Sex, Ethnicity, and Socioeconomic Deprivation," *Sleep* 27, 6 (2004): 1163–69.

154   **A study of insomnia in different occupations**   Markku Partinen et al., "Complaints of Insomnia in Different Occupations," *Scandinavian Journal of Work and Environmental Health* 10 (1984): 467–69.

154   **The lower your income**   Philip Moore et al., "Socioeconomic Status and Health: The Role of Sleep," *Psychosomatic Medicine* 64 (2002): 337–44. The authors suggest that it would be useful to know "the extent to which sleep is a determinant, or merely a reflection, of socioeconomic status and/or health."

154   **"The better educated you are"**   Tarja Porkka-Heiskanen, "Human Sex Difference in Sleep across the Life Span" (paper presented to the 20th Annual Meeting of the APSS, Salt Lake City, Utah, June 20, 2006), summarizing the findings of six different laboratories in Europe.

154   **"Studies that distinguished"**   Ohayon, and other studies.

154   **45 million Americans who are uninsured**   Dan Frosch, "Your Money or Your Life," *The Nation,* February 21, 2005.

154   **millions besides who are within a hairsbreadth**   Mueller, p. 13.

155   **"All it takes is a bit of bad luck"**   Paul Krugman, "Losing Our Country," *New York Times,* June 10, 2005. Whybrow observes that the gap between rich and poor is greater in the United States than in any other industrialized nation (p. 38).

155   **This . . . glaring inequality**   G. Kaplan et al., "Inequality in Income and Mortality in the United States: Analysis of Mortality and Potential Pathways," *British Medical Journal* 312 (1996): 995–1003.

157   "If you can't turn off the stress response"   Sapolsky, p. 16.

158   The 2006 National Sleep Foundation sleep survey   "America's Sleep-Deprived Teens Nodding Off at School, Behind the Wheel, New National Sleep Foundation Poll Finds," National Sleep Foundation, March 28, 2006, www.sleepfoundation.org/press.

159   television sets in their bedrooms   Philipson, p. 55.

159   it happens in rhesus monkeys   Golub.

159   "maturational changes greater in magnitude"   Feinberg.

159   Average sleep time drops from   Mary Carskadon and William Dement, "Sleepiness in the Normal Adolescent," in *Sleep and Its Disorders in Children,* ed. C. Guilleminault (Raven Press, 1987), pp. 53–66.

159   the loss of slow wave sleep . . . is precipitous   Feinberg and Carlson; also e-mail from Feinberg, April 19, 2007: "A paper with these data has been submitted to *Sleep* and we are awaiting a decision."

159   the brain loses a good deal of its plasticity   Schwartz and Begley, pp. 99–100.

159   It is thought that this loss of synaptic density   Feinberg.

160   deranged synaptic pruning   Ibid.

160   A study based on interviews of a thousand adolescents   Eric Johnson et al., "Epidemiology of DSM-IV Insomnia in Adolescence: Lifetime Prevalence, Chronicity, and an Emergent Gender Difference," *Pediatrics* 117, 2 (February 2006): 247–56, http://pediatrics.aappublications.org/cgi/content/full/117/2/e247?maxtoshow=&hits=10&hits=.

160   Estrogen "primes the body's stress response"   Ellen Leibenluft, "Why Are So Many Women Depressed?" *Scientific American* (June 1998), www.sciam.com/specialissues/0698leibenluft.html; Shors and Leuner.

160   Women have been found to have longer-lasting cortisol responses   Elizabeth A. Young, "Sex Differences and the HPA Axis: Implications for Psychiatric Disease," *Journal of Gender-Specific Medicine* 1, 1 (1998): 21–27.

160   hyperreactivity . . . "evolutionary adaptation"   George Chrousos quoted in Holden.

160–61   women are more vulnerable to affective disorders   Holden.

161   The difference arises at puberty   Rebecca Shansky et al., "Estrogen Mediates Sex Differences in Stress-Induced Prefrontal Cortex Dysfunction," *Molecular Psychiatry* 9 (2004): 531–38.

161   At menopause, women's sleep complaints more than double   Cecilia Bjorkelund et al., pp. 894–99; Landis and Moe.

161   hot flashes may disrupt sleep   Though many women actually sleep through them, or turn over and go back to sleep. Some studies find that hot flashes are not actually related to sleep disturbance. Joan Shaver et al., "Sleep Patterns and Stability in Perimenopausal Women," *Sleep* 11, 6 (1998): 556–61; Ann Clark, "Sleep Disturbance in Mid-life Women," *Journal of Advanced Nursing* 22 (1995): 562–68.

161   **"We hypothesize that it could reflect a behaviorally"**   Andrew Krystal et al., "Review Article: Sleep in Peri-menopausal and Post-menopausal Women," *Sleep Medicine Reviews* 2, 4 (1998): 243–53.

162   **rates of depression in women actually *decline* after menopause**   Joffe and Cohen.

162   **"midlife is not the predominant high-stress period for women"**   "The tendency to focus on women's reproductive role has led to the incorrect belief that menopause and the empty nest are central concerns, a belief not supported by empirical research"; the "peak 'age of stress' may be the twenties." Grace Baruch et al., "Isolation and Poverty," Women and Gender in Research on Stress (working paper no. 152, Wellesley College Center for Research on Women, 1985), p. 4, cited in Ruth Sidel, *On Her Own: Growing Up in the Shadow of the American Dream* (Viking, 1990), p. 189.

162   **Some researchers think it's the *fluctuations***   Shors and Leuner.

163   **an electric blanket**   Gilbert et al.

163   **hot bath, may facilitate**   Dorsey et al.

163   **the rapid dropping off of body temperature**   A rapid decline in core body temperature increases the likelihood of sleep initiation and may facilitate entry into the deeper stages of sleep. Murphy and Campbell.

163   **Women with PMS have higher**   Driver and Baker. They also have worse sleep at all stages of the menstrual cycle; Kathryn Lee et al., "Sleep Patterns Related to Menstrual Cycle Phase and Premenstrual Affective Symptoms," *Sleep* 13, 5 (1990): 403–9.

163   **women who take birth control pills**   Rebecca Burdick et al., "Oral Contraceptives and Sleep in Depressed and Healthy Women," *Sleep* 25 (2002): 347–49.

163   **a recent survey of the literature**   Moline et al.

164   **and many experienced insomnia**   "Insomnia was stated as a major, intolerable side effect of hormone therapy withdrawal for some women." Landis and Moe. For anecdotal evidence, see Jane Gross, "Strokes or Insomnia? A Woman's Hormone Quandary," *New York Times*, March 23, 2004.

164   **evidence that estrogen has a beneficial effect on memory**   Sherwin.

164   **that it may help buffer the hippocampus**   McEwen, "The Neurobiology of Stress"; McEwen and Lasley, p. 170.

164   **It enhances the action of GABA**   I. A. Antonijevic et al., "On the Gender Differences in Sleep-Endocrine Regulation in Young Normal Humans," *Neuroendocrinology* 70 (1999): 280–87.

164   **It enhances the action of serotonin**   Joffe and Cohen; Rubinow et al.

164   **estrogen lowers temperature**   Landis and Moe.

164   **Progesterone . . . raises temperature**   Ibid.

165   **"The harassed middle aged"**   Alvarez, p. 56.

165   **as high as 40 to 60 percent among the elderly**   Foley et al.

165   "Age-related changes in sleep are apparently independent"   Prinz et al.

165   Slow wave sleep . . . drops off   It becomes what one researcher calls a "functionally meaningless remnant." R. Spiegel et al., "Significance of Slow Wave Sleep: Considerations from a Clinical Viewpoint," *Sleep* 9 (1986): 66–79.

165   Age brings . . . a disturbance of the timing of sleep   It brings "an increasingly destabilized biologic rhythm or circadian system." Webb, "Age-Related Changes." Also, Michel Hofman and Dick Swaab, "Living by the Clock: The Circadian Pacemaker in Older People," *Ageing Research Reviews* 5 (2006): 33–51.

165   older subjects don't rebound like this   Bonnet and Rosa; Carskadon and Dement.

165   the nadir occurs earlier, and so also does the rise in temperature   Dorsey et al.

165   we wake up earlier   The circadian rise of cortisol occurs an hour and a half earlier in people over sixty-five, and temperature rises with it. There are reduced levels of growth hormone, elevated levels of cortisol, and a blunting of the cortisol rhythm—less cortisol in the morning and more of it in the evening—and a generally blunted circadian rhythm. Van Coevorden et al.

165   Body temperature . . . tends to be generally higher   Michael Vitiello et al., "Circadian Temperature Rhythms in Young Adult and Aged Men," *Neurobiology of Aging* 7 (1986): 97–100.

165   50 percent dampening of . . . prolactin   Van Cauter, p. 275.

165   general elevation of stress hormones   This includes levels of norepinephrine. Patricia Prinz et al., "Plasma Norepinephrine in Normal Young and Aged Men: Relationship with Sleep," *Journal of Gerontology* 39, 5 (1984): 561–67.

166   "unpredictable and highly variable"   Gaillard, "Chronic Primary Insomnia"; Dorsey and Bootzin, "Subjective and Psychophysiologic"; Dorsey, "Failing to Sleep."

166   "insomniacs exhibit significantly greater"   Karacan et al.

166   The unpredictability alone is sufficient to drive you nuts   "Unpredictability makes stressors much more stressful," writes Sapolsky in *Zebras* (p. 218). Loss of predictability, without any other stressor, is enough to trigger a stress response: if you want to watch an animal go to pieces, subject it to random and arbitrary shocks.

166   Gaillard   "Chronic Primary Insomnia" and "Is Insomnia a Disease of Slow-Wave Sleep?"

167   Scientists have long puzzled   Sonia Lupien et al., "Increased Cortisol Levels and Impaired Cognition in Human Aging: Implication for Depression and Dementia in Later Life," *Reviews in the Neurosciences* 10 (1999): 117–39.

167   "wear and tear . . . stress-responsive systems"   Van Cauter et al.,
         "Age-Related Changes."

167   "Chronic stress can accelerate"   Sapolsky et al.

167   "Decreased sleep quality . . . accelerates senescence"   Van Cauter et al.,
         "Effects of Gender and Age"; Van Cauter et al., "Age-Related Changes";
         Spiegel et al., "Impact of Sleep Debt."

167   In a survey of over nine thousand elderly persons   Foley et al.

167   The deterioration of sleep . . . may at least partially account   Miles
         and Dement. "I think it's not an unreasonable hypothesis," says Van
         Cauter, "that a lot of the effects of aging, including geriatric depression,
         could be ultimately traced to a sleep deficit": quoted in Klinkenborg.

167   "We can no more be cured of aging"   Sapolsky et al.

168   With all that cortisol coursing through his system   "A number of
         recent studies have reported deleterious effects of glucocorticoids
         upon cognition after a few days of a high-dose steroid regime in
         healthy volunteers. . . . Several studies have more closely linked
         learning and memory deficits with the hippocampus." McEwen and
         Sapolsky.

168   Elevated cortisol levels damage the hippocampus   Lupien et al. found
         impairments in the conscious or voluntary recollection of information,
         the type of memory known to be dependent on the hippocampus,
         and suggest that "if a certain threshold of hippocampal dysfunction is
         reached," there may be a spiraling effect.

168   "tons of glucocorticoids"   Sapolsky, p. 187.

168   "their hippocampi had shrunk"   M. Starkman et al., "Hippocampal
         Formation Volume, Memory Dysfunction, and Cortisol Levels in Pa-
         tients with Cushing's Syndrome," *Biological Psychiatry* 32 (1992):
         756–65.

168   "It's been known for decades"   Sapolsky, p. 187; Seeman and Rob-
         bins.

168   Some people with posttraumatic stress disorders   Sapolsky, pp. 192–93.

168   In the elderly, the size of the hippocampus   McEwen.

168   effects of Cushing's reversed   McEwen and Sapolsky.

168   "whatever is happening is not readily reversible"   Sapolsky, p. 193.

168   long believed that brain cells could not regenerate   McEwen and
         Lasley, p. 121.

168   sleep deprivation also arrests it   Ruben Guzman-Marin et al., "Sleep
         Deprivation Suppresses Neurogenesis in the Adult Hippocampus of
         Rats," *European Journal of Neuroscience* 22 (2005): 2111–16.

168   mice who ran on their exercise wheels   McEwen and Lasley, p. 138,
         cite H. Van Praag et al., "Running Increases Cell Proliferation and Neu-
         rogenesis in the Adult Mouse Dentate Gyrus," *Natural Neuroscience* 2
         (1999): 266–70.

169   **We say we do**   "In a four-city call-in study of 1383 respondents, a majority of untreated insomniacs reported that they . . . had trouble remembering (59%)." Walsh, "Clinical and Socioeconomic Correlates," cites M. B. Balter and E. H. Uhlenhuth, "The Beneficial and Adverse Effects of Hypnotics," *Journal of Clinical Psychiatry* 52, 7, suppl. (1991): 16–23.

169   **The few studies I find say we do**   Jutta Backhaus et al., "Impaired Declarative Memory Consolidation during Sleep in Patients with Primary Insomnia: Influence of Sleep Architecture and Nocturnal Cortisol Release," *Biological Psychiatry* 60, 12 (2006): 1324–30.

169   **sleep disturbances occur in 30 to 70 percent**   V. Rao and P. Rollings, "Sleep Disturbances Following Traumatic Brain Injury," *Current Treatment Options in Neurology* 2, 1 (2002): 77–87.

169   **Studies find a decrease in both REM and slow wave sleep**   M. Cohen et al., "Temporally Related Changes of Sleep Complaints in Traumatic Brain Injured Patients," *Journal of Neurology, Neurosurgery, and Psychiatry* 55 (1992): 313–15; Marie-Christine Ouellet et al., "Insomnia Following Traumatic Brain Injury: A Review," *Neurorehabilitation and Neural Repair* 18, 4 (2004): 187–98.

170   **many routes . . . to this place**   An insomniac described to me a conversation he'd had with his psychiatrist: *I told him all the stuff I have to do to sleep. "It seems crazy that I have to do and not do all these things, just to sleep," I complained. He replied, "When you think of the complicated chain of events necessary for sleep, it's hardly surprising that so many people have trouble sleeping. If one link is broken, anywhere in the chain, that's all it takes to spoil sleep."* Which seems very wise.

CHAPTER 7. ROCK, HARD PLACE

171   **Direct-to-consumer drug advertising**   Investigative journalists monitoring the evening newscasts of CBS, NBC, and ABC for a week in April 2005 found that viewers saw *each night* an average of sixteen commercials for prescription drugs and an average of eighteen for over-the-counter meds. Lieberman.

173   **"promiscuously prescribe"**   Styron, pp. 71–72.

173   **not actually well trained in pharmacology**   Cohen, p. 214.

173   **Drug companies spend about thirteen thousand dollars**   Moynihan, p. 9.

173   **"weapons of mass seduction"**   Moynihan and Cassels, p. 22.

173   **"The pressures to prescribe are enormous"**   Barry Meier, "Doctors, Too, Ask: Is This Drug Right?" *New York Times,* December 30, 2004.

173   **a Lilly rep on her way out**   Critser, p. 75.

173   **Physicians believe that they're beyond**   M. A. Steinman et al., "Of Principles and Pens: Attitudes and Practices of Medicine Housestaff toward

Pharmaceutical Industry Promotions," *American Journal of Medicine* 110 (2001): 551–57.

173 **hundreds of studies** Rodwin cites studies; Brian McMahon et al., "Developing and Implementing a Program of Grand Rounds for Internists That Is Free of Commercial Bias," *Annals of Internal Medicine* 139, 1 (July 1 2003): 77–78; there are many more.

174 **when they attend Continuing Medical Education events** A. Wazana, "Physicians and the Pharmaceutical Industry: Is a Gift Ever Just a Gift?" *Journal of the American Medical Association* 283, 3 (2000): 373–80; Angell, *Truth*, pp. 139, 141.

174 **"We physicians think"** Gerstein quoted in Moynihan, "Sweetening the Pill."

174 **"Doctors have been taught only too well"** Angell, *Truth*, p. 250.

174 **"Whatever the diagnosis—Librium"** *British Medical Journal* (March 1, 1969), cited in Medawar, "Doors of Deception."

174 **By 1972, it was the most frequently prescribed** Ingrid Waldron, "Increased Prescribing of Valium, Librium, and Other Drugs—an Example of the Influence of Economic and Social Factors on the Practice of Medicine," *International Journal of Health Services* 7, 1 (1977): 37–62. Hoffman-LaRoche, the manufacturer of both Valium and Librium, made enormous profits and fought regulation of these drugs; federal regulations limiting prescriptions to five refills were enacted only in 1975.

175 **most of the advertising aimed at women** Jonathan Metzl, "Selling Sanity through Gender: The Psychodynamics of Psychotropic Advertising," *Journal of Medical Humanities* 24, 1–2 (2003): 79–103.

175 **"Valiumania"** G. Cant, "Valiumania," *New York Times*, February 2, 1976, pp. 34–54.

175 **The barbiturates . . . implicated in . . . suicides** Borbely, p. 71.

175 **they, too, had been advertised as absolutely safe** Medawar, *Power and Dependence*, pp. 58–64.

175 **They increase receptor receptivity to GABA** Salomon Langer et al., "Symptomatic Treatment of Insomnia," *Sleep* 22, suppl. 3 (1999): S437–50.

175 **"a general quietening influence"** Ashton.

176 **they "do not induce natural sleep"** Ian Oswald, "Drugs and Sleep," *Pharmacological Reviews* 20, 4 (1968): 273–303.

176 **Kales was also finding** "Chronic Hypnotic Drug Use—Ineffectiveness, Drug-Withdrawal Insomnia and Dependence," *Journal of the American Medical Association* 227, 5 (February 4, 1974): 513–17.

176 **But the dependence risks** D. J. Greenblatt and R. I. Shade, "Dependence, Tolerance, and Addiction to Benzodiazepines: Clinical and Pharmacokinetic Considerations," *Drug Metabolism Reviews* 8, 1 (1978): 13–28.

176   Hospitals routinely prescribed   Medawar, *Power and Dependence,*
          pp. 41–42.

176   By the mid-1980s   Medawar, ibid., p. 202.

176   When Gordon told her psychiatrist   Gordon, *I'm Dancing,* p. 35.

176   London Broadcasting Company   Medawar, *Power and Dependence,*
          pp. 170–71.

176   A survey reported in *Woman's Own*   Ibid., pp.

176   The problem was particularly acute   Ibid., pp. 155–57.

177   "These painfully ignorant doctors"   Dr. Vernon Coleman, "The
          Nightmare Pills: How Millions Are Caught in the Tranquilliser Trap,"
          Today, May 7, 1986, www.benzo.org.uk/today1.htm.

177   "Evidence of benzodiazepine dependence"   Medawar, "The Antide-
          pressant Web," a twenty-thousand-word paper that can be downloaded
          from ADWEB, a Website run by Social Audit (socialaudit.org.uk) ded-
          icated to exposing the dangers of the SSRIs.

177   "patients tended to be patronized"   Medawar, *Power and Depen-
          dence,* p. 215.

177   believing the claims of the drug companies   "Benzodiazepines: Face
          the Facts," BBC Radio 4 (London), March 16, 1999.

177   "Where they might have expected"   David Healy, "SSRIs and With-
          drawal/Dependence," Briefing Paper: 20-06-2003, Social Audit,
          socialaudit.org.uk/58092-DH.htm.

177   "The abuse arises"   F. Ayd, "The Impact of Biological Psychiatry," in
          Discoveries in Biological Psychiatry, ed. B. Blackwell (Lippincott,
          1970), pp. 230–43; cited in Smith, p. 153. "There is little evidence that
          physical addiction to benzodiazepines is important though undoubt-
          edly in maladjusted individuals psychological dependence may occur."
          D. G. Grahame-Smith, "Self-Medication with Mood-Changing Drugs,"
          Journal of Medical Ethics 1 (1975): 132–37, cited in Medawar, *Power
          and Dependence,* p. 201.

177   Freud continued to believe   Medawar, *Power and Dependence,*
          pp. 32–33.

177   "True addiction is probably exceedingly unusual"   U.S. Senate, *Use
          and Misuse of Benzodiazepines: Hearing before the Subcommittee
          on Health and Scientific Research of the Committee on Labor and
          Human Resources,* 96th Cong., 1st sess., September 10, 1979, posted
          at Public Citizen, www.worstpills.org/member/page.cfm?op_id=20.
          An emeritus consultant in medicine for the Mayo Clinic, Dr. Walter
          Alvarez, acknowledged in 1956 that he had seen a few cases of bar-
          biturate addiction, but claimed that "all of them were undisciplined,
          somewhat psychotic persons before they got the drug. . . . They were
          lacking in self-control and had a poor nervous system." Rosenteur,
          p. 172.

178   **"Dependence liability relates to patient"**   Timothy Roehrs, "Benzodiazepine Receptor Agonist Safety" (paper presented to the NIH
Insomnia Conference, June 13, 2005).

178   *The doctors won't accept*   Statement by a woman interviewed for "Battle against Drug Addiction," *Good Housekeeping* (United Kingdom),
August 2003, posted at Benzo.org.uk, www.benzo.org.uk/ghaug.htm.

178   **"We thought only addictive personalities"**   Malcolm Lader, "Quota-
tions," Benzo.org.uk, www.benzo.org.uk/lader2.htm.

178   **"The Ativan Experience"**   Ad in *Medical Economics* (1978), cited in
Smith, p. 121.

178   **eleventh-most frequently prescribed medication for sleep**   Walsh,
"Drugs Used." The list of drugs approved by the FDA for sleep is interestingly different from the list of drugs most often *taken* for sleep.
Only four of the drugs approved as hypnotics are among the top twelve
medications used; the other six are sedating antidepressants, muscle relaxants, antihistamines—and lorazepam.

178   **"Angel Ativan"**   Lyn Strongin, *Indigo: A Poet's Memoir* (Publish
America, in press).

179   **Ativan was wiping out my deep sleep**   Benzodiazepines are "potent
suppressors of slow wave sleep." Mendelson, "Hypnotics," p. 411.

179   *I feel as if my own self*   Quoted on "Benzodiazepines: Face the Facts,"
BBC Radio 4 (London), March 16, 1999, Benzo.org.uk, www.benzo
.org.uk/facefax.htm.

179   **"a dangerous and unacceptable method"**   "FAQ: Benzodiazepines,"
part 1, www.benzo.org.uk.FAQ1.1.htm; benzo@egroups.com or
benzo@onelist.com.

180   **Dr. Heather Ashton**   Ashton "ran a benzodiazepine detoxification
clinic in Newcastle, England, between 1982 and 1994. During that
time, she detoxified over 300 patients, with a high rate of success."
"FAQ: Benzodiazepines," part 1.

180   **withdrawal syndrome from any drug**   Ashton.

181   **"recovery after long-term benzodiazepine use"**   Ibid.

181   **it's harder to withdraw from benzos than it is from barbiturates**
"FAQ: Benzodiazepines," part 1.

181   **"with heroin[,] usually the withdrawal"**   Malcolm Lader quoted on
"Benzodiazepines: Face the Facts," BBC Radio 4 (London), March 16,
1999.

182   **"When somebody comes into my office"**   Malcolm Lader quoted on
"Brass Tacks," BBC2, October 20, 1987. Ativan seems to be the most
problematic of the benzos. See W. Satzger et al., "Effects of Single
Doses of Alpidem, Lorazepam, and Placebo on Memory and Attention
in Healthy Young and Elderly Volunteers," *Pharmacopsychiatry* 23,
suppl. (1990): 114–19; Wallace Mendelson et al., "Adverse Reactions

to Sedative/Hypnotics: Three Years' Experience," *Sleep* 19, 9 (1996): 702–6.

183   **The physiology of addiction is not well understood**   "No one has any really clear idea why some people get bad drug withdrawal symptoms, others none," writes Charles Medawar, though those who suffer them used to be said to lack "moral fibre"; now they're more often described as having a "dependence-prone personality. . . . These are pretty sweeping assumptions in the light of the failure to analyze how individual metabolic differences may affect experience with drug withdrawal. It is well recognized that there are huge differences, from one person to another, in concentrations of drug in the body, and in rates of drug elimination. What isn't really known is how this influences what happens when drugs are withdrawn." "Beyond the Abstract," Social Audit, www.socialaudit.org.uk/5001-1.htm.

183   **One theory is that**   P. Tyrer et al., "Benzodiazepine Withdrawal Symptoms and Propanolol," *Lancet* 7 (March 1981): 520–22, cited in Medawar, *Power and Dependence*. The confusing results of such addiction studies as there are, says Medawar, "hardly support the conclusion" that it's "personality type" that makes one person become addicted to benzodiazepines, and another person not (pp. 202–3).

183   **Peter Hauri points out**   Quoted in Colligan, p. 90.

184   **"more than 40 percent of all benzodiazepines are prescribed to people over sixty-five"**   Olivera Bogunovic and Shelly Greenfield, "Practical Geriatrics: Use of Benzodiazepines among the Elderly," *Journal of the American Psychiatric Services* 53, 3 (March 2004): 233–35.

184   **And another 2004 study**   S. Iliffe et al., "Attitudes to Long-Term Use of Benzodiazepine Hypnotics by Older People in General Practice," *Aging and Mental Health* 8, 3 (2004): 242–48.

184   **so many older people take them**   "The five million elders in this country receive 35%–40% of the sedative hypnotics prescribed, despite the fact that they represent only 12% of the population." Michael Moran et al., "Sleep Disorders in the Elderly," *American Journal of Psychiatry* 145, 11 (1988): 1369–78.

184   **"We test drugs in young people"**   Peter Lamy quoted in "Nine Reasons Why Older Adults Are More Likely Than Younger Adults to Have Adverse Drug Reactions," in *Worst Pills, Best Pills*, excerpted in *Health Letter,* ed. Sidney Wolfe (21 February 2005): 2.

184   **A recent study of physicians who treat Medicare patients**   Public Citizen's Health Research Group, "The Causes of Misprescribing and Overprescribing," *Health Letter,* ed. Sidney Wolfe (May 12, 2005). Neither the author's name nor information about the study itself is supplied in this publication.

184   **It is known that sleep meds affect us differently**   Kaiser.

184   **Restoril "has a 73% longer half-life"**   Kimberly Yonkers and Jean Hamilton, "Sex Differences in Pharmacokinetics of Psychotropic

Mediations, Part II," in *Psychopharmacology and Women: Sex, Gender, and Hormones,* ed. Margaret Jensvold, Uriel Halbreich, and Jean Hamilton (American Psychiatric Press, 1996), p. 68.

184   **"more poorly to tricyclics"**   Susan Kornstein, "Gender Differences in Depression: Implications for Treatment," *Journal of Clinical Psychiatry* 58, suppl. 15 (1997): 12–18.

184   **Considering . . . that we're the primary consumers**   According to data from a pharmaceutical marketing database, women accounted for "two-thirds of the use of psychotropic drugs" in 1992. Wilma Harrison and Martha Brumfield, "Psychopharmacological Drug Testing in Women," in *Psychopharmacology and Women: Sex, Gender, and Hormones,* ed. Margaret Jensvold et al. (American Psychiatric Press, 1996), p. 374.

184   **Websites for benzodiazepine . . . withdrawal**   See Benzo.org.uk at www.benzo.org.uk. Also, benzo@egroups.com, or benzodiazepine@onelist.com, publishes an extremely informative FAQ on benzodiazepines. There is also the Council for Involuntary Tranquilliser Addiction, which has a helpline (though it's in Liverpool, England)—information about it is at benzo.org.uk or benzo@egroups.com. There are also numerous books: *The Accidental Addict,* by Di Porritt and Di Russell; *Prisoner on Prescription,* by Heather Jones; *Bitter Pills,* by Stephen Fried; *Life without Tranquillisers,* by Vernon Coleman.

185   **chronic use may "damage the sleep system"**   See *The Dark Side of Sleeping Pills,* an e-book by Daniel Kripke, at darksideofsleepingpills.org.

185   **Benadryl**   This is an over-the-counter antihistamine. The antihistamines were developed as allergy medications. Among their side effects was sleepiness, so the active ingredient, diphenhydramine, was put in over-the-counter sleep aids. Diphenhydramine was, in 2002—the last year for which I have information—the sixteenth-most frequently taken substance for sleep. (Walsh, "Drugs Used.") When I take Benadryl or Contac for a cold or allergies, it sometimes helps my sleep and sometimes not; it occasionally jazzes me up and often gives me a hangover (diphenhydramine stays in the system a long time). By the time I get to the end of a cold, it's lost whatever sleep effect it initially had; studies show that tolerance develops rapidly. But I know people who take antihistamines or over-the-counter sleep aids year after year, and swear they help their sleep.

185   **"Blurred vision and other complications related to the eyes"**   "FAQ: Benzodiazepines," part 1.

185   **they may affect the hormones released during deep sleep**   Lancel et al. The neuroendocrine effects of these drugs have not been much studied.

185   **More than one study links them**   B.L. Harlow et al., "Psychotropic Medication Use and Risk of Epithelial Ovarian Cancer," *Cancer Epidemiology Biomarkers and Prevention* 8 (August 1997): 697–702, among others. Also, Daniel Kripke, "Evidence That New Hypnotics Cause Cancer," August 15, 2006, eScholarship Repository, University of California, http://repositories.cdlib.org/ucsdpsych/3, 2006. I'm not sure what to make of this. In view of how widely these drugs have been used, it's likely that the cancer effect is quite small, or it would show up more; but this may be wishful thinking.

185   *anterograde amnesia*   Julien Biebuyck, "Benzodiazepines and Human Memory: A Review," *Anesthesiology* 72 (1990): 926–36.

185   **But in 1988, a legal action**   Medawar, *Power and Dependence,* p. 183; Medawar and Hardon, p. 43.

186   **benzo use increases the risk of falls**   Morin and Wooten.

186   **insomnia left untreated may lead to falls**   A. Y. Avidan et al., "Insomnia and Hypnotic Use, Recorded in the Minimum Data Set, as Predictors of Falls and Hip Fractures in Michigan Nursing Homes," *Journal of the American Geriatric Society* 53, 6 (2005): 955–62.

186   **A 1994 study of twenty-one . . . patients**   P. R. Tata et al., "Lack of Cognitive Recovery Following Withdrawal from Long-Term Benzodiazepine Use," *Psychological Medicine* 24 (1994): 203–13.

186   **"The impairment does not necessarily diminish with time"**   Teresa Rummans et al., "Learning and Memory Impairment in Older, Detoxified Benzodiazepine-Dependent Patients," *Mayo Clinic Proceedings* 68 (1993): 731–37.

186   **"cognitive impairment due to benzodiazepines"**   Ashton, "Benzodiazepines: The Skeleton in the Cupboard," April 24, 2004, Benzo.org .uk, www.benzo.org.uk/asholdm.htm.

186   **"I watched closely, amazed and appalled"**   Cohen, p. 153.

187   **In 2000, it was first on the list**   Truehope, "A Report on the Use of Psychiatric Medications, Their Safety and Efficacy" (Truehope, A Non-Profit Support for the Mentally Ill, July 23, 2003).

187   **In 2002, it was the tenth-most**   Walsh, "Drugs Used."

187   **"saw far more dependency"**   Cohen, p. 154.

187   **Kamen describes anxiety attacks so extreme**   Kamen, pp. 252–60.

187   **Medawar draws attention**   Medawar and Hardon, pp. 40–41.

187   **By 1989, it was "Upjohn's second biggest moneymaker"**   Cowley. And yet by 1987, it had already "racked up 8 to 30 times as many adverse-reaction reports as Dalmane and Restoril combined, even though it was still less widely used than either of them," according to a 1987 report by FDA staffers cited by Cowley.

187   **negative publicity began appearing**   W. E. Leary, "FDA Asks Stronger Label on Sleep Pill under Scrutiny," *New York Times,* September 23, 1989; report on Halcion, *MacNeil/Lehrer NewsHour,* September 1, 1989; "When Sleep Becomes a Nightmare," *20/20,* ABC News, February 17, 1989.

187   **In 1988, San Francisco writer**   Cindy Ehrlich, "Halcion Nightmare: The Frightening Truth about America's Favorite Sleeping Pill," *California* (September 1988): 60–67, 119.

188   **a Dutch psychiatrist, in a letter in *The Lancet***   Dr. Krees van der Kroef's letter shows the merest tip of the iceberg of the troubles Halcion

caused around the world, as described by Abraham and Sheppard, pp. 31–32.

188   **Halcion achieved real notoriety**   Styron, pp. 49, 71–72.

188   **"daytime rebound anxiety"**   K. Morgan and Ian Oswald, "Anxiety Caused by a Short-Life Hypnotic," *British Medical Journal* 284, 6320 (March 1982): 27.

188   **Three years later, Styron said**   "Prozac Days," *The Nation* (January 4–11, 1993): 18–20.

188   **"This is a very dangerous drug"**   Kales quoted in Cowley.

188   **In 1990, the FDA "tallied the numbers"**   Cowley.

188   **the best-selling benzodiazepine**   Medawar, *Power and Dependence,* p. 192.

188   **a 1997 review of Halcion**   Committee on Halcion, Institute of Medicine, *Halcion: An Independent Assessment of Safety and Efficacy Data* (National Academy of Sciences, 1997).

189   **By the end of the century, it had achieved**   Herper; Yi.

189   **they affect fewer receptor subtypes**   Norman Miller, "Benzodiazepines: Behavioral and Pharmacologic Basis of Addiction, Tolerance, and Dependence," *Essential Psychopharmacology* 2, 2 (1997): 119–45.

189   **When FDA approval of the drug was announced**   "Zolpidem for Insomnia," *The Medical Letter* 35, 895 (April 30, 1993): 35–38. Also, D. P. Brunner et al., "Effect of Zolpidem on Sleep and Sleep EEG Spectra in Healthy Young Men," *Psychopharmacology* 104, 1 (1991): 1–5.

189   **Spectral analysis of the EEG**   Irwin Feinberg et al., "Effects of Hypnotic on the Sleep EEG of Healthy Young Adults: New Data and Psychopharmacologic Implications," *Journal of Psychiatric Research* 34 (2000): 423–38.

190   **amnesic effects were described**   Bob Lobo and William Greene, "Zolpidem: Distinct from Triazolam," *Annals of Pharmacotherapy* 31 (May 1997): 625–31.

190   **now these effects are being described in the literature**   R. Goder et al., "Zolpidem: The Risk of Tolerance and Dependence," *Fortschritte der Neurologie-Psychiatrie* 69, 12 (2001): 592–99; M. Aragona, "Abuse, Dependence, and Epileptic Seizures after Zolpidem Withdrawal," *Clinical Neuropharmacology* 23, 5 (2003): 281–83.

190   **reports of people waking up to find**   J. M. Tsai et al., "A Novel Clinical Pattern of Visual Hallucination after Zolpidem Use," *Journal of Toxicology, Clinical Toxicology* 41, 6 (2003): 869–72.

190   **stories began appearing in the media**   Saul, "To Sleep, Perchance to Eat"; Stephanie Saul, "Sleeping Your Way to a Fuller You," editorial, *New York Times,* March 16, 2006.

190   **Sleep researchers knew about the sleep-eating**   Carlos Schenck et al., "Zolpidem Induces Amnesic Sleep-Related Eating Disorder in 19 Patients," in *Proceedings of the 19th Annual Meeting of the Associated*

Professional Sleep Societies (Associated Professional Sleep Societies, 2005), abstract 0773, p. 259.

190   **Ambien has been implicated in so many accidents**   Stephanie Saul, "A New Sleeping Sickness Is Haunting Highways," *New York Times,* March 8, 2006.

191   **A New York lawyer has filed a class-action suit**   Dowd.

191   **Early in 2007**   Saul, "U.S. Calls for Strong Warnings."

191   **"These drugs do things we do not understand"**   Ambien also does some positive things that are not understood. Physicians in England, South Africa, and the United States have been finding, in the past several years, that zolpidem may have miraculous effects on brain-damaged patients in a persistent vegetative state, awakening them to an awareness of their environment, allowing them to communicate, to move and even feed themselves, until the drug wears off. Wally Nel and Ralf Clauss published their findings in "Drug Induced Arousal from the Permanent Vegetative State," *NeuroRehabilitation* 21, 1 (2006): 23–28; and R. Clauss, M. Sathekge, and W. Nel, "Transient Improvement of Spinocerebellar Ataxia with Zolpidem," *New England Journal of Medicine* 351, 5 (2004): 511–12.

191   **Sonata . . . is (or it is claimed to be)**   Sonia Ancoli-Israel et al., "Zaleplon, a Novel Nonbenzodiazepine Hypnotic, Effectively Treated Insomnia in Elderly Patient without Causing Rebound Effects," *Primary Care Companion to the Journal of Clinical Psychiatry* 1, 4 (1999): 114–20.

192   **As the use of benzos fell off**   Walsh, "Ten-Year Trends."

192   **drugs most prescribed**   Walsh, "Drugs Used."

193   **I'd just read a study**   Regenstein and Reich.

193   *I am a different person now*   Posted on "Julie's Health Club," May 5, 2006, featuresblogs.chicagotribune.com/features_julieshealthclub/2006/sleep_aids.html.

194   **The speakers at the sleep conferences**   Wallace Mendelson, "A Review of the Evidence for the Efficacy and Safety of Trazodone in Insomnia," *Journal of Clinical Psychiatry* 66, 4 (2005): 469–76.

194   **"regulatory-based . . . medicine"**   Walsh, "Drugs Used."

194   **I'm skeptical**   A *New York Times* op-ed piece by Daniel Carlat points out that "trazodone-bashing" is often done by authors "paid by Sepracor, Sanofi-Aventis or Takeda, the companies that stand to gain from trazodone's downfall." "Generic Smear Campaign," May 9, 2006.

194   **"And then something just kind of changed in me"**   Elizabeth Wurtzel, *Prozac Nation* (Houghton Mifflin, 1994), p. 329.

194   **it was a "media event"**   Healy, *Anti-Depressant Era,* p. 226.

194   **"bottled sunshine"**   James Kingsland, "The Rise and Fall of the Wonder Drugs," *New Scientist* (July 3, 2004): 36–40.

194   **"personality pill"**   A. Toufexis, "The Personality Pill," *Time* (October 11, 1993): 53.

195 **They are given for . . . getting through the holidays** Warren St. John and Alex Williams, "High for the Holidays," *New York Times,* November 28, 2004.

195 **most heavily marketed category of drugs** David Kirkpatrick, "Inside the Happiness Business," *New York Magazine,* March 24, 2002, www.newyorkmag.com.

195 **by 2001, they were the best-selling drug category** "Prescription Drug Expenditure in 2001: Another Year of Escalating Costs," National Institute for Health Care Management, May 6, 2002, www.nihcm.org/ spending2001.pdf.

195 **four years later, it moved up to fourteenth** Yi.

195 **Americans spent more than $9 billion** Scott Garrison, "Prozac Nation," *North Carolina Society of Anesthesiologists* 12, 1 (Winter 2003): 3.

195 **"It is estimated," says a 2005 study** Richard Kadison, "Getting an Edge—Use of Stimulants and Antidepressants in College," *New England Journal of Medicine* 353 (September 15, 2005): 1089–91.

195 **"Antidepressant prescriptions to children"** Julie Zito quoted in Ellen Barry, "Students' Prescriptions Worry Health Counselors," *Boston Globe,* September 26, 2002.

195 **"Preschoolers . . . are now the fastest growing group"** James Gorman, "The Altered Human Heart Is Already Here," *New York Times,* April 6, 2004.

195 **"Fundamentally," says Dr. Thomas Kramer** Kramer, "Mechanisms of Action," *Medscape Mental Health* 6, 1 (2001).

196 **In 1997, thirteen-year-old Matt Miller** Jonathan Mahler, "The Antidepressant Dilemma," *New York Times Magazine* (November 21, 2004).

196 **"Common to all of them"** Critser, p. 203.

196 **(Forty percent of Prozac users require sleep medication.)** Cohen, p. 44.

197 **Sleep specialists recommend such cocktails** Lisa Lustberg and Charles Reynolds III are among the many who do. "Depression and Insomnia: Questions of Cause and Effect," *Sleep Medicine Reviews* 4, 3 (2000): 253–62.

197 **many studies . . . significant withdrawal problems** Healy, "Psychopharmacology."

197 **a problem most of us hadn't known was a medical disorder** Critser, pp. 66–68.

197 **"at least 25% [of those who take Paxil]"** Medawar, e-mail, September 17, 2006.

197 ***My brain has turned into liquid*** Ljohnson31, June 13, 2001, forums .about.com.n.mb.message.

197 **"history has been repeating itself"** Medawar, *Power and Dependence,* p. 10.

198   "doctors have been prescribing"   Medawar and Hardon, p. 1.

198   "a pattern of error"   Medawar, *Power and Dependence*, p. 5.

198   "one drug after another"   Medawar and Hardon, p. 1.

198   "The clear message of history is to beware"   Medawar, "Doors of Deception."

198   the number of prescriptions filled in the United States rose   Greider, p. 3.

198   "In the last seven years"   Dan Shapiro, "Drug Companies Get Too Close for Med School's Comfort," *New York Times,* January 20, 2004.

198   By 2004, drug companies were spending   Critser, p. 6.

198   "I tell my patients"   Brian Strom quoted by Kathleen Kerr, "Drug Must Prove Itself in Crowded Insomnia-Remedy Market," Newsday .com, Sept. 21, 2005.

198   People assume that FDA approval   Breggin, pp. 361–62.

198   New drugs are becoming even more dangerous   Angell, *Truth,* p. 209.

198   Within a twenty-five-year period, 20 percent   Karen Lasser et al., "Timing of New Black Box Warning and Withdrawals for Prescription Medications," *Journal of the American Medical Association* 287 (2002): 2215–20.

198   "It's a form of Russian roulette"   Wolfe quoted by Denise Grady, "Study Finds New Drugs May Carry Extra Hazards," *New York Times,* May 1, 2002; Karen Lasser et al., "Timing of New Black Box Warnings and Withdrawals for Prescription Medications," *Journal of the American Medical Association* 287 (2002): 2215–20.

199   Internet was "groaning with evidence"   Medawar and Hardon, pp. 2–3.

199   A mutation that makes women . . . redheaded   Kaiser.

200   "like depression before Prozac"   Southwell quoted in Marsa.

200   "There is such a huge, untapped market"   Southwell quoted in Wells.

200   The marketing analyst group Spectra Intelligence   "Global Market for Sleep-Wake Disorders, 2005–2012," www.piribo.com/publications/dis eases_conditions/cns/global_market_sleep_wake_disorder.html. This is an advertisement for the book *Global Market for Sleep-Wake Disorders, 2005–2012,* on sale for a mere $2,020 (that's not a typo).

200   The discovery of the most important drugs   Relman and Angell.

200   "me-toos," modified versions of older drugs   Angell, *Truth,* pp. 16–17.

201   people have to be persuaded   Ibid., p. 133.

201   the industry spends close to $54 billion   Ibid., p. 122.

201   more drug-company lobbyists than there are members of Congress   Relman and Angell.

201   in 1990, a brand-name prescription cost around twenty-seven dollars   Greider, p. 6.

201   the most profitable in the nation   The most profitable "by a long shot," as Angell says. *Truth,* p. 3.

201   "under-penetrated market"   Gershell.

201   Drug makers spent $298 million advertising   Stephanie Saul, "Record
        Sales of Sleeping Pills Are Causing Worries," *New York Times,* Febru-
        ary 7, 2006.

201   "an advertising effort that industry watchers say"   Jewell.

201   "one of the epic marketing battles"   "Insomnia Programs Reviewed by
        Neuroinvestment," Marketwire, September 7, 2005, www.marketwire
        .com/mw/release.

201   "a taboo in the use of sleeping pills had been broken"   Andrew Pol-
        lack, "With New Sleeping Pill, New Acceptability?" *New York Times,*
        December 17, 2004.

202   "Within two months of its launch"   Gershell.

202   Sepracor had spent $500 million on advertising   Saul, "U.S. Calls
        for Strong Warnings," citing the research firm TNS Media Intelli-
        gence.

202   Lunesta's performance "massively exceeded"   "Sleep Drug Wakes Sepra-
        cor," Red Herring.com: The Business of Technology, January 31, 2006,
        www.redherring.com/Article.aspx?a=15539&hed=Sleep+Drug+Wakes+
        Sepracor.

202   "In the twelve years I've been in practice"   Statement by David Cla-
        man, director of the U.C. San Francisco Sleep Disorders Center, quoted
        in Lazarus.

202   "people come in all the time"   Daniel Carlat quoted in Deidre Hen-
        derson, "The Big Sleep," *Boston Globe,* June 11, 2006, www.boston
        .com/business/healtcare/articles/2006/06/11.

202   Zopiclone bears much the same baggage   A.M. Holbrooke et al.,
        "Meta-analysis of Benzodiazepine Use in the Treatment of Insomnia,"
        Canadian Medical Association Journal 162, 2 (2000): 225–33.

202   "another carriage"   "Zopiclone: Another Carriage on the Tranquilliser
        Train," *Lancet* 335 (March 3, 1990): 507–8.

202   the Drug Enforcement Administration's announcement   "Proposed
        Rules," *Federal Register* 70, no. 27 (February 14, 2005): 7449–51,
        from the Federal Register Online via GPO Access, wais.access
        .gpo.gov.

202   The main difference between Lunesta   "DO NOT USE."

202   "complex sleep-related behaviors"   "FDA Requests Label Change for
        All Sleep-Disorder Drug Products," *FDA News,* March 14, 2007,
        www.fda.gov/bbs/topics/NEWS/2007/NEW01587.html.

202   The FDA *Pink Sheet Daily*   "Sepracor Lunesta Cancer Risk at Cen-
        ter of FDA Approvability Debate," *Pink Sheet Daily* 17, 157, no.
        013 (August 16, 2005), www.fdcreports.net/fdcreports/ppv/view
        item.doc.

203   less receptor specificity   Daniel Kripke, letter to the editor, *Sleep* 28,
        3 (2005): 370.

203   **Ambien CR**   This doesn't get me past my three-hour wake-up call, though it does make it easier to get back to sleep after I wake up.

204   **ramelteon increased total sleep . . . might raise levels of prolactin** "DO NOT USE until July 2012 Ramelteon (Rozerem)—an Unimpressive New Sleeping Pill," *Worst Pills, Best Pills Newsletter,* January 2006; B. Silverman, "Takeda Rozerem: Clinical Significance Debated in FDA Review," *Pink Sheet Daily* 18, 14 (January 23, 2006).

205   **It was said to increase sleep pressure**   Stefan Mathias et al., "The GABAa Agonist Gaboxadol Improves the Quality of Post-nap Sleep," *Psychopharmacology* 157 (2001): 299–30.

205   **Harvard sleep researcher Clifford Saper speculated**   Saper, "Effects of GABAa Drugs on the Wake/Sleep System" (paper presented to the 19th Annual Meeting of the APSS, Denver, June 22, 2005).

205   **Merck canceled the project**   Stephanie Saul, "Merck Cancels Work on a New Insomnia Medication," *New York Times,* March 29, 2007.

205   **Actelion is announcing success with animal and human studies**   Randolph Schmid, "Researchers Make Progress with Insomnia," Washingtonpost.com, January 28, 2007, www.washingtonpost.com/wp-dyn/content/article/2007/01/28/AR2007012800532_pf.html.

205   **At least one company is at work on melatonin agonists**   "New Drug Class to Broaden Treatment Options for Insomnia," Pharmaceutical Business Review Online, May 18, 2007, www.pharmaceutical-business-review.com/article_featureprint.asp?guid=45222020-7ASF-4C5A-9FOC-EB5CA84CB045.

206   **French researcher Henri Laborit**   Laborit lists "very low toxicity" as one of the "principal elements" of GHB's pharmacology. "Sodium 4-Hydroxybutyrate," *International Journal of Neuropharmacology* (Great Britain), 3 (September 1964): 433–52. It has been used in Europe as an anesthetic, and in Italy as a treatment for alcohol withdrawal. L. Gallimberti et al., "Gamma-Hydroxybutyric Acid in the Treatment of Alcohol Dependence: A Double-Blind Study," *Alcoholism—Clinical and Experimental Research* 16 (1992): 673–76.

206   **it is thought to work**   S. Nishino and Mignot, "Pharmacological Aspects of Human and Canine Narcolepsy," *Progress in Neurobiology* 52 (1998): 27–78.

206   **attracting the attention**   Eve Van Cauter et al., "Simultaneous Stimulation of Slow-Wave Sleep and Growth Hormone Excretion by Gamma-Hydroxybutyrate in Normal Young Men," *Journal of Clinical Investigation* 100, 3 (August 1997): 745–53.

207   **But in November 1990**   Ward Dean et al., *GHB: The Natural Mood Enhancer: The Authoritative Guide to Its Responsible Use* (Smart Publications, 1997), p. 7.

207   **the media were full of scare stories**   Patrick Roger and Peter Katel, "The New View from on High," *Newsweek* (December 6, 1993); Christine Gorman, "Liquid X," *Time* (September 30, 1996); M. Cooper, "A

New Danger in Drug World Is Spelled GHB," *New York Times,* September 29, 1996.

207   **Nobody actually knows**   O. Carter Snead III and K. Michael Gibson, "G-Hydroxybutyric Acid," *New England Journal of Medicine* 352, 26 (June 30, 2005): 2721–32.

207   **taken with . . . alcohol**   Alcohol is actually the substance most often associated with sexual assault. I. Hindmarch and R. Brinkmann, "Trends in the Use of Alcohol and Other Drugs in Cases of Sexual Assault," *Human Psychopharmacology* 14, 4 (1999): 225–31.

208   **Bob Cloud . . . describes what cataplexy feels like**   U.S. Food and Drug Administration.

208   **Scharf studied the drug**   Martin Scharf, telephone interview by author, February 22, 2006.

208–9   **Meyers organized patient advocates**   Abbey Myers, "History of the American Orphan Drug Act," Rarediseases.org, February 18, 2000, www.rarediseases.org/news/speeches/span2.

209   **new law provided financial incentives**   David Duffield Rohde, "The Orphan Drug Act: An Engine of Innovation? At What Cost?" *Food and Drug Law Journal* 55 (2000): 125–43.

209   **advocates from the Narcolepsy Network testified**   Schedule III specifies that GHB has medical use but also has a potential for abuse, and it imposes tight controls (Schedule III includes drugs like Ritalin and Dexedrine). Schedule I imposes even more severe penalties for illegal use. David Fuller and Carl Hornfeldt, "From Club Drug to Orphan Drug: Sodium Oxybate for the Treatment of Cataplexy," *Pharmacotherapy* 23, 9 (November 9, 2003): 1205–9.

209   **So GHB was designated a Schedule III agent**   Matthew Herper, "Former Street Drug Takes on Narcolepsy," *Forbes* (September 16, 2002).

210   **The "risk management plan"**   Patti Engel, Orphan representative, quoted in U.S. Food and Drug Administration; David Fuller et al., "The Xyrem Risk Management Program," *Drug Safety* 27, 5 (2004): 293–306; Ariel Neuman, "GHB's Path to Legitimacy: An Administrative and Legislative History of Xyrem" (paper submitted to Professor Peter Barton Hutt in satisfaction of the course requirement for Food and Drug Law, Harvard Law School, Winter 2004).

210   **"steel-reinforced"**   David Fuller, "Xyrem Risk Management Program," *Drug Safety* 27 (2004): 293–306.

210   **"favorable side effect/efficacy profile"**   Mignot, "Commentary."

210   **FDA has issued an "import alert"**   "FDA Strengthens Controls, Issues Consumer Alert on Importing Certain Prescription Drugs," FDA News, December 9, 2002, www.fda.gov/bbs/topics/NEWS/2002/NEW00856.html.

210   **"unexpected that a medication"**   Jed Black said this in the congressional hearing "Peripheral and Central Nervous System Drugs." See U.S. Food and Drug Administration.

211   **best bet for finding a doctor**   The Advocatesforsleep Website, at Talk
       aboutsleep.com, may be able to help you find a doctor, I've heard.

212   **works wonders with the pain of fibromyalgia**   Martin Scharf et al.,
       "The Effect of Sodium Oxybate on Clinical Symptoms and Sleep Pat-
       terns in Patients with Fibromyalgia," *Journal of Rheumatology* 30, 5
       (2003): 1070–74.

212   **average annual wholesale price**   Mark Mahowald, "What? Influenced
       by Industry? Not Me!" editorial, *Sleep Medicine* 6 (2005): 389–90.

213   **What especially . . . interests the researchers**   O. Lappiere et al., "The
       Effect of Gamma-Hydroxybutyrate on Nocturnal and Diurnal Sleep of
       Normal Subjects," *Sleep* 3, 1 (1990): 24–30.

213   **This is where the restorative processes . . . are thought to take place**
       Growth hormone is important not only because it keeps muscles toned
       but also because it "has a well established role in fostering cellular im-
       munity." Patricia Prinz, "Age Impairments in Sleep, Metabolic, and Im-
       mune Functions," *Experimental Gerontology* 39 (2004): 1739–43.

213   **"The sinister purpose of the ads"**   Avorn quoted in Marsa.

214   **Sanofi-Aventis "pumped $55 million"**   Arlene Weintraub, "I Can't
       Sleep," BusinessWeek.Online, January 26, 2004.

214   **For the $350 million Sanofi-Aventis put into advertising**   Saul, "U.S.
       Calls for Strong Warnings."

214   **The use of sleep meds in the United States doubled**   Gardiner Harris,
       "Youths Using More Sleep Aids," *New York Times,* October 19, 2005.

214   **it's not happening in the European Union**   There, "the market for in-
       somnia therapeutics" was, as of 2005, "stagnating." Holzinger.

215   **how to minimize the damage**   Public Citizen recommends oxazepam
       (Serax) as the only kind of benzo an elderly person should take, because
       it has a short half-life and minimal memory impairment; and, given that
       there's nothing to distinguish the nonbenzos from the shorter-acting
       benzos, "the drug with the lowest purchase cost . . . should be pre-
       scribed." Public Citizen, www.worstpills.org/member/drugprofile.cfm?
       m_id=89. I have no personal experience of this drug, nor have I heard
       about it from insomniacs.

216   **"When it comes to their own values"**   Avorn, p. 167.

216   **"As someone who has taken cocktails"**   Jennifer Kaplan, letter to the
       editor, *New York Times,* November 20, 2005.

217   **"Read, ask, think"**   Cohen, p. 246. Reliable Websites are WebMD
       and PDRhealth. Consumer Reports offers a free online site, www.Con
       sumerReports.org/cro/health-fitness/index.htm, to help with decisions.
       Wikipedia also has good information on drugs.

CHAPTER 8. CHANGE YOUR ATTITUDE, CHANGE YOUR WAYS

218   **Get a life, Ben**   Bishop and Levy, p. 162.

218   **a drug-driven culture**   The term is Michael Irwin's, quoted in "Behavior Changes Can Help Seniors Sleep without Drugs," Health Behavior News Service, December 15, 2005, www.newswise.com/articles.

219   **"When the stressors fade away"**   Morin, *Relief from Insomnia*, p. 68.

219   **This is the view enshrined in the DSM-IV**   *Diagnostic and Statistical Manual*, p. 601.

219   **what Morin calls "mild sleep deprivation"**   "Psychological and Behavioral," p. 727. This article gives one of the clearest descriptions of behavioral modification.

220   **success with support groups**   Manber and Kuo. I've talked to people who've been helped by the groups they run at Stanford.

220   **"not many people are using CBT"**   This and other remarks by Morin are from "Insomnia" (paper presented to the 18th Annual Meeting of the APSS, Philadelphia, June 8, 2004).

220   **"Given that behavioral treatments"**   Stepanski, "Behavioral Therapy," p. 651.

221   **satisfaction is "significantly enhanced"**   Morin et al., "Nonpharmacologic Treatment."

221   **Morin guesses that 70 to 80 percent are helped**   Ibid.

221-22 **How representative are these subjects?**   "Those who are less enthusiastic note that many studies of non-pharmacologic therapy use a highly selected set of patients, often show benefits on only some sleep variables[,] . . . sometimes present data only for those who completed treatment, and often do not have parallel placebo groups." Mendelson et al., "The Treatment of Chronic Insomnia."

223   **Gregg Jacobs . . . assures us**   Jacobs, p. 79.

223   **"Doctors are stunningly casual"**   Kamen, p. 44.

224   **Hauri and others say it's okay to take . . . a nap**   Hauri, "Consulting"; Leah Friedman et al., "An Actigraphic Comparison of Sleep Restriction and Sleep Hygiene Treatments for Insomnia in Older Adults," *Journal of Geriatric Psychiatry and Neurology* 13 (Spring 2000): 17–27.

224   **"This ceiling effect suggests"**   Morin and Azrin.

224   **subjects' moods and daytime functioning aren't much improved**   Jacobs et al.; Morin et al., "Nonpharmacologic Treatment."

224   **The two meanings of *significant***   James Horne also makes this distinction. *Sleepfaring*, p. 40.

224   **you stay slightly sleep-deprived**   Bonnet and Arand, "Caffeine Use" and "Consequences of a Week."

226   **"Insomnia in Aged Found Treatable"**   Erica Goode, *New York Times*, March 17, 1999.

226   *New York Times* mention   John O'Neil, "Think Before You Sleep,"
       New York Times, October 5, 2004.

227   **This is a question that haunts**   Jack Edinger et al., "Does Cognitive-
       Behavioral Insomnia Therapy Alter Dysfunctional Beliefs about Sleep?"
       Sleep 24, 5 (2001): 591–99. Charles Reynolds III comments, "It is one
       thing to show the efficacy of a psychopharmacological, psychosocial,
       or psychoeducational intervention in a specialty research clinic; it is
       very much more challenging to demonstrate efficacy or effectiveness in
       a real-world general medical setting." "Improving Evidence-Based
       Practice in the Treatment of Chronic Insomnia: A Commentary on
       'Chronic Hypnotic Use: Deadly Risks, Doubtful Benefits,'" *Sleep Med-
       icine Reviews* 4, 1 (2000): 21–23.

227   **"None of the studies"**   Harvey and Tang.

227   **they often contradict the subjective accounts**   Stepanski, "Behavioral
       Therapy," p. 652.

227   **Most of the behavioral modification studies**   Ibid.

227   **Doctors in military field hospitals**   Dylan Evans, pp. 1, 24.

227   **two types of biofeedback**   Hauri, "Treating Psychophysiologic
       Insomnia."

227–28 **In a follow-up study**   Hauri et al., "The Treatment of Psychophysio-
       logic Insomnia."

228   **why alternative approaches have high success rates**   Evans, p. 157.

228   **ranked as not having a "high degree of clinical certainty"**   Andrew
       Chesson et al., "Practice Parameters for the Nonpharmacologic Treat-
       ment of Chronic Insomnia," *Sleep* 22 (1999): 1128–33.

229   **"few studies have demonstrated superior efficacy"**   Drake et al. An-
       other study, also published in 2003, found that "the wide popularity
       of sleep hygiene recommendations by sleep specialists appears to be out
       of proportion to the available data demonstrating the efficacy of this
       approach." Stepanski and Wyatt.

229   **AASM states as its official position**   "Sleep hygiene, behavioral ther-
       apies, and prescription sleep aids are the best ways to treat insomnia.
       They are widely available and highly effective": "Insomnia Cures,"
       Clinical Practice Review Committee, Sleepeducation.com, April 8,
       2005, sleepeducation.com/Topic.aspx?is=28.

230   **"we need to explain why some improve"**   Morin et al., "Nonphar-
       macologic Treatment."

230   **"one study has directly examined"**   Morin et al., "Psychological
       Treatment of Insomnia: A Clinical Replication Series with 100 Pa-
       tients," *Behavioral Therapy* 25 (1994): 159–77.

230   **A 1997 study observed**   Jack Edinger, "Searching for the Dose-Response
       Curve in Behavioral Insomnia Therapy," *Sleep Research* 26 (1997): 356.

230   **A study of paradoxical intention**   Colin Espie and William Lindsay,
       "Paradoxical Intention in the Treatment of Chronic Insomnia: Six Case

Studies Illustrating Variability in Therapeutic Response," *Behavioral Research Therapy* 23, 6 (1985): 703–9.

231   **Two studies headed by Stephen Haynes**   Haynes et al., "The Stimulus Control Paradigm in Sleep-Onset Insomnia: A Multimethod Assessment," *Journal of Psychosomatic Research* 26, 3 (1982): 333–39; Haynes et al., "Insomnia: Sleep Patterns and Anxiety Levels," *Journal of Psychosomatic Research* 18 (1974): 69–74.

232   **A 1997 study of 348 patients**   Gagne Bastien and Charles Morin, "Precipitating Events of Insomnia," *Sleep Research* 26 (1997): 363, abstract.

232   **"Quite frankly, there isn't much evidence"**   Lichstein, "Psychological Models of Chronic Insomnia" (paper presented to the NIH Insomnia Conference, Bethesda, Md., June 13, 2003). "There has been surprisingly little research confirming the hypothesized mechanisms responsible for its [stimulus control therapy's] efficacy, namely the extinction of conditioned associations with the bedroom environment." Drake et al. "The central tenets of the stimulus control model . . . have never been evaluated empirically," say Michael Perlis et al., "Etiology and Pathophysiology of Insomnia," in *Principles and Practice of Sleep Medicine*, ed. Meir Kryger et al. (2000; reprint, Saunders, 2005), pp. 714–25.

232   **look at the way they sleep away from home**   Some insomniacs sleep better in the clinic, as Hauri and Olmstead found. "Reverse First Night Effect."

232–33 **studies that have looked . . . have been "equivocal"**   Drake et al.

233   **Wehr placed fifteen subjects**   Wehr et al.

234   **"an altered state"**   Quoted in Ekirch, "Sleep We Have Lost"; Wehr et al.

234   **"a state not terribly familiar to modern sleepers"**   Quoted in Klinkenborg.

234   **Prolactin . . . stimulated by meditation**   R. Jevning et al., "Plasma Prolactin and Growth Hormone during Meditation," *Psychosomatic Medicine* 40 (1978): 329–33.

234   **"Perhaps . . . what those who meditate"**   Wehr quoted in Angier.

234   **"an extended period of quiet wakefulness"**   Wehr, "The Impact of Changes."

234   **Wehr speculates that this may be why**   Ibid.

234   **animals, whose sleep "occurs in multiple bouts"**   Wehr et al.

234   **"compresses and consolidates . . . artifact of modern lighting"**   Wehr, "In Short Photoperiods."

235   **"There is every reason to believe"**   Ekirch, "Sleep We Have Lost."

235   **"Families rose from their beds"**   Ibid.

235   **"After the first sleep," people "have more enjoyment"**   Sixteenth-century French physician Laurent Joubert quoted in ibid.

235   Through the seventeenth century   Wright, p. 18.

235   "In travellers' tales"   Ibid, p. 125.

236   "demanded a transformation of human nature"   Thompson, pp. 362, 357.

236   "They were not enthusiastic"   Keyes, pp. 21–22.

236   Sunday sermons . . . denounced "the slumbers of sin"   Thompson, p. 409.

236   "There is really no reason"   Edison quoted in Martin, p. 334.

236   Sleep, by the end of the nineteenth century   "The subject of sleeplessness is once more under public discussion. The hurry and excitement of modern life is quite correctly held to be responsible for much of the insomnia of which we hear: and most of the articles and letters are full of good advice to live more quietly and of platitudes concerning the harmfulness of rush and worry. The pity of it is that so many people are unable to follow this good advice and are obliged to lead a life of anxiety and high tension." Editorial, *British Medical Journal* (September 29, 1894): 719.

237   (except for Sweden)   Barbara Welles-Nystrom, "Co-sleeping as a Window into Swedish Culture: Considerations of Gender and Health Care," *Scandinavian Journal of Caring Sciences* 29 (2005): 354–60.

237   "By sleeping next to its mother"   James McKenna, "Babies Need Their Mothers Beside Them," World Health, March–April 1996, www .naturalchild.com/james_mckenna; Lysa Parker, "From Primates to Late Nights: One Researcher's Path to Sleep Studies," interview with James McKenna, www.gentlebirth.org/archives/sleepMcKenna.html.

237   McKenna sees enforced separation   McKenna and Thomas McDade, "Why Babies Should Never Sleep Alone: A Review of the Co-sleeping Controversy in Relation to SIDS, Bedsharing, and Breast Feeding," *Pediatric Respiratory Reviews* 6 (2005): 134–52. They note that "25– 45% of otherwise healthy infants and children in western societies are said to suffer from 'sleep disturbances,'" but such disturbances "are greatly reduced, if reported at all" with cosleeping.

238   expressions like "caught napping"   Martin, p. 341.

238   the changes currently taking place in Mediterranean   Renwick McLeanthe, "Spaniards Dare to Question the Way the Day Is Ordered," *New York Times*, January 12, 2005. I wonder if there will now be a higher incidence of sleep disorders.

238   "In China recently"   Hodgkinson, p. 83.

239   Not all of Wehr's subjects reverted   Wehr et al.

239   Studies of shift workers   L. Weibel et al., "Twenty-Four-Hour Melatonin and Core Body Temperature Rhythms: Their Adaptation in Shift Workers," *American Journal of Physiology* 272 (1997): 948–54.

239   One of Wehr's subjects "became profoundly depressed"   Wehr et al.

239   E. P. Thompson sees the preindustrial rhythm   Keyes, p. 17.

240   **whole range of stages between**   Non-Western cultures may have greater awareness that "sleep behaviorally, and perhaps conceptually, may lie on a continuum" that includes "disengaged semialert, to somnolence or drowsing, to dozing, to napping," modes that may be "more tolerated and perhaps more prevalent" in these cultures, write Worthman and Melby.

240   **"We're going to have to reconceptualize"**   Wehr quoted in Bruce Bower, "Slumber's Unexplored Landscape," *Science News Online*, September 25, 1999, www.sciencenews.org/sn_arc99/9_25?99/bob2.htm. "The fluid nature of sleep-wake boundaries, absence of strict bedtimes, and long periods of involuntary inactivity that we report for traditional human societies and which likely characterized human history, suggest the need to reconsider definitions of 'normal' rest and sleep patterns, reassess the standard model of sleep architecture, and review the potential value of somnolent resting states," say Worthman and Melby.

240   **"When modern humans find . . . sleep is fragmented"**   Wehr, "Impact of Changes."

240   **"it gets harder to override it"**   Wehr quoted in Klinkenborg.

241   **"The self-management approach"**   Morin, *Relief from Insomnia*, p. 52.

241   **self-help and recovery programs**   Wendy Kaminer, *I'm Dysfunctional, You're Dysfunctional: The Recovery Movement and Other Self-Help Fashions* (Addison Wesley, 1992), pp. 46–47, 65.

241   **"Last night you didn't sleep well"**   Wiedman, pp. 145, 169–70.

242   **"nothing more than a bad habit"**   Ibid., p. 103.

242   **"faulty causal attribution"**   Morin, "Psychological and Behavioral," p. 728.

242   **"For insomniacs, the erroneous belief"**   Morin, *Relief from Insomnia*, p. 51.

243   **"Even though a particular intervention is efficacious"**   Morin and Wooten.

243   **a person . . . in chronic pain**   A physician who works with patients in chronic pain commented, at a lunch session during one of the conferences, that "the CBT advice we give our patients who have chronic pain doesn't work well. They can't get out of bed and do sleep restriction—when they restrict their sleep, their pain gets worse."

243   **"Telling someone whose life is disorganized"**   Dr. Merril Mitler quoted in Daniel Goleman, "Can't Sleep? Changes in Behavior May Be More Effective Than Pills," *New York Times*, August 26, 1992.

245   *I was averaging maybe five*   Quoted in "Sleep Clinics: Treating the Exhausted," *Tennessee Medicine* (July 2005): 325–28.

246   **Joyce Wasleben**   Wasleben and Baron-Faust, p. 23.

246   **Deepak Chopra advises**   Chopra, p. 21. "The mere act of remaining motionless with your eyes closed, even if you're feeling anxious, actually provides the body with significant benefits," he writes (p. 16).

246   **"Since the mid-eighties, the etiology"**   Perlis et al., "Psychophysiological Insomnia."

246   **behavioral theory is a "top-down theory"**   Nofzinger, "Advancing the Neurobiology."

247   **"they seem to work best for the most seriously ill patients"**   S.R., interview by author, August 31, 2002: "People with insomnia caused by or associated with a major mental illness improve considerably with behavioral treatment, but those without an obvious cause (or maybe with primary insomnia)—who have been classically labeled as neurotic—are not helped so much. My experience flies in the face of the criticisms of Morin's work, whose studies are attacked for including only the 'cleanest' of patients."

247   **not much more effective than placebo**   "It appears from these reviews that behavioral treatments of insomnia are clearly better than placebo, but that the improvement of insomnia after behavior therapy still is not very impressive." Hauri et al., "The Treatment of Psychophysiologic Insomnia."

CHAPTER 9. ASLEEP AT THE SWITCH

248   **Sleep like other Things**   Nicholas Boileau, quoted in Ekirch, "Sleep We Have Lost."

251   **"sleep state misperception"**   This does not have a separate category in the DSM-IV, but in the *International Classification of Sleep Disorders* it is defined (under its new name, "paradoxical insomnia") as "a complaint of severe insomnia that occurs without evidence of objective sleep disturbance." *International Classification of Sleep Disorders*, p. 9.

255   *obstructive apnea*   This is different from *central apnea*, where the brain fails to signal the muscles to breathe and you actually stop breathing.

256   **administering ten milligrams of Ambien**   Christopher Lettieri et al., "Does Zolpidem Enhance the Yield of Polysomnography?" *Journal of Clinical Sleep Medicine* 1, 2 (2005): 129–31. But some clinics insist that the decision to medicate be made "on a case-by-case basis." Stephen Kramer, "Testing under the Influence," *Sleep Review* (May–June 2006), www.sleepreviewmag.com/issues/articles/2006-05_06.asp.

257   **"I wouldn't be surprised if I have a breathing problem"**   I have since tried to sleep with a CPAP machine, but I found that the air forced into me was enormously energizing. After a half hour of what felt like hyperventilating, I wanted to get up and run around the block. This was with a top-of-the-line model, too, which adjusted itself to my breathing, not the kind where the breath rate is preset. I had to stay up for several hours before I even attempted to sleep again. The machine went in the closet.

258   **"a super booming industry"**   "Sleep Centers—A Super Booming Industry."

258   **"on the sizzling size of hot"**   "New Careers Driven by Personal Interests, Market Forces," TMCnet, January 8, 2006, www.tmcnet.com/usubmit/2006/jan/1269163.htm.

258   **"a monster market"**   Peter Farrell, chief executive of ResMed, quoted in Wells.

258   **"a large number of patients"**   Stuart Menn quoted in "Sleep Centers—a Super Booming Industry."

258   **part owner of Pacific Sleep Medicine**   Wells.

259   **ResMed, which makes CPAPs**   Jack Hough, "More Profits in Snore," SmartMoney.com, April 26, 2006, www.smartmoney.com/stockscreen/index.ctm?story=20060426intro.

259   **By some reckonings**   Press release, SleepTech.com, May 10, 2004, www.sleeptech.com/text/pressrel.

259   **A business analyst says**   This is the projection of Frost and Sullivan, "Sleep Market Projected to Grow," "Industry News," *Sleep Review* (July–August 2006), www.sleepreviewmag.com/issues/articles/2006-7_04.asp.

259   **Another analyst estimates**   Ted Griffith, "Newton Firm Vows Improved Sleep-Disorder Treatments," *Boston Business Journal,* March 5, 1999, bizjournals.com.

259   **they weren't moneymakers**   "I know of no sleep clinic that makes money. They lose money. We're losing money all the time—it's expensive to run the centers," Hauri told Goldberg and Kaufman, p. 246.

259   **a sleep center for every 113,000 people**   In 2004, "2,515 sleep laboratories were available to the public," 850 of which were accredited sleep labs, according to the American Academy of Sleep Medicine. Katherine Shariq, "Sleep Centers in the US Reach 2,515 in 2004," *Sleep* 28 (2005): 145–46.

259   **"The number of accredited sleep centers"**   *Sleep Disorders and Sleep Deprivation.*

259   **There's now a clinic within 150 miles of you**   Dana Points, "Better Sleep from As to Zs," *Reader's Digest,* www.rd.com/content/tips-for-better-sleep/.

259   **"The number of sleep specialists"**   *Sleep Disorders and Sleep Deprivation.*

260   **The sleep business is keenly aware of itself as a business**   Tony Ramos, "Spreading the Word," *Sleep Review* (September 2005), www.sleepreviewmag.com/issues/articles/2005-09_07.asp: "No sleep practice can grow unless it markets and promotes itself within the health care community."

260   **A "Sleep Center Management Institute"**   Michael Breus, "The Management Side of Sleep," *Sleep Review* (July 2001), www.sleepreviewmag.com/issues/articles/2001-07_11.asp.

260   **a preface that reads like "a promotional message"** Pam Ryan, review of *Sleep Lab Compliance and the Law,* 2007, Advance NewsMagazine for Sleep.com, www.sleep-medicine.advanceweb.com/common/ editorial/ editorial.aspx?cc=37500.

260   **Physicians are encouraged** "Sleep Centers—a Super Booming Industry."

260   **SleepTech Solutions, "the largest company to focus"** From www .sleeptech.com/text/pressrel, May 10, 2004.

260   **"The first couple of years are often a financial struggle"** Epstein quoted in "Sleep Centers—a Super Booming Industry."

261   **"very much like a hotel business"** Paul Valentine quoted in Sean McFadden, "Wake-Up Call," *Boston Business Journal,* December 10, 2004, www.bizjournals.com.

261   **Israeli entrepreneur David Barone** Barone once addressed a venture forum on "turning brains to bucks." I hope that predatory phrase was the writer's, not his. Phyllis Hanlon, "Crossing the Pond to Turn Brains into Bucks," WPI Venture Forum (Worcester Polytechnic Institute), news release, January 24, 2001.

261   **"one-stop shop for sleep disorders"** Carol Daus, "A Model for Success," *Sleep Review* 4, 3 (May–June 2003), www.sleephealth.com/ PDF_files/sleepreviewamodelforsuccess.pdf.

262   **Sleep clinics diagnose 93 to 95 percent** Don Pantino, "Advances in Dental Sleep Medicine" (paper presented to the 19th Annual Meeting of the APSS, Denver, June 19, 2005).

262   **"What helps private companies improve"** "Sleep Centers—a Super Booming Industry."

262   **with a "possible net profit of between \$800 and \$1,000"** Michael Breus, "Reimbursement: What's New for CPAP?" *Sleep Review* (March–April 2003), www.sleepreviewmag.com/issues/articles/2003-3_03.asp.

262   **"15% of sleep centers sell masks"** "Market Forecast Good to Sleep Industry," *Sleep Review* (March–April 2006), www.sleepreviewmag .com/issues/articles/2006-3_09.asp.

262   **Columnist Mark Hayter** *The Pasadena Citizen,* May 12, 2005, www.hcnonline.com/site/news.cfm?newssid=14509691&BRD=1574 &PAG=461&dept_id=532207&rfi=8.

262   **treatment with CPAP** Jose Marin et al., "Long-Term Cardiovascular Outcomes in Men with Obstructive Sleep Apnoea-Hypopnoea with or without Treatment with Continuous Positive Airway Pressure," *Lancet* 365 (2005): 1046–53.

262   **"I'm a new woman now"** Amy Storer, "While You Were Sleeping," TherapyTimes.com, November 15, 2005, www.therapytimes.com/ content=5401J64C485E8C841.

262   **"I had no energy, no motivation"** David Markiewicz, "Reporter Snoozes in a Sleep Lab," ajc.com, June 19, 2005.

263   **the number of women they treat tends to be small**   James Rowley, "Gender: Does It Make a Difference in the Diagnosis and Management of Sleep Disorders?" (paper presented to the 20th Annual Meeting of the APSS, Salt Lake City, June 21, 2006). "I don't see a lot of insomniacs in my practice," Rowley said.

263   **"Insomnia has not become a well-established"**   Dement, "A Personal History."

264   **"In 1999, the majority of individuals"**   Tiago Moreira, "Sleep, Health, and the Dynamics of Biomedicine," *Social Science Medicine* 63, 1 (July 2006): 54–63.

264   *twice as many publications about apnea*   Richardson and Roth.

264   **At an interactive session**   B. Phillips et al., "Sleep Medicine Practices, Training and Attitudes: A Wake-Up Call for Pulmonologists," *Chest* 117 (2000): 1603–7.

266   **Daniel Kaufman**   Goldberg and Kaufman, p. 261.

266   **Bill Hayes**   Hayes, p. 290.

266   **"A big uvula"**   Ibid., pp. 289–90.

267   **nine-month follow-up study**   Hauri et al., "Effectiveness of a Sleep Disorders Center."

267   **His general assessment**   Quoted in Rubenstein, p. 54.

267   **a principle of suggestibility**   Hauri et al., "Effectiveness of a Sleep Disorders Center."

267   **patients are more likely to exaggerate their insomnia**   Hauri calls this a "hello–good-bye effect." "Consulting."

267   **Hobson describes how, when he volunteered**   *Sleep*, p. 149.

268   **Atul Gawande**   "The Bell Curve," *New Yorker,* December 6, 2004, www.newyorker.com/fact/content/articles/041206fa_fact?041206fa_fact.

269   **"I can't say for certain that the *amount*"**   Hayes, p. 294.

269   **Dr. Vipin Garg**   George Wiley, "Sleep Testing Multiculturally," *Sleep Review* (March–April 2006), www.sleepreviewmag.com/issues/articles/2006-3_02.asp. Sleep researcher Mark Mahowald fears that "some facilities are skimming off the most profitable part of the business—diagnosis—while leaving the actual care to others." Chen May Yee, "Their Business Is Putting You to Sleep," Startribune.com, January 28, 2007, wwwstartribune.com/535/story/964357.html.

270   **The American Academy of Sleep Medicine explains**   Littner et al.

270   **"Patients with psychophysiological insomnia"**   Hauri and Olmstead, "Reverse First Night Effect."

270   **"less than 22% of the time"**   Bonnet and Rosa. Hauri writes, "Based on current data, one might even claim that the amount of EEG defined sleep that people get is nearly *irrelevant* to whether they call themselves insomniacs." "Cognitive Deficits in Insomnia Patients," *Acta Neurologica Belgica* 97 (1997): 113–17.

270   insomniacs who complain . . . are more neurotic   Dorsey and Bootzin.

270   Quality of sleep . . . is "in the eye of the beholder"   Edinger et al.

270   A. Alvarez . . . describes a night he spent in a sleep clinic   Alvarez,
       pp. 80–81.

271   Puzzling, indeed   As Bonnet and Rosa observe, "A substantial per-
       centage of those with poor EEG sleep do not report a sleep problem."

271   "I sat down with her and went over the EEG"   Dement and Vaughan,
       p. 146. "Many severe insomniacs need a listener who has patience enough
       to discover that they are not insomniacs after all," write Luce and Segal,
       p. 31.

271   "They feel groggy, they do poorly"   Hauri and Linde, p. 241. Bonnet
       and Arand find that the twenty-four-hour metabolic rates of subjective
       insomniacs are "as high as those of objective insomniacs." "Physio-
       logical Activation in Patients with Sleep State Misperception," Psy-
       chosomatic Medicine 59 (1997): 533–40.

271   Other investigators find   Jeffrey Sugerman et al., "Daytime Alertness
       in Subjective and Objective Insomnia: Some Preliminary Findings," Bi-
       ological Psychiatry 20 (1985): 741–50: There are "events that are not
       reflected in PSG recordings."

271   Hauri also finds that the "misperceivers" have more motor activity
       Hauri and Joyce Wisbey, "Wrist Actigraphy in Insomnia," Sleep 15
       (1992): 239–301.

271   what our hormones are up to while we're "misperceiving"   Kirstine
       Adam and her colleagues at Royal Edinburgh Hospital found that, al-
       though there was only about a half-hour difference in sleep time be-
       tween insomniacs and normal sleepers, insomniacs had higher levels of
       stress hormones and "woke up twice as often in the first five hours of
       sleep. . . . It would seem that they are not mere complainers," that their
       feelings of unrestorative sleep "probably reflect biochemical events."
       "Physiological and Psychological Differences between Good and Poor
       Sleepers," Journal of Psychiatric Research 20, 4 (1986): 301–16.

272   "The physician should always be on guard"   T. R. Harrison, Principles
       of Internal Medicine, cited in Martin Reite et al., "The Use of Polysomnog-
       raphy in the Evaluation of Insomnia," Sleep 18, 6 (1995): 58–70.

272   "Hence one viewpoint is that such individuals"   Holzinger.

272   women complain more than men about their sleep   C. Schubert et al.,
       "Prevalence of Sleep Problems and Quality of Life in an Older Popula-
       tion," Sleep 25, 8 (2002): 48–52.

272   A more nuanced view   Charles Reynolds and his colleagues suggest
       that elderly women may find sleep deprivation to be more mood-
       disturbing. Reynolds et al.

272   "Subjective experience is so problematical"   Hobson, "Sleep Is of the
       Brain."

272   Seventy percent of people with apnea are not conscious of waking up
       Don Watenpaugh, in conversation. He also told me that a significant

number of people with restless legs syndrome don't know they have it, though their bodies register the effects of sleep loss.

273   like "great ocean swells"   Dement and Vaughan, p. 20.

273   a "third state . . . as different from sleep"   Jouvet, p. 5.

273   "prevents memories from being stored"   Empson, p. 45.

273   But insomniacs do remember   Perlis et al., "Mesograde Amnesia"; Bonnet, "Memory for Events Occurring during Arousal from Sleep," *Psychophysiology* 20 (1983): 81–87.

273   when awakened from nonREM   Rechtschaffen, "Polygraphic Aspects of Insomnia," in H. Gastaut et al., pp. 62–73.

273   When awakened from REM   Wallace Mendelson et al., "Experience of Insomnia."

273   In 1982, Irwin Feinberg and T.C. Floyd   Feinberg and Floyd. They cite David Foulkes, "Dream Reports from Different Stages of Sleep," *Journal of Abnormal and Social Psychology* 65 (1962): 14–25, on "the continuous mental activity."

274   they simply wipe out *memory* of sleep disturbances   Mendelson, "Do Studies of Sedative/Hypnotics"; Perlis et al., "Psychophysiological Insomnia."

274   more beta persists   Michael Perlis et al., "Beta/Gamma Activity"; Mercia et al. As Rechtschaffen surmised in 1968, insomniacs "are physiologically closer to wakefulness than good sleepers." "Polygraphic Aspects of Insomnia," in H. Gastaut et al., pp. 62–73.

274   "some regions of the brain aren't deactivating. . . . Maybe they aren't crazy"   Nofzinger, "Brain Imaging in Sleep and Sleep Disorders" (paper presented to the 19th Annual Meeting of the APSS, Denver, June 29, 2005); Nofzinger et al., "Functional Neuroimaging for Hyperarousal in Insomnia," *American Journal of Psychiatry* 161, 11 (November 2004): 2126–28.

274   there is often a "weak fit"   Sewitch.

275   "a sleep/wake discrimination difficulty"   Edinger and Andrew Krystal, "Subtyping Primary Insomnia: Is Sleep State Misperception a Distinct Clinical Entity?" *Sleep Medicine Reviews* 7, 3 (2001): 201–14.

275   you need to be taught to improve the accuracy   Insomniacs have "a perceptual discrimination problem," but "sleep-wake discrimination can be learned." Sewitch.

275   Sleeping pills . . . help "improve insomniacs' accuracy"   W. Vaughn McCall, "Pharmacologic Treatment of Insomnia," in *Sleep Medicine,* ed. Teofilo Lee-Chiong Jr. et al. (Elsevier, 2002), p. 171.

275   "the misperception . . . may be more in our tools"   Buysse, "Treatment Efficacy" (paper presented to the 17th Annual Meeting of the APSS, Chicago, June 7, 2003). Also, Mendelson, "Do Studies of Sedative/ Hypnotics."

275   "There is for me a state"   Sewitch.

276   Sleepwalkers . . . "wake up enough"   Dement and Vaughan, pp. 211–12.

276   Hobson describes how   *Sleep,* p. 149.

276   our word *wakefulness*   "Entering the language in the seventeenth century, this mouthful of a word has a contrived academic ring to it." Schiller.

276   This "kaleidoscopic sequence of rapidly morphing images"   Naiman, p. 48.

277   the line between sleep and wakefulness is not a clear demarcation   Pioneer sleep researcher Rosalind Cartwright writes, "When subjects are asked to lie awake in bed during the day and are then interrupted periodically for a report, their reports also have a fairly high proportion of regressed thoughts or hallucinatory images. It appears that throughout all three states—waking, quiet sleep, and active sleep—the mind has several styles of cognitive behaviors that can be going on: organized, logical thought; regressed thought that is less organized; and imagistic thought. Their distribution at any one time is a matter of degree, rather than an either/or affair" (p. 17).

277   there may be this toggling back and forth   Nathaniel Kleitman, the father of sleep medicine, describes this in his 1939 book *Sleep and Wakefulness:* "Whereas it is easy to distinguish between the conditions of alertness, or being wide-awake, and definite sleep, the passage from one to the other involves a succession of intermediate states, part wakefulness and part sleep in varying proportions—what is designated in Italian as *dormivegia,* or sleep-waking" (p. 71). "Ambiguous sleep" is another term I come across (in Mahowald and Schenck) to describe what John Spiro calls "curious states that combine aspects of both sleep and wakefulness"; "Introduction: Sleep," *Nature* 437 (October 2005): 1253.

278   "living without life"   "A Renaissance professor of poetry at Helmstedt," referred to by R. Wittern (of the University of Erlangen), "Sleep Theories in the Antiquity and in the Renaissance," *Sleep '88,* ed. J. Horne (Gustav Fischer Verlag, 1989), pp. 11–22. Wittern is paraphrasing Heinrich Meibom, "Sleep, oh come . . . / Without life, how sweet to live, Without death, to die." Quoted in Schiller.

278   in 1975, an NIH grant was not renewed   Dement and Vaughan, p. 112.

278   "The evolution of sleep research"   Jouvet, pp. 168–69.

280   "People with problems sleeping are . . . a desperate group"   Kimberley Cote, quoted in Karen von Hahn, "So You Haven't Slept in Weeks? Join the 4 AM Club," Globeandmail.com, January 28, 2006.

CHAPTER 10. ALTERNATIVES

281   "Successful patients search out possibilities"   Weil, p. 308.

282   About half of all Americans   Ernst.

282   **more than $27 billion annually**   A.R. White and E. Ernst, "Economic Analysis of Complementary Medicine: A Systematic Review," *Complementary Therapies in Medicine* 8 (2000): 111–18.

282   **Consumer satisfaction "tends to be very high"**   Dylan Evans, p. 154.

282   **compared to the seven or so minutes**   Margaret Talbot, "The Placebo Prescription," *New York Times Magazine* (January 9, 2000).

282   **the more actively involved**   S. Greenfield et al., "Assessing the Effects of Physician-Patient Interactions on the Outcomes of Chronic Disease," *Annals of Internal Medicine* 27, suppl. 3 (1989): S110–27.

282   **"Modern care . . . lacks the human touch"**   Atul Gawande, "The Computer and the Hernia Factory," in *Complications,* p. 45.

283   **pioneer sleep researcher Eliot Weitzman**   Goldberg and Kaufman, p. 249.

283   **it seems presumptuous to dismiss them**   Root-Bernstein and Root-Bernstein, p. 3.

284   **"there is solid research evidence"**   Hauri and Linde, p. 118.

284   **one of the few self-help books**   Goldberg and Kaufman also have a chapter on diet.

284   **anything . . . too spicy**   Martin, p. 159.

284   **Tryptophan is easily depleted**   Ross, *Mood Cure,* p. 29.

285   **a minimum of four ounces of protein food per meal**   Ibid., pp. 28–30.

285   **others claim that carbohydrates are what's essential**   Arne Lowden et al., "Performance and Sleepiness during a 24 Hour Wake in Constant Conditions Are Affected by Diet," *Biological Psychology* 65 (2004): 251–63.

285   **The advice given to insomniacs in *Alternative Medicine***   Goldberg, p. 924.

285   **"Low blood sugar, or hypoglycemic distress"**   Ross, *Diet Cure,* pp. 41–42.

286   **hypoglycemia "does exist"**   Hauri and Linde, p. 123.

286   **Grethe Birketvedt and her colleagues**   Grethe Birketvedt et al., "Hypothalamic-Pituitary-Adrenal Axis in the Night Eating Syndrome," *American Journal of Physiology, Endocrinology, and Metabolism* 282, 2 (February 2002): E366–69.

286   **Leptin levels normally rise**   J.M. Mullington et al., "Sleep Loss Reduces Diurnal Rhythm Amplitude of Leptin in Healthy Men," *Journal of Neuroendocrinology* 15 (2003): 851–54.

287   **relation between adrenal fatigue and erratic**   Ross, *Diet Cure,* p. 46.

287   **adrenal fatigue . . . as key to a constellation**   Ibid.

287   **Alcohol "acts just like a sugar biochemically"**   Ross, *Mood Cure,* pp. 272–73.

287   ***tyrosine* and *tyramine***   Hirshkowitz and Smith, p. 138.

288   **we need calcium and magnesium to convert**   Ross makes a powerful argument for a "nutrient rich" diet as the means to weight control and mental health. *Mood Cure,* p. 29 and throughout. Also see Fugh-Berman and Cott.

288   **Brewer's yeast . . . "a virtual wonder food"**   Goldberg and Kaufman, p. 133.

288   **Our diets may be deficient**   Freinkel.

288   **Hauri found it to be effective**   Hauri and Linde, p. 128.

289   **Alternative health practitioners are bitter about this**   Goldberg, p. 48.

289   **5-HTP . . . is as good as or better than tryptophan**   Ross, *Mood Cure,* pp. 42–43; Fugh-Berman and Cott.

289   **it doesn't work for everyone**   Ross, *Mood Cure,* p. 44.

289   **One study found that in a group of fifteen to twenty people**   Roger Williams, *Biochemical Individuality* (University of Texas Press, 1980), cited in Goldberg, p. 14.

289   **which makes the search for a "recommended daily allowance"**   William Walsh, "Biochemical Individuality and Nutrition," Health Research Institute, 2004, hriptc.org/biochemical_individuality.html.

289   *orthomolecular medicine*   Goldberg, pp. 406–12.

289   **"The brain is a chemical factory"**   Walsh, "Biochemical Individuality and Nutrition." Also, Freinkel.

289   **landmark study of bipolar depression**   W. E. Severus et al., "Omega 3 Fatty Acids—The Missing Link?" *Archives of General Psychiatry* 54, 6 (April 1999): 380–81.

290   **the worst disease a person can get**   "Once the sufferer can no longer sleep, a downward progression ensues, as he loses his ability to walk or balance. Perhaps most tragic, the ability to think remains intact." Max, p. xv.

290   **"DF," as he was called in the case study**   Joyce Schenkein and Pasquale Montagna, "Self-Management of FFI. Part 2: Case Report," *Medscape General Medicine* 8, 2 (2006), medscape.com. "Later in his illness, DF added what he referred to as massive, but unspecified doses of octoconosal (a spinach derivative prepared with long-chain alcohols). Of all supplements, he found this to be most effective and quick-acting in masking symptoms of fatigue following long periods of sleeplessness."

291   **SAM-e**   Ross, *Mood Cure,* p. 47.

291   **others find that it speeds them up**   Fugh-Berman and Cott.

291   **injection of SAM-e into certain parts of a rat's brain**   C. G. Charlton and J. Mack, "Substantia Nigra Degeneration and Tyrosine Hydroxylase Depletion Caused by Excess S-Adenosylmethionine in the Rat Brain," *Molecular Neurobiology* 9, 11–3 (August–September 1994): 149–61.

291   **even from a computer monitor**   S. Higuchi et al., "Effects of VDT Tasks with a Bright Display at Night on Melatonin, Core Temperature,

Heart Rate, and Sleepiness," *Journal of Applied Physiology* 94, 5 (2003): 1173–76.

292   vendors couldn't keep enough of it on the shelves   Jacobs, p. 9.

292   evidence for its effectiveness . . . is "mixed"   Rod Hughes et al., "The Role of Melatonin and Circadian Phase in Age-Related Sleep-Maintenance Insomnia: Assessment in a Clinical Trial of Melatonin Replacement," *Sleep* 21, 1 (1998): 52–68.

292   There may be some risk to taking melatonin   Wallace Mendelson, "The Many Faces of Insomnia," *Sleep Medicine Reviews* 4, 3 (2000): 225–28.

292   wear glasses or use lightbulbs   Both have been developed by a group of John Carroll University physicists, headed by Richard Hansler, and are available at Lowbluelights.com. Some people say they've helped their sleep.

292   if your pineal gland is calcified   Dieter Kunz et al., "A New Concept for Melatonin Deficit: On Pineal Calcification and Melatonin Excretion," *Neuropsychopharmacology* 21 (1999): 765–72.

292   **Bronson, a nutritional-biochemical consultant**   Goldberg, pp. 411–12.

293   **"nutrients in overload"**   Ibid., p. 803.

293   **Emperor Shennong**   Goldberg and Kaufman, p. 175.

293   **Pliny the Elder . . . Ficino**   Dannenfeldt cites *Natural History,* bks. 20–23, and Ficino, whose recipes were directed especially to men of letters whose "brains became dried out."

293   **nutmeg oil**   Hauri and Linde, p. 118; Martin, p. 167.

293   **A current folk remedy**   Goldberg and Kaufman, p. 174.

293   **"Then scientists learned how to extract and synthesize"**   Arnold Relman, "A Trip to Stonesville: Some Notes on Andrew Weil," *New Republic* (December 14, 1998).

293   **still used the ways they were traditionally**   Dylan Evans, p. 150; Goldberg, p. 252.

293   **In the United States, a 1999 survey**   Fugh-Berman and Cott.

293   **Herbs known to help sleep**   Ross et al., pp. 163–68.

294   **"odiferous root"**   Goldberg, p. 266.

294   **"the safest sedative I know"**   Weil, p. 238; Ross et al., p. 163.

294   **it's said to outsell Prozac**   Ross, *Mood Cure,* p. 46.

294   **"Both are members of the Papaveraceae family"**   Natural Medicines Comprehensive Database at www.naturaldatabase.com.

295   **A cautionary note**   "Among the questions consumers should consider asking manufacturers of herbals supplement are: Have the ingredients been thoroughly researched, with reliance on authoritative sources . . . ? How are the raw materials chosen? . . . How are the herbs extracted? Are only natural processes used? Are independent labs used for testing? . . . Are potentially harmful additives included in

the final product? Does the product come with warnings, cautions, ingredients, and expiration dates on each container, like pharmaceuticals?" Samuel Benjamin, "A Focus on Complementary and Alternative Medicine," *Patient Care* (January 15, 2000): 36–43. Web pages to know about include http://sis.nlm.nih.gov/enviro/dietarysupplements/html, quackwatch.com, and www.ncahf.org (National Council Against Health Fraud). Standard references are V. E. Tyler, *Rational Phototherapy: A Physician's Guide to Herbal Medicine* (Springer, 1998); and C. Newall, *Herbal Medicine: A Guide for Health-Care Professionals* (Pharmaceutical Press, 1996).

295   Ayurvedic medicine   Ross et al., p. 113.

296   as Weil says, "one of the oldest medical systems"   Weil, p. 295.

296   integral part of medical practice . . . in India   Patricia Leigh Brown, "Ayurvedic Spas in Southern India Find That Spiritual Enlightenment Is a Hot Tourist Draw," *New York Times,* August 13, 2006.

296   "therapeutic value . . . might be worth exploring"   Weil, pp. 295, 290.

296   Today, it is estimated   Goldberg, p. 62.

296   "In conventional western medicine, two insomniacs"   Ross et al., pp. 116–17.

297   acupuncture is effective with pain   Goldberg, pp. 62, 64, 923; P. H. Richardson and C. A. Vincent, "Acupuncture for the Treatment of Pain," *Pain* 24 (1986): 1540–49.

297   studies that say it helps sleep   S. R. Sok et al., "Effects of Acupuncture Therapy on Insomnia," *Journal of Advanced Nursing* 44, 4 (2003): 375–84.

297   based on the principle that "like cures like"   Ross et al., pp. 168–69.

297   it is practiced worldwide   Goldberg, p. 270.

297   1991 study in the *British Medical Journal*   J. Kleignen et al., "Clinical Trials of Homeopathy," *British Medical Journal* 302 (February 1991): 316–23, cited in Goldberg, p. 273.

298   success with aromatherapy   I. S. Lee and G. J. Lee, "Effects of Lavender Aromatherapy on Insomnia and Depression in Women College Students," *Taehan Kanho Hakhoe Chi* (Journal of the Korean Academy of Nursing) 36, 1 (2006): 136–43.

298–99   according to Dr. Weil, x rays confirm that the cranial bones do move   Weil, p. 35.

299   A recent study suggests   Michael Cutler et al., "Cranial Manipulation Can Alter Sleep Latency and Sympathetic Nerve Activity in Humans: A Pilot Study," *Journal of Alternative and Complementary Medicine* 11, 1 (2005): 103–8.

299   I hear about a cathode ion collector dish   Bill Stremmel, e-mail, Herb foods.com.

299   One study that was double-blinded and placebo-controlled   Raniere Pelka et al., "Impulse Magnetic-Field Therapy for Insomnia: A

Double-Blind, Placebo-Controlled Study," *Advances in Therapy* 18, 4 (July–August 2001): 174–80.

299 **silver lollipop** Nora Zamichow, "Lullaby Lollipop," *Los Angeles Times,* September 29, 1991; B. Pasche et al., "Effects of Low Energy Emission Therapy in Chronic Psychophysiological Insomnia," *Sleep* 19 (1996): 327–36.

299 **Transcranial magnet stimulation** Innateintelligence.com. Matthew Kirkcaldie and Saxy Pridmore, "A Bright Spot on the Horizon: Transcranial Magnetic Stimulation in Psychiatry," Medical University of South Carolina, www.musc.edu/tmsmirror/intro/layintro.html. This article was written for *Open Mind: The Journal of the Tasmanian Association for Mental Health.*

299 **"With a single pulse, we were able"** Tononi quoted in "Understanding the Function of Sleep Comes One Step Closer," *Medical News Today,* May 4, 2007, www.medicalnewstoday.com/medicalneds.php?newsid=6961. His study is Marcello Massimini et al., "Triggering Slow Waves by Transcranial Magnetic Stimulation," *Proceedings of the National Academy of Sciences,* May 4, 2007, 10.1073/pnas.0702495104.

300 **cranial electrotherapy stimulation** Marc Weiss, "The Treatment of Insomnia through the Use of Electro Sleep: An EEG Study," *Journal of Nervous and Mental Disease* 157, 2 (1973): 108–20; Rosalind Cartwright and Marc Weiss, "The Effects of Electro Sleep on Insomnia Revisited," *Journal of Nervous and Mental Disease* 161, 2 (1975): 134–37.

300 **"Brain Music Therapy for Treatment of Insomnia and Anxiety"** Leonid Kayumov et al., "Brain Music Therapy for Treatment of Insomnia and Anxiety," in *Proceedings of the 16th Annual Meeting of the Associated Professional Sleep Societies* (Associated Professional Sleep Societies, 2002), abstract 327L, p. 241.

300 **brain music by other Russian researchers** Ya. I. Levin, "Brain Music in the Treatment of Patients with Insomnia," *Neuroscience and Behavioral Physiology* 28, 3 (1998): 330–35.

300 **music . . . as a sleep tool** Hui-Ling Lai and Marion Good, "Music Improves Sleep Quality in Older Adults," *Journal of Advanced Nursing* 49, 3 (2005): 234–44.

301 **forty thousand therapists** *ABC News,* June 19, 2002.

301 **"EMDR's oscillating stimulation"** Solomon, pp. 140–41.

301 **Clinical psychologist John Preston** Preston, pp. 23–24.

302 **Proponents of these claim . . . a "theta state"** Michael Hutchison, "MegaBrain Report," from *MegaBrain Report,* 1, 2, online; also, Brad Hicks, "Mind Machine Frequently Asked Questions," February 2, 1999, www.us-shamanics.com/mm-faq.html.

302 **Practitioners of biofeedback claim success** Goldberg, pp. 97–99.

303 **The techniques are promising . . . and need much more research** Jim Robbins, "On the Track with Neurofeedback," *Newsweek* (June 11, 2000).

303 **When people talk about meditation** Weil, p. 247.

304   "similar to those . . . in highly trained experts"   Wallace and Benson.

305   some of the same things happen in meditation   Goldberg and Kaufman, pp. 77–83.

305   "The vibratory frequencies of these sounds"   Ibid., pp. 82–83.

305   Benson . . . teaches "a demystified form of meditation"   Jane Brody, "Relaxation Method May Aid Health," *New York Times,* August 2, 2006.

306   it might . . . improve your sleep   Goldberg and Kaufman, p. 78; Robert Woolfolk et al., "Meditation Training as a Treatment for Insomnia," *Behavior Therapy* 7 (1976): 359–65.

306   One study found that only eight sessions of meditation   Richard Davidson et al., "Alterations in Brain and Immune Function Produced by Mindfulness Medication," *Psychosomatic Medicine* 65, 4 (July–August 2003): 546–70.

306   people whose EEG shows greater activity in the left frontal cortex   H.L. Urry et al., "Making a Life Worth Living: Neural Correlates of Well-Being," *Psychological Science* 15, 6 (2004): 367–72; and many other studies.

306   an ancient yogi technique, breathing through the right nostril   D. Shannahoff-Khalsa et al., "The Effects of Unilateral Forced Nostril Breathing on Cognition," *International Journal of Neuroscience* 57, 3–4 (April 1991): 239–49, cited in Flaherty, p. 139.

306   One study found that vigorously grinning   Bernard Schiff and Mary Lamon, "Inducing Emotion by Unilateral Contraction of Facial Muscles: A New Look at Hemispheric Specialization and the Experience of Emotion," *Neuropsychologia* 27, 7 (1989): 923–35.

307   I've read that "placebos are ineffective"   Woolfolk et al.

307   the Feldenkrais method   The practitioner who claims success with it is Michael Krugman, *The Insomnia Solution* (Warner Books, 2005). Another method I'd like to check out is qigong. This is a slow-movement, stress-reduction method, or set of methods, that includes yoga as well. "Qigong devotees report better sleep, less anxiety and increased energy," reports Nora Isaacs. "Exercisers Slow It Down with Qigong," *New York Times,* April 5, 2007.

308   thyroid problems . . . affect many more women than men   Lois Verbrugge, "Gender and Health: An Update on Hypotheses and Evidence," *Journal of Health and Social Behavior* 26 (September 1985): 156–82.

308   alternative practitioners are better at picking up   Ross, *Diet Cure,* pp. 60–64.

309   Until the 1940s, says Julia Ross   Ibid., p. 64.

309   Other tests they do are for T4 and T3   Ross also recommends two antibody tests, a thyroid-releasing hormone test, and a temperature and reflex test. *Mood Cure,* p. 309.

309   **"Most Americans . . . would probably jump"**   Ralph Snyderman and Andrew Weil, "Integrative Medicine: Bringing Medicine Back to Its Roots," *Archives of Internal Medicine* 162 (2002): 395–97.

310   **I've found the merest trickle**   To find a physician trained in alternative healing, see the American Holistic Medicine Association, www.holisticmedicine.org, and the American Board of Holistic Medicine, www.holisticboard.org/roster.html.

CHAPTER 11. BEDDING DOWN WITH THE BEAST

311   **Jane Kenyon, "Insomnia at the Solstice"**   In *Acquainted with the Night: Insomnia Poems,* ed. Lisa Spaar (Columbia University Press, 1999), pp. 51.

313   **would their insomnia go away?**   James Horne actually looked at whether sensory stimulation would enhance sleep: "When I studied this in a systematic way, by sending people off on a supervised sightseeing tour when they expected to spend the day in the dull laboratory, not only were they more sleepy in the evening, but their sleep was deeper with more slow waves." *Sleepfaring,* p. 137. A study by University of Wisconsin researchers suggests that visual stimulation that leads to exploratory behavior in rats increases sleep pressure. Rego Huber et al., "Exploratory Behavior, Cortical BDNF Expression, and Sleep Homeostasis," *Sleep* 30, 2 (2007): 129–39.

313   **a woman in the luteal phase . . . on birth control pills**   M.J. Arnaud, "Metabolism of Caffeine and Other Components of Coffee," in *Caffeine, Coffee, and Health,* ed. Silvio Garattini (Raven Press, 1993), p. 49.

314   **Most cups of tea contain less caffeine**   A cup of tea contains about 60 to 75 milligrams of caffeine to coffee's 100 to 150; Gillin et al., p. 1351.

314   **tea has something in it**   Possibly flavonoids, or possibly theanine, an amino acid found in tea. Andrew Steptoe et al., "The Effects of Tea on Psychophysiological Stress Responsivity and Post-stress Recovery," *Psychopharmacology* 190 (2007): 81–89. The consumption of coffee is associated with myocardial infarction, whereas the consumption of tea is not. Arthur Klatsky et al., "Coffee Use Prior to Myocardial Infarction," *American Journal of Epidemiology* 132, 3 (1990): 479–88.

314   **People have wildly different responses**   "The biochemical protection of alcohol-destroying enzymes is not conferred equally among individuals. . . . Alcohol dehydrogenase [which breaks down alcohol] is manufactured according to blueprints stored in DNA. Since everyone's DNA is unique, individuals vary, sometimes strikingly, in the efficiency and activity of their alcohol dehydrogenase." In women, this enzyme is less efficient than in men, although after age fifty, the situation reverses; Braun, pp. 30–31.

314   **it's the substance most frequently used**   Gillin et al.

314   **it stimulates the stress system**   Zarcone, p. 660.

314   **If a pregnant woman drinks**   M. Akay and E. J. Mulder, "Acute Maternal Alcohol Consumption Disrupts Behavioral State Organization in
the Near-Term Fetus," *Pediatric Research* 44, 5 (1998): 774–79.

314   **Even after alcoholics have abstained**   Sean Drummond et al., "The
Sleep of Abstinent Pure Primary Alcoholic Patients: Natural Course
and Relationship to Relapse," *Alcoholism—Clinical and Experimental
Research* 22 (1998): 1796–1802.

314   **"From nature's point of view"**   Braun, p. 37.

315   **(white, that is, not red)**   Red wine is more likely than white wine to
disturb my sleep, and more likely to give me a headache. "Histamines
are 20–200% higher in red wine than in white." "Red Wine Headache
vs Sulfite Allergy," www.beekmanwine.com/prevtopbd.htm. But some
people find that red wine helps sleep. One study shows that some vari-
eties of grapes used in red wine, particularly in cabernet sauvignon and
merlot, are rich in melatonin. M. Iriti and F. Faoro, "Grape Phyto-
chemicals: A Bouquet of Old and New Nutraceuticals for Human
Health," *Medical Hypotheses* 67, 4 (2006): 833–38. Also, the tannins
in red wine cause the release of serotonin.

315   **some complex, invisible vagary of the inner weather**   "A transient
change in the chemical profile of your internal milieu, brought about by
factors as diverse as your state of health, diet, weather, hormonal cycles,
how much or how little you exercised that day[:] . . . the change would
be substantial enough to engender some response and alter your body
state," though you might not be aware of it. Damasio, *Feeling,* p. 48.

316   **A recent review of many studies**   Driver and Taylor.

316   ***The harder I exercise***   There's such a thing as overtraining syndrome:
S. R. Taylor et al., "Effects of Training Volume on Sleep, Psychological,
and Selected Physiological Profiles of Elite Female Swimmers," *Medicine and Science in Sports and Exercise* 29 (1997): 688–93.

316   **Studies suggest that exercise is most likely to help**   Driver and Taylor.

316   **studies don't show that this actually makes a difference**   Ibid.

317   **make a barrier between the day and the bed**   Zarcone, p. 659.

318   **even a short nap can be reinvigorating**   Amber Books and Leon Lack,
"A Brief Afternoon Nap Following Nocturnal Sleep Restriction: Which
Nap Duration Is Most Recuperative?" *Sleep* 29, 6 (2006): 831–40.

319   **extremities need to be warm**   The warmer your hands and feet, the
cooler your body temperature; the dilation of blood vessels in the extremities allows heat to escape. K. Krauchi et al., "Warm Feet Promote
the Rapid Onset of Sleep," *Nature* 401 (1999): 36–37.

319   **20 percent of couples sleep apart**   Lauri Githens Hatch, "Growing
Number of Couples Slumbering Separately," IndyStar.com, December
25, 2005.

320   **silk jacquard eye mask**   Ruth La Ferla, "Sleep, the Final Luxury,"
        New York Times, December 11, 2000; Steven Klein, "Sleep Invest-
        ments," *Vogue* (May 2005): 168–80; Natasha Singer, "Hey, Sleepy,
        Want to Buy a Good Nap?" *New York Times,* February 1, 2007.

320   **A blogger, European**   Circadiana, February 2005, http://circadiana
        .blogspot.com/2005/01/everything-you-always-wanted-to-know.html.

322   **"pre-sleep cognitive activity" . . . "negatively toned"**   Harvey.

322   **"excessive rumination about sleeplessness"**   Harvey and Greenall.

322   **"People with insomnia"**   Harvey.

322   **"*ruminative* thinking of guilt, fear of death"**   Weitzman et al.

323   **"thoughts leapfrog like evil imps"**   Bishop and Levy, p. 52.

323   **Catastrophize***   Harvey and Greenall.

323   **As Allison Harvey says, "The tendency"**   "Pre-sleep Cognitive Activ-
        ity: A Comparison of Sleep-Onset Insomniacs and Good Sleepers,"
        British Journal of Clinical Psychology 39 (2000): 275–86.

323   **It comes from the Latin verb**   Schwartz and Begley, p. 55.

324   **"Consciousness then resembles a rat trap"**   De la Mare, p. 46. Any-
        one plagued by this kind of racing mind might try one of the "mind ma-
        chines" discussed in the previous chapter.

325   **"Only dolts and drudges sleep"**   Isak Dinesen quoted by Boxer.

325   **Billy Collins . . . "Insomnia"**   *Sailing Alone around the Room: New
        and Selected Poems* (Random House, 2001), pp. 142–43.

327   **"We talk to ourselves all the time"**   Hobson, *Sleep,* p. 69.

328   **"Left to its own devices, my mind"**   Anne Lamott, *Bird by Bird: Some
        Instructions on Writing and Life* (Anchor Books, 1994), p. 26.

328   **"the lifelong dialogue"**   Carol Shields, *Unless* (Fourth Estate, 2002),
        p. 144.

328   **Lamott compares her inner chattering**   *Plan B: Further Thoughts on
        Faith* (Riverhead Books, 2005), p. 259.

329   **"Observe the breath"**   Weil, pp. 255–59.

329   **sources besides Bob**   One "theory of schizophrenic auditory halluci-
        nations" says that they are "a misattributed inner voice," and "when
        schizophrenics wear a simple device that prevents them from subvocal-
        izing (mumbling under their breath), their hallucinations dramatically
        decrease." Flaherty, p. 240. I wonder if such a device would help quiet
        an insomniac's racing mind. A study by A. B. Levey et al. had success
        with "engag[ing] the vocal apparatus in a very simple way which pre-
        cludes concurrent thought." "Auditory Suppression and the Treatment
        of Insomnia," *Behavior Research and Therapy* 29, 1 (1991): 85–89.

330   **"repeating some well-known rhyme"**   Wright, p. 190.

330   **If you have any talent for visualization**   One study found that "treat-
        ments employing visual focusing were superior to somatic-focusing
        treatments in reducing the number of nocturnal awakenings." Robert

Woolfolk and Terence McNulty, "Relaxation Treatment for Insomnia: A Component Analysis," *Journal of Consulting and Clinical Psychology* 51, 4 (1983): 495–503.

332   *Nocturia*   Bliwise, p. 27.

332   **"bladder training"**   This involves urinating at set intervals, whether you want to or not, and then gradually lengthening those intervals. I've heard it works.

333   **According to Yoga philosophy**   Weil, p. 257.

333   **One study found that babies snugly blanketed**   P. Franco et al., "Influence of Swaddling on Sleep and Arousal Characteristics of Healthy Infants," *Pediatrics* 115, 5 (May 2005): 1307–11.

333   **a "swaddler/sleep sack"**   Advertised in *Sleep Review* (September–October 2005), sleepreviewmag.com/issues/articles/2005-09_13.asp.

335   **"I find those meditation thingys very distracting"**   Eric Zorn, "Insomnia Cure: Take Your Buds to Bed," *Chicago Tribune,* May 5, 2006, blogs.chicagotribune.com/news_columnists_ezorn/2006/05/insomnia _cure_t.html.

335   **the Golf Channel**   Vic Reato, "One Man's Cure for Insomnia," October 23, 2006, suburbanchicagonews.com/heraldnews/sports/107371,4_ 2_Jo23_VICCOL_SI.articleprint.

336   **I'll be a tapeworm**   I wish I could claim that line, but it's David Sedaris's. Can't tell you where it's from, though, because I heard it on tape.

336   **"a good snoozy story"**   M.P. Dunleavey, "Dream Works: Never Underestimate the Ability of a Good Snoozy Story to Help Lull a Child to Sleep," *New York Times,* May 15, 2005.

336   **what Anne Lamott calls "the listening child"**   *Plan B,* p. 188.

337   **she "stopped sleeping, partly from a permanently blocked nose"**   Lorna Sage, *Bad Blood* (Fourth Estate, 2000), pp. 109, 219–20.

338   **In "The Haunted Mind"**   Hawthorne quoted in Ekirch, "Sleep We Have Lost."

339   **"I have been one acquainted with the night"**   Robert Frost, in *Acquainted with the Night: Insomnia Poems,* ed. Lisa Spaar (Columbia University Press, 1999), p. 32.

339   **"When the house is dark"**   Joyce Carol Oates, preface to *Night Walks: A Bedside Companion* (Ontario Review Press, 1982), p. xiii. She calls "this wakefulness . . . a region of profound revelations."

339   **"The middle of the night is my special haven"**   Alan Berliner, *Director's Statement* (56th Internationale Filmfestspiele, Berlin, 2006), pamphlet.

CHAPTER 12. MAKING CHANGE

342   **"how are you supposed to get better"**   Martin Miller, "Not Exactly a Quiet Zone," *Los Angeles Times,* March 8, 2004.

342   **Nighttime noise levels**   S.L. Krachman et al., "Sleep in the Intensive
        Care Unit," *Chest: The Cardiopulmonary and Critical Care Journal*
        107 (1995): 1713–20; Cheryl Ann Cmiel, "Noise Control: A Nursing
        Team's Approach to Sleep Promotion," *American Journal of Nursing*
        104, 2 (February 2004): 40–48.

342   **55 decibels, . . . with spikes up to 80**   Mark Opp, "Sleep and the Im-
        mune System" (lecture delivered at "A Primer of Sleep Research," Sleep
        Research Society, February 11, 2006, La Jolla, Calif.).

342   **better hours for residents**   Debra Weinstein, "Duty Hours for Resi-
        dent Physicians: Tough Choices for Teaching Hospitals," *New England
        Journal of Medicine* 347, 16 (2002): 1275–78.

342   **"the new self-imposed rules"**   Czeisler quoted in Lambert.

343   **"Physicians aren't being trained"**   A.Y. Avidan and R.D. Chervin,
        "Sleep Medicine Content of Medical Textbooks—a Follow-Up Study,"
        in *Proceedings of the 19th Annual Meeting of the Associated Profes-
        sional Sleep Societies* (Associated Professional Sleep Societies, 2005),
        abstract 993, p. 337.

343   **The National Sleep Foundation has campaigned**   Amy Wolfson,
        "Bridging the Gap between Research and Practice: What Will Adoles-
        cents' Sleep-Wake Patterns Look Like in the 21st Century?" in *Adoles-
        cent Sleep Patterns: Biological, Social, and Psychological Influences,* ed.
        Mary Carskadon (Cambridge University Press, 2002), pp. 212–13.

343   **Long-haul drivers**   Atul Gawande, "Drowsy Docs: If Tired Truckers
        Are a Threat, What about Those Sleep-Deprived Medical Residents,"
        Slate, October 10, 1997, www.slate.com/id/2666/.

343   **"the transportation system is really out to lunch"**   "In decisions that
        had the support of the White House, the motor carrier industry has
        eased the rules on truckers' work hours," reports Stephen Labaton.
        "the trucking industry has provided some of the Republican party's
        most important fund-raisers." "As Trucking Rules Are Eased, a Debate
        on Safety," *New York Times,* December 3, 2006.

343   **tsunami of aging**   Avorn, p. 123. UN statistics on aging cited in Pietro
        Gareri et al., "Conventional and New Antidepressant Drugs in the
        Elderly," *Progress in Neurobiology* 61 (2000): 353–96.

343   **"Aging in place"**   Fred Turek, "Collapse: Economic Impact of Aging
        and Sleep on Modern Societies," *Sleep* 28, 10 (2005): 1223–24.

344   **insomnia is not seen as a disability**   There are too many millions of us for
        it to be defined as a disability, and there isn't even agreement about what
        "it" is. Yet a screening of over five hundred patients in fourteen countries
        showed that "persons with sleep problems reported a degree of disability
        in the performance of their daily activities and social role" (*disability* was
        defined as "any restriction or lack of capacity to perform an activity
        in a manner or within a range considered normal for a human being").
        T.B. Ustun et al., "Form, Frequency, and Burden of Sleep Problems in
        General Health Care," *European Psychiatry* 11, suppl. 1 (1996): S5–10.

345   "It's the early bird"   Schur, p. 119.

345   Some night owls absolutely cannot adjust   S. J. Paine et al., "The Epidemiology of Morningness/Eveningness: Influence of Age, Gender, Ethnicity, and Socioeconomic Factors in Adults (30–49 Years)," *Journal of Biological Rhythms* 21, 1 (2006): 68–76.

346   "Academia is a good place"   DePaulo quoted in St. John and Williams.

349   and post it on the Web   NIH *State-of-the-Science Conference Statement on Manifestations and Management of Chronic Insomnia in Adults,* June 13–15, 2005, http://consensus.nih.gov/2005/2005Insomnia SOS026html.htm.

349   Comorbid conditions often accompany insomnia   Ibid.

349   "This sounds like a small matter"   Buysse, "Report on NIH Conference" (presented to the 19th Annual Meeting of the APSS, Denver, June 21, 2005); Buysse, "Insomnia, State of the Science: An Evolutionary, Evidence-Based Assessment," editorial, *Sleep* 28, 9 (2005): 1045–46.

349   a "stand-alone disorder"   Ben Harder describes this "shifting paradigm on sleeplessness" and quotes Thomas Roth, who calls it "critically important. . . . It redefined our view of insomnia." Harder, "Staring into the Dark," *Science News Online,* November 26, 2005, www.sciencenews.org/articles/20051126/bob9.asp.

350   A U.K. researcher wrote in 2005   Holzinger.

350   NIH presentations that addressed possible neurological etiologies   Gary Richardson, "Physiological Models of Chronic Insomnia," and Clifford Saper, "Neurobiology of Insomnia" (papers presented to the NIH Insomnia Conference, Bethesda, Md., June 13, 2003).

351   Also puzzling to me was the press release   "Panel Calls for a New Look at Treatments Commonly Used for Chronic Insomnia," NIH News, June 15, 2005, www.nih.gov/news/pr/jun2005/od-15.htm.

351   "Insomnia Sufferers Need Better Care, Experts Say"   *American Journal of Health-System Pharmacists News* (August 1, 2005). "NIH has expressed concern over their widespread use of many medications to manage chronic insomnia that have not been studied for that indication." "Treating Chronic Insomnia," *Journal of the American Medical Association* 294, 4 (July 27, 2005): 418.

352   I'd have quoted Daniel Buysse   "Rational Pharmacotherapy for Insomnia."

352   I'd have quoted Marcia Angell   *Truth,* p. 22.

352   "Fundamental advances"   Gershon, pp. 309.

352   "The money always goes to the quick fixes"   Hauri, interview by author, May 16, 2003. An analysis of NIH funding in 1998 found that "fully half of sleep grants were clinical in nature, while 30% addressed basic research. . . . Basic sleep science . . . was substantially underrepresented." Martha Gillette et al., "NIH Funding of Sleep Research: A Prospective and Retrospective View," *Sleep* 22, 7 (1999): 956–58.

352   "The lonely beacon of the insomniac"   Forner.

353   "barriers of secrecy and shame"   Ehrenreich, "Body Politic."

353   "A group of us in the late 1960s"   Jane Pincus, "How a Group of
       Friends Transformed Women's Health," *Women's eNews*, March 13,
       2002, www.womensenews.org/article.cfm/dyn/aid/844.

354   "we . . . are the best experts"   Boston Women's Health Book Collec-
       tive, p. 653.

354   "We discovered that every one of us had a 'doctor story'"   Judy Nor-
       sigian et al., "The Boston Women's Health Book Collective and *Our
       Bodies, Ourselves*: A Brief History and Reflection," Our Bodies, Our-
       selves, www.ourbodiesourselves.org/about/jamwa.asp, originally pub-
       lished in *Journal of the American Medical Women's Association* (Win-
       ter 1999).

354   In 1969, Barbara Seaman   Mann.

354   "by 1975, nearly 2,000"   Cynthia Pearson quoted in Mann.

355   "When I think of the beginnings"   Ehrenreich, "Body Politic."

355   "inequities in women's health"   Vivian Pinn, "Women's Health Re-
       search," *Journal of the American Medical Association* 268, 14 (1992):
       1921–22; Angell, "Caring."

355   Healy launched the Women's Health Initiative   Angell, "Caring."

355   By 1997, about a third of hospitals   Francine Nichols, "History of the
       Women's Health Movement in the 20th Century," *Journal of Obstet-
       ric, Gynecologic, and Neonatal Nursing* 29, 1 (2000): 56–64. By 2000
       there were thirty-six hundred women's health centers, according to
       Naomi Rogers, review of *Into Our Own Hands: The Women's Health
       Movement in the U.S., 1969–1990*, by Sandra Morgen, *Journal of the
       History of Medicine* 58 (April 2003): 244–46.

355   legs that "have minds of their own"   Virginia Wilson, p. 191.

356   Utley recounts   Utley, p. 114.

356   Over time, as lawyer and patient advocate Bob Cloud says   Cloud,
       "Do Sleep Centers and Patient Groups Really Need Each Other?" *Sleep
       Review* (July–August 2002), www.sleepreviewmag.com/issues/2002-
       07.asp.

356   She made up a questionnaire   Virginia Wilson, pp. 82–84, 280–81.

356   first International Symposium on Restless Legs Syndrome   Ibid.,
       p. 158.

357   sufferers can find "someone else in the world"   Utley, p. 143.

357   "Join an RLS support group"   Wilson, p. 252.

357   "The great majority of patients with frequent insomnia"   Nalaka
       Gooneratne, "Treatment Epidemiology" (paper presented to the NIH
       Conference, Bethesda, Md., June 13, 2005).

358   learn from the National Organization for Rare Disorders   Mary Dun-
       kle, "How Do You Spell 'Hope'?" *MetDESK News: Information and*

Support for the Special Needs Community, no. 2 (April–May 2003), www.metlife.com/WPSAssets/13446976851086204205V1F03%20A pr-May%20Newsletter.pdf.

359   **Patient groups are useful to drug companies**   Healy, "Psychopharmacology," p. 241.

359   **about two-thirds of patient advocacy groups accept**   Moynihan and Cassels, pp. 73–74.

359   **"Put this in your book, IN BIG LETTERS"**   Daniel Kripke, interview by author, November 17, 2003.

359   **"It's a massive revolution"**   Charon quoted in Kolata.

359–60   **But doctors who attend . . . One physician says**   Quoted in Kolata.

360   **the seven-minute shuffle**   Peter Salgo, "The Doctor Will See You for Exactly Seven Minutes," *New York Times,* March 22, 2006.

360   **"You can't sit and talk"**   Physician quoted in Jan Hoffman, "Awash in Information, Patients Face a Lonely, Uncertain Road," *New York Times,* August, 14, 2005.

360   **"Patients are goldmines of information"**   Walker, p. 42.

361   **History offers a long line of physician-observers**   The stories of Edward Jenner and William Withering and others are told in Root-Bernstein and Root-Bernstein, pp. 6–10.

362   **if what we say collides with existing theoretical models**   Harvey and Tang.

362   **"better define which research questions should be studied"**   Heymann.

362   **"certain personality types—as established by questionnaire"**   Jerome Burne, "The Rebranding of a Disease," *New Statesman,* March 11, 2002, www.biopsychiatry.com/bigpharma/index.html.

362   **In 1972, Ismet Karacan**   Karacan et al.

363   **"Variability has been largely overlooked"**   Hans Van Dongen et al., "Individual Differences in Adult Human Sleep and Wakefulness: Leitmotif for a Research Agenda," *Sleep* 28, 4 (2005): 479–95.

363   **"One often-neglected issue"**   Hauri et al., "The Treatment of Psychophysiologic Insomnia."

363   **"There are 'lumpers' and 'splitters'"**   Hauri, e-mail, May 29, 2003.

363   **"Sleep researchers need to make greater efforts"**   Fred Turek, "Gender (Sex) and Sleep: Shh . . . Not in Front of the Children," *Sleep* 29, 1 (2006): 21–22.

364   **The depression study I described in chapter 6**   Caspi et al.

364–65   **a study of chronic fatigue syndrome**   Suzanne Vernon and William Reeves, "The Challenge of Integrating Disparate High-Content Data: Epidemiological, Clinical, and Laboratory Data Collected during an In-Hospital Study of Chronic Fatigue Syndrome," *Pharmacogenomics* 3 (2006): 341–43.

365 **The afflicted are overwhelmed by fatigue . . . and insomnia** "'Unrefreshing sleep' and rest is a hallmark of chronic fatigue syndrome," reports Wikipedia; also, Nancy Klimas, "Wake-Up Call," *Ms* (summer 2006): 53–55.

365 **"We've brought together a whole bunch"** Quoted by Amanda Gardner, "Genetics May Drive Chronic Fatigue Syndrome," Healthfinder .gov, 2006, www.healthfinder.gov/news/newsstory.asp?docID=532266.

365 **William Reeves . . . "an underlying biologic basis"** "Press Briefing on Chronic Fatigue Syndrome," Centers for Disease Control, April 20, 2006, www.cdc.gov/od/oc/media/transcripts/t060420.htm.

365 **the autoimmune connections I keep finding** "In some people, ongoing stress does not impair the immune system: it has the opposite effect, goading the immune system until it attacks targets that don't really pose a threat[,] . . . initiating an allergy or asthma attack . . . or an autoimmune disease," where "the immune cells actually fail to distinguish self from nonself and begin attacking healthy tissue." McEwen and Lasley, p. 99.

366 **damage found by Baron Von Economo** Siegel, "Brain Mechanisms."

366 **I find one study that describes** Ferdinand Zizi et al., "Sleep Complaints and Visual Impairment among Older Americans: A Community-Based Study," *Journal of Gerontology: Medical Sciences* 57, 10 (2002): M691–4. I find a few studies that connect Ambien use with visual problems, but they don't quite describe my symptoms.

366 **"There has been an avalanche"** Mignot quoted by Rob Stein, "Lack of Sleep Linked to Major Illnesses," *Washington Post,* October 10, 2005.

367 **four hundred times as much melatonin** Regina Patrick, "Melatonin and Irritable Bowel Syndrome," *Focus: Journal for Respiratory Care and Sleep Medicine* (January–February 2006): 12.

367 **Its workings are closely coordinated with sleep** Sandra Blakeslee, "Mystery of Sleep Yields as Studies Reveal Immune Tie," *New York Times,* August 3, 1993; Blakeslee, "Complex and Hidden Brain in the Gut Makes Cramps, Butterflies, and Valium," *New York Times,* January 23, 1996.

367 **"decreased small intestinal motility"** D. A. Gorard et al., "Migrating Motor Complex and Sleep in Health and Irritable Bowel Syndrome," *Digestive Diseases and Sciences* 40, 11 (November 1995): 2283–89.

367 **REM has "immediate stimulatory effects on colonic motility"** Yoshiyiki Furukawa et al., "Relationship between Sleep Patterns and Human Colonic Motor Patterns," *Gastroenterology* 107 (1994): 1372–81.

367 **"The information content of the messages"** Gershon, pp. 216–17.

367 **An estimated 26 to 55 percent of people with irritable bowel syndrome** Patrick.

367 **They also seem to have more REM** D. Kumar et al., "Abnormal REM Sleep in the Irritable Bowel Syndrome," *Gastroenterology* 103

(1992): 12–17; William Orr et al., "Sleep and Gastric Function in Irritable Bowel Syndrome: Derailing the Brain-Gut Axis," *Gut* 41 (1997): 390–93.

368   **"All NIH is suffering from the prioritizing of war over life"**   Michael Irwin, interview by author, April 27, 2005. "Whereas national defense spending has reached approximately $1,600 per capita, federal spending for biomedical research now amounts to about $97 per capita," writes Joseph Loscalzo, noting that young researchers "increasingly opt for alternative career paths, shrinking the pipeline of future investigators." "The NIH Budget and the Future of Biomedical Research," *New England Journal of Medicine* 354 (2006): 1665–67.

368   **"The innovative approaches that are really pushing the envelope"**   Irwin's comments remind me of Dr. Susan Love's castigation of cancer research: "If you have a wild idea or a completely new paradigm, forget about it." What we get is a lot of research about "better ways of doing the same thing": what we need are "wild ideas to get us out of the rut of doing the same thing better." Love, "To Break the Disease, Break the Mold," *New York Times,* April 1, 2007.

368   **"The U.S. is losing its dominance in the sciences"**   William Broad, *New York Times,* June 3, 2004.

368   **"We are sorry to announce"**   *The Network* newsletter, spring 2005.

369   **Dermatology is suddenly hot**   "Other specialties also enjoying a surge in popularity are radiology, anesthesiology and even emergency room medicine," which "all allow doctors to put work behind them when their shifts end." Matt Richtel, "Young Doctors and Wish Lists: No Weekend Calls, No Beepers," *New York Times,* January 7, 2004.

370   **"It's a vital field"**   A less optimistic view is stated by Allan Pack and Phyllis Zee in a 2006 editorial in *Sleep:* "The very limited pipeline of investigators in sleep research is a crisis." Clinical practice is a more attractive choice for someone going into the sleep field, since "both clinical demand for sleep specialists and economic incentives are high," but "where are the career opportunities for . . . young investigators" when "so few of our leading institutions have vibrant academic programs in sleep medicine? . . . If the current situation is not remedied, there could be no field of sleep research in 15 years." "The Pipeline of Investigators for Sleep Research—a Crisis!" *Sleep* 29, 10 (2006): 1260–61. Bonnet nevertheless maintains that "exciting work is starting to be done in areas relevant to insomnia, and because such work is new and important, I think much of it will continue to be funded" (e-mail, December 4, 2006). Let's hope he's right.

Glossary

AASM See **American Academy of Sleep Medicine.**

adenosine A neurotransmitter associated with sleepiness, it accumulates during our waking hours and dissipates during sleep. Caffeine promotes wakefulness by blocking its action, acting as an adenosine receptor **antagonist.**

adrenaline See **epinephrine.**

adrenals A small gland on top of each kidney. When we need sudden energy, whether for an emergency or just for exercise, the **hypothalamus** alerts the **pituitary,** which causes the adrenals to pour out stress hormones (cortisol). See **hypothalamic-pituitary-adrenal axis (HPA)** and **sympathetic nervous system.**

agonist A substance that enhances the effects of a neurotransmitter, as benzodiazepines augment the action of **GABA.**

American Academy of Sleep Medicine The AASM was founded in the 1970s for professionals interested in sleep. It made itself responsible for setting standards of practice related to the study and treatment of sleep and for the accreditation of sleep clinics.

antagonist A substance that inhibits the effect of a neurotransmitter, often by blocking the receptor for it.

antihistamine A chemical that inhibits the action of the wake-up neurotransmitter histamine. Antihistamines were developed as allergy medications. Among their side effects is sleepiness, so the active ingredient *diphenhydramine* became the basis for over-the-counter sleep aids.

apnea (Literally, *without breath.*) A cessation of breathing during sleep, lasting ten seconds or more.

APSS See **Association of Professional Sleep Societies.**

Association of Professional Sleep Societies (APSS) A joint venture of the **AASM** and the Sleep Research Society, this organization holds the annual meetings of sleep professionals. The name was streamlined to "Sleep" in 2006.

barbiturates The class of drugs used for insomnia until benzodiazepines came along in the 1960s. The best known are phenobarbital, Nembutal, and Seconal. Like the benzodiazepines, barbiturates augment the action of **GABA.** Long thought to be perfectly safe, they turned out to be seriously addictive and were implicated in many overdoses. Today they're used mainly to sedate patients prior to surgery and to treat certain forms of epilepsy.

behavioral modification   See **cognitive behavioral therapy.**

benzodiazepines   The class of drugs that supplanted the barbiturates in the early 1960s. Librium and Valium were the first of this category, which is sometimes referred to as the "minor tranquilizers." They accentuate the action of **GABA,** the main braking system of the brain (they're also referred to as benzodiazepine receptor agonists, BzRAs). Shorter-acting versions such as Xanax and Restoril are preferred today to longer acting forms like Dalmane.

biofeedback   Monitoring devices that feed back information about physiological processes of which we're normally unaware, such as heart rate, breathing, blood pressure, muscle tension, to teach us to consciously regulate involuntary functions.

blood-brain barrier   A mechanism that stops the passage of large, potentially dangerous molecules from the bloodstream into the brain.

cataplexy   Episodes of muscle paralysis that sometimes accompany narcolepsy. The muscles go limp and the person is plunged, while still conscious, into the sleep paralysis and dream state of REM.

CBT   See **cognitive behavioral therapy.**

circadian   (Literally, "around a day.") The circadian cycle is the twenty-four-hour cycle of light and dark. Our peak and slump times are keyed to this clock, 6 to 10 A.M. being a peak, and 3 to 4 A.M. being a slump.

circadian clock   A biological timing mechanism that regulates the twenty-four-hour cycle, controlled by the **suprachiasmic nucleus.**

CME   See **Continuing Medical Education.**

cognitive behavioral therapy (CBT)   A system of therapies based on the assumption that distorted or dysfunctional thinking and maladaptive behavior are the causes of insomnia, and that, since such attitudes and habits have been learned, or conditioned, they can be unlearned. Treatments aim at reforming maladaptive attitudes and modifying behavior by means of **stimulus control therapy, sleep hygiene,** and **sleep restriction.**

Continuing Medical Education   Health care professionals are required to attend a certain number of hours of educational medical activities each year to keep their licenses current.

continuous positive airways pressure (CPAP) machine   A mask fitted over the nose that delivers pressured air to keep the airways open during sleep and allow normal breathing.

control group   In a scientific study or clinical trial, one group of subjects receives the treatment or drug that's being tested, and the other group receives the standard treatment or no treatment (**placebo**). The comparison group is the control group, sometimes called the case controls.

controlled substances   Drugs whose possession, use, manufacture, and distribution are regulated by the Controlled Substances Act and which come under the jurisdiction of the Drug Enforcement Administration. They're classified, or scheduled, according to potential for abuse and medical use, from class I through V, the worst being Schedule I (the benzodiazepines and nonbenzodiazepines are class IV). It's "important to note that these classifications are not necessarily scientifically-based, but rather can be based on political priorities (alcohol and nicotine are placed in no categories despite their health risks and addiction potentials)," says Wikipedia.

CPAP (Pronounced "see-pap.") See **continuous positive airways pressure.**

deep sleep In stages 3 and 4 sleep, sometimes called **delta** or **slow wave sleep,** breathing and heart rate are slow and regular and muscle relaxation becomes complete. This is where the restorative processes of sleep are thought to take place.

delta sleep Stages 3 and 4 sleep, or **deep sleep,** so termed for the delta waves that become prevalent or dominant on the EEG, slow, large, and regular waves with a frequency less than four hertz, or cycles, per second.

double blind A type of clinical trial or scientific study in which neither the subjects nor those who are administering the study know who is receiving which treatment. "Blinding" the participants is intended to eliminate the bias that might result when participants expect certain outcomes.

DSM-IV The *Diagnostic and Statistical Manual of Mental Disorders,* fourth edition, 1994. This is the American Psychiatric Association's compendium of definitions of behaviors deemed abnormal enough to be described as mental disorders. (That insomnia is included here prejudges it as a "mental disorder.") DSM terms and categories are recognized by insurance companies, funding agencies, and government entities such as Medicare.

EEG (electroencephalogram) Electrodes, tiny silver disks, are attached to the skull to measure the electrical impulses of the brain. "They pick up brain waves largely from the cortex, rather than from deeper inside the brain" (Horne, *Sleepfaring,* p. 128).

endocrine, endocrinal Pertaining to the endocrine system. Endocrine glands (which include the adrenals, the pituitary, and the thyroid) secrete **hormones** that circulate through the bloodstream to control crucial physiological processes.

endogenous Originating or produced internally, within the brain or body.

epidemiology The study of how diseases begin and progress.

epinephrine (Also called **adrenaline.**) A hormone released by the adrenal glands to speed the heart, step up the breathing, and get blood to the muscles to prepare us for fight or flight.

etiology Cause or origin.

FDA See **Food and Drug Administration.**

fibromyalgia A chronic disorder characterized by muscle pain, fatigue, and sleep disturbance.

Food and Drug Administration The U.S. federal agency responsible for approving new drugs and ensuring their safety and efficacy; also responsible for the safety of food products, medical devices, and much else.

GABA (gamma-aminobutyric acid) The major inhibitory neurotransmitter in the brain, it slows down the firing of excitatory neurons. Most sleep medications enhance its action.

generic Drug companies are granted patents for twenty years, during which time they can market the drug exclusively and charge what they want. After this, competitors are allowed to sell unbranded versions (generics), which are chemically equivalent copies, for a fraction of the original price.

genes Pieces of DNA that contain information about hereditary characteristics. Most traits are defined by several genes working together.

GHB (gammahydroxybutyric acid) A substance that naturally occurs in the brain. Approved by the FDA in 2002 (in the form of sodium oxybate) for the cataplexy associated with narcolepsy, and in 2005 for "excessive daytime sleepiness," Xyrem is now available as a short-acting drug that gives deep sleep.

growth hormone (GH) A hormone released in deep sleep by the pituitary gland. It controls growth in children and adolescents and stimulates muscle and bone growth throughout adulthood. We produce less of it as we age and lose the capacity for deep sleep.

half-life Time it takes for the concentration of a substance to be reduced to half its original level.

hippocampus A part of the brain critical to forming memories. It plays a crucial role in restraining the production of the stress hormone cortisol. It may be damaged by prolonged or excessive exposure to cortisol, brought on by stress.

histamine A neurotransmitter associated with wakefulness.

homeostatic sleep pressure The drive for sleep that builds up in the course of time spent awake and dissipates during sleep.

hormone A chemical substance released into the body by the endocrine glands.

HPA See **hypothalamic-pituitary-adrenal axis.**

hyperarousal Elevated heart rate, temperature, blood pressure, and levels of stress hormones that are often associated with insomnia, as though "the idle's too high." Evidence of an overactive stress system.

hypersomnia Opposite of insomnia: tendency to excessive sleepiness.

hypnotics Sleep medications, named after Hypnos, the Greek god of sleep.

hypocretin A wake-up neurotransmitter, also called *orexin*. Postmortem examinations of narcoleptics' brains found that the cells that make hypocretin were completely missing, or if any cells remained, they were not producing the neurotransmitter, which is why narcoleptics have difficulty staying awake.

hypothalamic-pituitary-adrenal axis (HPA) When we need to move quickly, as in an emergency and in exercise, the **hypothalamus** alerts the **pituitary,** which causes the **adrenals** to pour out stress hormones (cortisol). The HPA, together with the **sympathetic nervous system,** speeds the heart, steps up breathing, and gets blood to the muscles, preparing us for fight or flight.

hypothalamus A tiny structure about the size of a grape at the base of the brain, it regulates heart rate, appetite, water balance, blood sugar, temperature, and the release of crucial hormones: thyroid, growth hormone, stress hormones. It is the key center for regulating sleep and wakefulness, containing the ventrolateral preoptic nucleus and suprachiasmic nucleus.

insulin resistance When cells become unresponsive to the effects of insulin— the hormone that controls levels of sugar, or glucose, in the blood—blood sugar levels remain abnormally high. This happens in adult-onset diabetes and prediabetic states—and with sleep deprivation.

International Classification of Sleep Disorders (ICSD)   This is the classification system used by sleep specialists. It is produced by the **American Academy of Sleep Medicine**, in association with the Sleep Research Society of the U.S. and other countries. It has more diagnostic categories and a greater specificity than the **DSM-IV**. It was first published in 1990, and revised in 2004–05.

longitudinal study   A long-term study that follows peoples' habits and behavior over many years, looking for development or change with respect to certain variables. These kinds of studies are needed with insomnia.

melatonin   The hormone secreted by the **pineal gland** in response to darkness, melatonin is known as "the hormone of darkness." Levels begin to rise a few hours before sleep and remain elevated through the night, declining just prior to awakening.

mentation   The stream of mental activity, thoughts, images, dreams that is now believed to run through all stages of sleep.

MMPI (Minnesota Multiphasic Personality Inventory)   One of the most frequently used personality tests.

multifactorial   Having many contributory factors—as insomnia has.

narcolepsy   Narcoleptics experience extreme daytime sleepiness and, in some cases, episodes of muscle paralysis (**cataplexy**) accompanied by hypnagogic hallucinations.

neuroendocrine, neuroendocrinal   The parts of the **endocrine** system that are keyed to the workings of the brain or nervous system, including the hormones that are released by the prompts of the **hypothalamus** or **pituitary**.

neurogenic   Having its origins or causes in neurobiology.

neuron   A brain cell that has the ability to transmit information.

neurotransmitter   A brain chemical that passes nerve impulses from one neuron to the next.

NIH   The National Institutes of Health is made up of twenty separate institutes and centers in Bethesda, Maryland, just outside Washington, D.C. It funds most biomedical research in this country, not only at the institutes, but by grants to researchers at universities and medical schools throughout the country.

nonbenzodiazepines   Like the benzodiazepines, these work by accentuating the action of GABA, though they're chemically different from benzodiazepines and shorter-acting. They're sufficiently similar to all be termed benzodiazepine receptor agonists, or BzRAs. They include Ambien, Sonata, Lunesta, and indiplon.

nonREM sleep   The part of sleep that's not **REM**—about 80 percent of it—and that includes the lighter stages 1 and 2 as well as the deeper stages 3 and 4. (Some researchers say this terminology gives REM exaggerated importance.) Muscles are relaxed in nonREM sleep, though there is some muscle activity, unlike in REM, where there is none.

norepinephrine   (Also called **noradrenaline**.) Both a neurotransmitter and a hormone. As a hormone, it's released by the adrenals and works alongside **epinephrine** (adrenaline) to prime the body to respond to stress. Some studies have found elevated norepinephrine levels in insomniacs.

nucleus   A bundle of **neurons** specialized for a particular activity.

off-label use   The FDA allows doctors to prescribe drugs off-label—that is, for purposes other than what the FDA has approved.

opiate   A class of drugs derived from the opium poppy or produced synthetically to have opium-like effects, dulling the senses, relieving pain, inducing sleep. These include heroin, methadone, codeine. There are also opiates produced by the body (endorphins and enkephalins) that are natural painkillers and that create a sense of well-being. (The term *opioid* refers to all of the above.)

paradoxical insomnia   In 2004, the term **sleep state misperception** was changed to *paradoxical insomnia,* "so as not to imply that it's the patient's fault," though it was changed only in the **International Classification of Sleep Disorders,** the system used by sleep specialists, and not in the more widely used **DSM-IV.**

paradoxical intention   Sometimes used as part of behavioral modification therapy, this treatment asks the patient to engage in the most feared behavior, which, for an insomniac, is (supposedly) staying awake, on the theory that insomniacs have "performance anxiety" associated with sleep and fall asleep most easily when they're trying not to.

paradoxical sleep   A term for **REM sleep,** so used because the body is paralyzed but the brain is as aroused as during wakefulness.

parasympathetic nervous system   This counteracts the sympathetic nervous system, dampening the stress response, slowing breathing, and restoring normal heart rate.

personalized medicine   A hoped-for medical practice in which treatment will be tailored to the individual's genetics.

pharmacogenomics   A science that studies how our individual genetic codes affect our responses to drugs. When more is known about this, the age of **personalized medicine** will be here.

pituitary gland   A small gland about the size of a pea at the base of the brain. It is crucial to the stress response, stimulating the adrenals to produce cortisol.

pineal gland   A small gland about the size of a pea near the center of the brain; secretes **melatonin.**

placebo   (From the Latin, *I will please.*) A treatment or therapy that has no therapeutic value but which is administered as if it did, to test the role of psychological factors.

plasticity   The ability of the brain to reconfigure itself in response to new stimuli, to lay down new neural pathways. The process continues throughout adulthood as we evolve and adapt to new environments.

polysomnogram (PSG)   The recordings used in sleep studies. These include the **EEG,** the EOG (electrooculograph, which measures eye movements); the EMG (electromyograph, which measures muscle activity); and the ECG (electrocardiograph, which monitors heartbeat and rhythm).

primary insomnia   This is the **DSM-IV** term for insomnia that is not **secondary** to another condition, to a mental or a medical problem such as apnea, restless legs syndrome, or pain. It is defined as difficulty initiating or maintaining sleep (DIMS) or nonrestorative sleep that goes on more than a month. Only in 1994 was it acknowledged that insomnia might actually be a primary disorder; before this, it was assumed to be **secondary** to or symptomatic of some other condition—and many people continue to see it this way, to this day.

prolactin   A sleep-promoting hormone released in sleep by the **pituitary.**

PSG   See **polysomnogram.**

psychogenic   Originating in—or "generated by"—the psyche or psychology of the sufferer.

psychophysiological insomnia   A catchall diagnosis for insomnia that cannot otherwise be explained. Used synonymously with **primary insomnia.**

RBD   See **REM behavior disorder.**

receptors   Sites on the surfaces of neurons. When a neurotransmitter binds to a receptor, it acts like a key opening a lock, stimulating the cell to activity.

REM behavior disorder   Normally in REM, the body is paralyzed, but with RBD, signals get through from the brain to the body, the muscles react, and the dreamer tries to act out his dreams (most people with this disorder are male). This was once assumed to be a psychological problem but is now known to be a malfunction of the part of the brain that causes muscle paralysis (atonia) during REM.

REM (rapid eye movement) sleep   The stage of sleep associated with rapid eye movements and the most vivid kind of dreaming. The body is paralyzed during this stage, except for the eyes, which dart back and forth, yet the brain is as active as during wakefulness.

restless legs syndrome (RLS)   A creepy-crawly feeling that creates an overwhelming desire to move the legs that's disruptive of sleep. Once thought to be **psychogenic,** it is now understood to have a physiological basis.

secondary insomnia   Insomnia that is caused by some other condition, such as depression or illness. Until very recently, all insomnia was said to be of this type.

selective serotonin reuptake inhibitors   SSRIs are the class of antidepressants that replaced tricyclics as the main treatment for depression. SSRIs are thought to inhibit the reabsorption of **serotonin,** so that more serotonin remains available. They include Prozac, Zoloft, and Paxil, the SSRI most frequently prescribed for sleep.

serotonin   A neurotransmitter also known as 5-hydroxytyrptamine (5-HT), a derivative of tryptophan. Important in regulating mood, body temperature, and sleep. Deficiencies are associated with depression and anxiety.

sleep architecture   Sleep proceeds in **sleep cycles** of ninety minutes, from nonREM stages 1 through 4, to REM, then back again, through 4 to 6 cycles (in normal sleep), with nonREM predominating during the first part of the night and REM predominating during the second part of the night.

sleep cycle   The progress of sleep through nonREM (stages 1, 2, 3, 4) and REM; it takes about ninety minutes.

sleep debt   "The cumulative effect of not getting enough sleep," says Wikipedia. Nobody quite knows how it works, but it doesn't seem to build up indefinitely.

sleep efficiency   Ratio of total sleep time to time spent in bed. Ninety percent sleep efficiency—that is, 90 percent of time in bed spent asleep—is optimal.

sleep hygiene   The avoidance of substances and behaviors likely to undermine sleep (alcohol, caffeine, big meals, stimulating activities) close to bedtime, and the cultivation of sleep-promoting activities, such as adhering to a regular schedule, getting regular exercise.

sleep restriction therapy   Part of behavioral modification therapy aimed at getting insomniacs to sleep in a single, consolidated block, by limiting the time spent in bed to the time spent sleeping.

sleep state misperception   The notion that insomniacs are asleep when they believe they're awake. Insomniacs' complaints are often—usually—uncorroborated by the EEG. The term was changed, in 2004, to **paradoxical insomnia.**

slow wave sleep   Stage 3 and 4 sleep. See **deep sleep** and **delta sleep.**

somnolence   Sleepiness or drowsiness.

spectral power analysis   A finer-grained, computer-aided analysis of the EEG that looks at the microstructure of sleep.

SSRIs   See **selective serotonin reuptake inhibitors.**

stimulus control therapy   A behavioral modification strategy that aims at getting insomniacs to associate the bed with sleep by discouraging use of the bed for anything but sleep and sex and encouraging adherence to a regular sleep-wake schedule.

stress system   The biochemical system that prepares us to react to difficult or threatening situations. See **hypothalamic-pituitary-adrenal axis** and **sympathetic nervous system.**

suprachiasmic nucleus   A cluster of neurons located in the **hypothalamus** at the point where the nerves from our eyes cross on the way to opposite sides of the brain. It synchronizes brain activity with the cycles of light and dark, sending signals, at the prompt of darkness, to the nearby **pineal** gland to create melatonin.

sympathetic nervous system   The part of the nervous, system that primes bodily systems for hardship or danger. It works in seconds by means of nerve cells. A second line of defense, which works in minutes by means of hormones flowing through the blood, is the **HPA.**

synapse   The junctions between neurons, by which they communicate.

thalamus   A large bundle of nerve cells in the center of the brain that connects various parts of the brain and connects the brain to the body and sensory organs. It plays a crucial role in regulating sleep and wakefulness.

tricyclics   A class of antidepressants that came on the market in the 1950s. The name derives from their molecular structure, which contains three rings of atoms.

upper airway resistance syndrome (UARS)   A type of obstructive apnea caused by an anatomical obstruction in the nose, mouth, or throat.

ventrolateral preoptic nucleus   A tiny bunch of neurons in the hypothalamus called "the sleep switch." Whereas most neuronal systems in the brain are active when we're awake and become quiescent with the onset of sleep, these neurons fire about twice as fast during sleep and inhibit the neurotransmitters involved in wakefulness. Elderly people have been found to have 50 percent fewer of these neurons.

Selected Bibliography

Abraham, John, and Julie Sheppard. 1999. *The Therapeutic Nightmare: The Battle over the World's Most Controversial Tranquilizer.* Earthscan.

Abramson, John. 2004. *Overdosed America: The Broken Promise of American Medicine.* HarperCollins.

Alvarez, A. 1995. *Night: Night Life, Night Language, Sleep, and Dreams.* Norton.

Angell, Marcia. 1993. "Caring for Women's Health—What Is the Problem?" *New England Journal of Medicine* 329, 4: 271–72.

———. 2004. *The Truth about the Drug Companies.* Random House.

Angier, Natalie. 1995. "Modern Life Suppresses Ancient Body Rhythm." *New York Times,* March 14.

Armour, Richard. 1982. *Anyone for Insomnia? A Playful Look at Sleeplessness by a Blear-Eyed Insomniac.* Woodbridge Press.

Aronoff, Michael. 1991. *Sleep and Its Secrets.* Plenum Press.

Ashton, Heather. 2002. "Benzodiazepines: How They Work and How to Withdraw." Rev. August. www.benzo.org.uk/manual/index.htm.

Avorn, Jerry. 2004. *Powerful Medicines: The Benefits, Risks, and Costs of Prescription Drugs.* Knopf.

Baddiel, David. 1996. *Time for Bed.* Warner.

Baron-Faust, Rita, and Jill Buyon. 2002. *The Autoimmune Connection.* Contemporary Books.

Bastien, Celyne, and Charles Morin. 2000. "Familial Incidence of Insomnia." *Journal of Sleep Research* 9: 49–54.

Billiard, Michel, and Alison Bentley. 2004. "Is Insomnia Best Categorized as a Symptom or a Disease?" *Sleep Medicine* 5, suppl. 1: S35–40.

Bishop, Deborah, and David Levy. 2001. *Hello Midnight: An Insomniac's Literary Bedside Companion.* Touchstone.

Bjorkelund, Cecilia, et al. 2002. "Women's Sleep: Longitudinal Changes and Secular Trends in a 24-Year Perspective: Results of the Population Study of Women in Gothenburg, Sweden." *Sleep* 25, 8: 894–99.

Bliwise, Donald. 2000. "Normal Aging." In *Principles and Practice of Sleep Medicine,* ed. Meir Kryger et al., pp. 26–42. Saunders.

Bonnet, Michael, and Donna Arand. 1992. "Caffeine Use as a Model of Acute and Chronic Insomnia." *Sleep* 15: 526–36.

———. 1995. "24-Hour Metabolic Rate in Insomniacs and Matched Normal Sleepers." *Sleep* 18, 7: 581–88.

———. 1996. "The Consequences of a Week of Insomnia." *Sleep* 19: 453–61.

———. 1997. "Review Article: Hyperarousal and Insomnia." *Sleep Medicine Reviews* 1, 2: 97–108.

———. 1998. "Heart Rate Variability in Insomniacs and Matched Normal Sleepers." *Psychosomatic Medicine* 60, 5: 610–15.

Bonnet, Michael, and Roger Rosa. 1987. "Sleep and Performance in Young Adults and Older Normals and Insomniacs during Acute Sleep Loss and Recovery." *Biological Psychology* 25: 153–72.

Borbely, Alexander. 1986. *The Secrets of Sleep.* Basic Books.

Borkovec, T. D. 1982. "Insomnia." *Journal of Consulting and Clinical Psychology* 50, 6: 880–95.

Boston Women's Health Book Collective. 1992. *The New Our Bodies, Ourselves.* Touchstone.

Boxer, Sarah. 2003. "Art/Architecture: How Louise Bourgeois Draws Herself to Sleep." *New York Times,* July 27.

Braun, Stephen. 1996. *Buzz: The Science and Lore of Alcohol and Caffeine.* Penguin Books.

Breggin, Peter. 1999. *Toxic Psychiatry.* St. Martin's Press.

Brown, Chip. 2003a. "The Stubborn Scientist Who Unraveled a Mystery of the Night." *Smithsonian* (October).

———. 2003b. "The Man Who Mistook His Wife for a Deer." *New York Times Magazine* (February 2).

Brown, Megan. 2004. "Taking Care of Business: Self-Help and Sleep Medicine in American Corporate Culture." *Journal of Medical Humanities* 25, 3: 173–87.

Buysse, Daniel. 2000. "Rational Pharmacotherapy for Insomnia: Time for a New Paradigm." *Sleep Medicine Reviews* 4, 6: 521–27.

Buysse, Daniel, and Michael Perlis. 1996. "The Evaluation and Treatment of Insomnia." *Journal of Practical Psychology and Behavioral Health* (March): 80–93.

Buysse, Daniel, et al. 2004. "Regional Brain Glucose Metabolism during Morning and Evening Wakefulness in Humans: Preliminary Findings." *Sleep* 27, 7: 1245–54.

Carey, Thomas, et al. 2005. "Focusing on the Experience of Insomnia." *Behavioral Sleep Medicine* 3, 2: 73–86.

Carskadon, Mary, ed. 1993. *Encyclopedia of Sleep and Dreaming.* Macmillan.

———, ed. 2002. *Adolescent Sleep Patterns: Biological, Social, and Psychological Influences.* Cambridge University Press.

Carskadon, Mary, and William Dement. 1985. "Sleep Loss in Elderly Volunteers." *Sleep* 8: 207–21.

Cartwright, Rosalind. 1978. *A Primer on Sleep and Dreaming.* Addison-Wesley.

Caspi, Avshalom, et al. 2003. "Influence of Life Stress on Depression: Moderation by a Polymorphism in the 5-HTT Gene." *Science* (July 18): 386–89.

Chopra, Deepak. 1994. *Restful Sleep.* Random House.

Coe, Jonathon. 1999. *The House of Sleep.* Vintage.

Cohen, Jay. 2001. *Overdose: The Case against the Drug Companies.* Tarcher/Putnam.

Coleman, Richard M. 1986. *Wide Awake at 3:00 A.M.: By Choice or by Chance?* W.H. Freeman.

Colligan, Douglas. 1978. *Creative Insomnia.* McGraw Hill.

Coren, Stanley. 1996. *Sleep Thieves.* Free Press.

Cowley, Geoffrey. 1991. "Sweet Dreams or Nightmare?" *Newsweek* 118 (August 19): 8.

Critser, Greg. 2005. *Generation Rx: How Prescription Drugs Are Altering American Lives, Minds, and Bodies.* Houghton Mifflin.

Damasio, Antonio. 1999a. *The Feeling of What Happens.* Harcourt.

———. 1999b. "How the Brain Creates the Mind." *Scientific American* 281, 2 (December): 112–18.

Dannenfeldt, Karl. 1986. "Sleep: Theory and Practice in the Late Renaissance." *Journal of the History of Medicine and Allied Sciences* 41, 4: 415–41.

Dauvilliers, Yves, et al. 2005. "Family Studies in Insomnia." *Journal of Psychosomatic Research* 58: 271–78.

Davies, Ruth. 1986. "Countercontrol Treatment of Sleep-Maintenance Insomnia in Relation to Age." *Psychology of Aging* 1: 233–38.

Davis, Gail. 2003. "Improved Sleep May Reduce Arthritis Pain." *Holistic Nursing Practice* (May–June): 128–33.

Dean, Ward, et al. 1997. *GHB: The Natural Mood Enhancer: The Authoritative Guide to Its Responsible Use.* Smart Publications.

de la Mare, Walter. 1939. *Behold This Dreamer! Of Reverie, Night, Sleep, Dream, Love-Dreams, Nightmare, Death, the Unconscious, the Imagination, Divination, the Artist, and Kindred Subjects.* Faber and Faber.

Dement, William. 1990. "A Personal History of Sleep Disorders Medicine." *Journal of Clinical Neurophysiology* 7, 1: 17–47.

———. 2003. "Knocking on Kleitman's Door: The View from 50 Years Later." *Sleep Medicine Reviews* 7, 4: 289–92.

Dement, William, with Christopher Vaughan. 1999. *The Promise of Sleep.* Delacorte Press.

Dewdney, Christopher. 2004. *Acquainted with the Night: Excursions through the World after Dark.* Bloomsbury.

Diagnostic and Statistical Manual. 2000. 4th ed. American Psychiatric Association.

Diamond, Edwin. 1967. "Long Day's Journey into the Insomniac's Night." *New York Times Magazine* (October 1).

Dinges, David, et al. 1995. "Sleep Deprivation and Human Immune Function." *Advances in Neuroimmunology* 5: 97–110.

Dixon, Katharine, et al. "Insomniac Children." *Sleep* 14 (1981): 313–18.

"DO NOT USE Eszopiclone (Lunesta): A Not-So-New Sleeping Pill." 2005. *Worst Pills, Best Pills News* (July). Public Citizen's Health Research Group.

Dorsey, Cynthia. 1991. "Failing to Sleep: Psychological and Behavioral Underpinnings of Insomnia." In *Sleep, Sleepiness, and Performance,* ed. Timothy Monk, pp. 223–47. John Wiley and Sons.

Dorsey, Cynthia, and Richard Bootzin. 1997. "Subjective and Psychophysiologic Insomnia: An Examination of Sleep Tendency and Personality." *Biological Psychiatry* 41: 209–16.

Dorsey, Cynthia, et al. 1999. "Core Body Temperature and Sleep of Older Female Insomniacs before and after Passive Body Heating." *Sleep* 22, 7: 891–98.

Dowd, Maureen. 2006. "Valley of the Rolls." *New York Times*, March 18.

Drake, Christopher, et al. 2003. "Insomnia Causes, Consequences, and Therapeutics: An Overview." *Depression and Anxiety* 18: 163–76.

Driver, Helen, and Fiona Baker. 1998. "Menstrual Factors in Sleep." *Sleep Medicine Reviews* 2, 4: 213–29.

Driver, Helen, and Sheila Taylor. 2000. "Exercise and Sleep." *Sleep Medicine Reviews* 4, 4: 387–402.

Drucker-Colin, Rene, et al. 1979. *The Functions of Sleep*. Academic Press.

Drummond, Sean, et al. 2004. "Functional Imaging of the Sleeping Brain: Review of Findings and Implications for the Study of Insomnia." *Sleep Medicine Reviews* 8: 227–42.

Durmer, Jeffrey, and David Dinges. 2005. "Neurocognitive Consequences of Sleep Deprivation." *Seminars in Neurology* 25, 1: 117–29.

Edinger, Jack, et al. 2000. "Insomnia and the Eye of the Beholder: Are There Clinical Markers of Objective Sleep Disturbances among Adults with and without Insomnia Complaints?" *Journal of Consulting and Clinical Psychology* 68, 4: 586–93.

Ehrenreich, Barbara. 2001. *Nickel and Dimed: On (Not) Getting By in America*. Henry Holt.

———. 2002. "Body Politic: The Growth of the Women's Health Movement." *Ms.* (Spring): 49–50.

Ekirch, A. Roger. 2001. "Sleep We Have Lost: Pre-industrial Slumber in the British Isles." *American Historical Review* 106, 2: 343–85.

———. 2005. *At Day's Close: Night in Times Past*. Norton.

Empson, Jacob. 1989. *Sleep and Dreaming*. Palgrave, 2002.

Ernst, E. 2003. "Obstacles to Research in Complementary and Alternative Medicine." *Medical Journal of Australia*, www.mja.com.au/public/issues/179_06_150903/ern10442_fm-1.htm.

Evans, Dylan. 2004. *Placebo: Mind over Matter in Modern Medicine*. Oxford University Press.

Evans, Peter. 1983. *Landscapes of the Night: How and Why We Dream*. Ed. Christopher Evans. Viking.

Feinberg, Irwin. 1982–83. "Schizophrenia: Caused by a Fault in Programmed Synaptic Elimination during Adolescence?" *Journal of Psychiatric Research* 17, 4: 319–34.

Feinberg, Irwin, and V. R. Carlson. 1968. "Sleep Variables as a Function of Age in Man." *Archives of General Psychiatry* 18: 239–50.

Feinberg, Irwin, and T. C. Floyd. 1982. "The Regulation of Human Sleep: Clues from Its Phenomenology." *Human Neurobiology* 1: 185–94.

Fichten, Catherine, et al. 1995. "Poor Sleepers Who Do Not Complain of Insomnia: Myths and Realities about Psychological and Lifestyle Characteristics of Older Good and Poor Sleepers." *Journal of Behavioral Medicine* 18, 2: 189–223.

Flaherty, Alice. 2004. *The Midnight Disease: The Drive to Write, Writer's Block, and the Creative Brain.* Houghton Mifflin.

Foley, Daniel, et al. 1995. "Sleep Complaints among Elderly Persons: An Epidemiologic Study of Three Communities." *Sleep* 18, 6: 425–32.

Ford, D. E., and D. B. Kamerow. 1989. "Epidemiological Study of Sleep Disturbances and Psychiatric Disorders: An Opportunity for Prevention?" *Journal of the American Medical Association* 262: 1479–84.

Forner, Aminatta. 2004. "About Last Night." *London Observer Magazine* (May 30).

Frankel, Bernard, et al. 1976. "Recorded and Reported Sleep in Chronic Primary Insomnia." *Archives of General Psychiatry* 33: 615–23.

Franken, Paul, et al. 2001. "The Homeostatic Regulation of Sleep Need Is under Genetic Control." *Journal of Neuroscience* 21, 8: 2610–21.

Freedman, Robert, and Howard Sattler. 1982. "Physiological and Psychological Factors in Sleep-Onset Insomnia." *Journal of Abnormal Psychology* 94, 5: 380–89.

Freinkel, Susan. 2005. "Vitamin Cure." *Discover* 26, 5 (May).

Fugh-Berman, Adriane, and Jerry Cott. 1999. "Dietary Supplements and Natural Products as Psychotherapeutic Agents." *Psychosomatic Medicine* 61: 712–28.

Gaillard, Jean-Michel. 1976. "Is Insomnia a Disease of Slow-Wave Sleep?" *European Neurology* 14: 473–84.

———. 1978. "Chronic Primary Insomnia: Possible Physiopathological Involvement of Slow-Wave Sleep Deficiency." *Sleep* 1, 2: 133–47.

Gaillard, Jean-Michel, et al. 1994. "Clinical Observations in Psychophysiological and Idiopathic Insomnia." *Journal of Sleep Research* 3, suppl. 1: S84.

Garattini, Silvio. 1993. *Caffeine, Coffee, and Health.* Raven Press.

Gastaut, H., et al., eds. 1968. *The Abnormalities of Sleep in Man.* Gaggi.

Gawande, Atul. 2002. *Complications.* Holt.

Gershell, Leland. 2006. "From the Analyst's Couch: Insomnia Market." *Nature* 5 (January): 15–16, www.nature.com/nrd/journal/v5/n1/full/nrd1932.html.

Gershon, Michael. 1998. *The Second Brain: A Groundbreaking New Understanding of Nervous Disorders of the Stomach and Intestine.* HarperPerennial.

Gilbert, Saul, et al. 2004. "Thermoregulation as a Sleep Signaling System." *Sleep Medicine Reviews* 8: 81–93.

Gillin, J. Christian, et al. 2005. "Medication and Substance Abuse." In *Principles and Practice of Sleep Medicine,* ed. Meir Kryger et al., pp. 1345–58. Saunders.

Gleick, James. 1999. *Faster.* Random House.

Goldberg, Burton. 2002. *Alternative Medicine: The Definitive Guide.* Celestial Arts.

Goldberg, Philip, and Daniel Kaufman. 1979. *Natural Sleep.* Rodale.

Golub, Mari, et al. 2002. "Nutrition and Circadian Activity Offset in Adolescent Rhesus Monkeys." In *Adolescent Sleep Patterns: Biological, Social, and Psychological Influences,* ed. Mary Carskadon, pp. 50–68. Cambridge University Press.

Gordon, Barbara. 1979. *I'm Dancing as Fast as I Can.* Harper and Row.

Greene, Gayle. 1999. *The Woman Who Knew Too Much: Alice Stewart and the Secrets of Radiation.* University of Michigan Press.

Greider, Katharine. 2002. *The Big Fix: How the Pharmaceutical Industry Rips Off American Consumers.* Public Affairs.

Groopman, Jerome. 2001. "Eyes Wide Open: Can Science Make Regular Sleep Unnecessary?" *New Yorker* (December 3): 52–57.

Guilleminault, C., and E. Lugaresi, eds. 1983. *Sleep/Wake Disorders: Natural History, Epidemiology, and Long-Term Evolution.* Raven Press.

Hajak, Goran. 2000. "Insomnia in Primary Care." *Sleep* 23, suppl. 3: S54–63.

Harrison, Yvonne, et al. 2000. "Prefrontal Neuropsychological Effects of Sleep Deprivation in Young Adults—A Model for Healthy Aging?" *Sleep* 23, 8: 1067–73.

Harvey, Allison. 2002. "A Cognitive Model of Insomnia." *Behaviour Research and Therapy* 40: 869–93.

Harvey, Allison, and Emmiline Greenall. 2003. "Catastrophic Worry in Primary Insomnia." *Journal of Behavior Therapy and Experimental Psychiatry* 34, 1: 11–23.

Harvey, Allison, and Nicole Tang. 2003. "Cognitive Behaviour Therapy for Primary Insomnia: Can We Rest Yet?" *Sleep Medicine Reviews* 7, 3: 237–62.

Hauri, Peter. 1981. "Treating Psychophysiologic Insomnia with Biofeedback." *Archives of General Psychiatry* 38 (July): 752–58.

———. 1983. "A Cluster Analysis of Insomnia." *Sleep* 6, 4: 326–38.

———, ed. 1991. *Case Studies in Insomnia.* Plenum.

———. 1993. "Consulting about Insomnia: A Method and Some Preliminary Data." *Sleep* 16, 4: 344–50.

———. 2000. "Primary Insomnia." In *Principles and Practice of Sleep Medicine,* ed. Meir Kryger et al., pp. 633–39. Saunders.

———. n.d. "Insomnia Manual and Reference." www.talkaboutsleep.com/sleep-disorders/archives/insomnia_manual.htm.

Hauri, Peter, and Joan Fisher. 1986. "Persistent Psychophysiologic (Learned) Insomnia." *Sleep* 9, 1: 38–53.

Hauri, Peter, and Shirley Linde. 1990. *No More Sleepless Nights.* John Wiley and Sons.

Hauri, Peter, and Elaine Olmstead. 1980. "Childhood-Onset Insomnia." *Sleep* 3, 1: 59–65.

———. 1989. "Reverse First Night Effect in Insomnia." *Sleep* 12: 97–105.

Hauri, Peter, et al. 1982a. "The Treatment of Psychophysiologic Insomnia with Biofeedback: A Replication Study." *Biofeedback and Self-Regulation* 7, 2: 223–35.

———. 1982b. "Effectiveness of a Sleep Disorders Center: A 9-Month Follow-Up." *American Journal of Psychiatry* 139: 663–66.

Hayes, Bill. 2001. *Sleep Demons: An Insomniac's Memoir.* Washington Square Press.

Healy, David. 1997. *The Anti-Depressant Era.* Harvard University Press.

———. 2004. "Psychopharmacology at the Interface between the Market and the New Biology." In *The New Brain Science: Perils and Prospects,* ed. D. Rees and S. Rose, pp. 232–48. Cambridge University Press.

Herper, Matthew. 2004. "Sleep on Demand." Forbes.com, July 22, www.forbes
.com/healthcare/2004/12/16/cx_mh_1216sepr.html?partner=rss.

Heymann, Jody. 1995. "Patients in Research: Not Just Subjects but Partners."
Science 269 (August): 797–98.

Hirshkowitz, Max, and Patricia Smith. 2004. *Sleep Disorders for Dummies.*
Wiley.

Hislop, Jenny, and Sara Arber. 2003a. "Sleepers Wake! The Gendered Nature of
Sleep Disruption among Mid-life Women." *Sociology* 37, 4: 695–711.

———. 2003b. "Understanding Women's Sleep Management: Beyond
Medicalization-Healthicization." *Sociology of Health and Illness* 25, 7:
815–37.

Hobson, J. Allan. 1989. *Sleep.* Scientific American Library.

———. 2005. "Sleep Is of the Brain, by the Brain, and for the Brain." *Nature*
437: 1254–56.

Hobson, J. Allan, and Jonathan A. Leonard. 2001. *Out of Its Mind: Psychiatry
in Crisis.* Perseus.

Hodgkinson, Tom. 2005. *How to Be Idle.* HarperCollins.

Holden, Constance. 2005. "Sex and the Suffering Brain." *Science* 308 (June 10):
1574–77.

Holzinger, Erik. 2005. "Insomnia." *Drugs* 8, 5: 410–15.

Horne, James. 1988a. "Sleep Loss and 'Divergent' Thinking Ability." *Sleep* 11,
6: 528–36.

———. 1988b. *Why We Sleep: The Functions of Sleep in Humans and Other
Mammals.* Oxford University Press.

———. 1991. "Dimensions to Sleepiness." In *Sleep, Sleepiness, and Performance,* ed. Timothy Monk, pp. 170–96. John Wiley and Sons.

———. 1993. "Human Sleep, Sleep Loss, and Behaviour." *British Journal of
Psychiatry* 162: 413–19.

———. 2006. *Sleepfaring: A Journey through the Science of Sleep.* Oxford University Press.

International Classification of Sleep Disorders: Diagnostic and Coding Manual.
2005. 2nd ed. American Academy of Sleep Medicine.

Irwin, Michael, et al. 1994. "Partial Sleep Deprivation Reduces Natural Killer
Cell Activity in Humans." *Psychosomatic Medicine* 56: 493–98.

———. 2006. "Sleep Deprivation and Activation of Morning Levels of Cellular
and Genomic Markers of Inflammation." *Archives of Internal Medicine* 166:
1756–62.

Jacobs, Gregg. 1998. *Say Good Night to Insomnia.* Owl Books.

Jacobs, Gregg, et al. 2004. "Cognitive Behavior Therapy and Pharmacotherapy
for Insomnia." *Archives of Internal Medicine* 164: 1888–96.

Jensvold, Margaret, et al. 1996. *Psychopharmacology and Women: Sex, Gender,
and Hormones.* American Psychiatric Press.

Jewell, Mark. 2005. "Ad War Looms in Crowded Sleep Aid Market." *Business
Week* (July 19), www.businessweek.com/ap/financialnews.

Joffe, Hardine, and Lee S. Cohen. 1998. "Estrogen, Serotonin, and Mood Disturbance: Where Is the Therapeutic Bridge?" *Biological Psychiatry* 44, 9:
798–811.

Jouvet, Michel. 1993 [1999]. *The Paradox of Sleep: The Story of Dreaming.* MIT Press.

Kaiser, Jocelyn. 2005. "Gender in the Pharmacy: Does It Matter?" *Science* (June 10): 1172–74.

Kales, Anthony, ed. 1969. *Sleep: Physiology and Pathology; A Symposium.* Lippincott.

Kales, Anthony, and Joyce Kales. 1984 [1990]. *Evaluation and Treatment of Insomnia.* Oxford University Press.

Kamen, Paula. 2005. *All in My Head.* Perseus.

Karacan, Ismet, et al. 1973. "Insomniacs: Unpredictable and Idiosyncratic Sleepers." In *Sleep: Physiology, Biochemistry, Psychology, Pharmacology, Clinical Implications,* ed. W.P. Koella and P. Levin, pp. 120–32. S. Karger.

Kassirer, Jerome. 2005. *On the Take: How Medicine's Complicity with Big Business Can Endanger Your Health.* Oxford University Press.

Keyes, Ralph. 1991. *Timelock.* HarperCollins.

Kiley, James. 1999. "Insomnia Research and Future Opportunities." *Sleep* 22, 1, suppl. 2: S344–45.

Kleitman, Nathaniel. 1939 [1963]. *Sleep and Wakefulness.* University of Chicago Press.

Klinkenborg, Verlyn. 1997. "Awakening to Sleep." *New York Times Magazine* (January 5).

Kolata, Gina. 2000. "Web Research Transforms Visit to the Doctor." *New York Times,* March 6.

Kripke, Daniel. 2000. "Chronic Hypnotic Use: Deadly Risks, Doubtful Benefit." *Sleep Medicine Reviews* 4, 1: 5–20.

Kryger, Meir, et al., eds. 2000 [2005]. *Principles and Practice of Sleep Medicine.* Saunders.

Lambert, Craig. 2005. "Deep into Sleep." *Harvard Magazine* (July): 25–33.

Lancel, Marike, et al. 2001. "Effect of the GABAa Agonist Gaboxadol on Nocturnal Sleep and Hormone Secretion in Healthy Elderly Subjects." *American Journal of Physiology, Endocrinology, and Metabolism* 281, 1: E130–37.

Landis, Carol, and Karen Moe. 2004. "Sleep and Menopause." *Nursing Clinics of North America* 39: 97–115.

Lavie, Peretz. 1996. *The Enchanted World of Sleep.* Yale University Press.

Lazarus, David. 2006. "Sleep Aids a Booming Business." *San Francisco Chronicle,* March 3.

Lee-Chiong, Teofilo, Jr., et al., eds. 2002. *Sleep Medicine.* Elsevier.

Leger, Damien, et al. 2001. "Evaluation of Quality of Life in Severe and Mild Insomniacs Compared with Good Sleepers." *Psychosomatic Medicine* 63: 49–55.

Leproult, Rachel, et al. 1997. "Sleep Loss Results in an Elevation of Cortisol Levels the Next Evening." *Sleep* 20, 10: 865–70.

Lieberman, Trudy. 2005. "Bitter Pill." *Columbia Journalism Review.* Rednova, July 13, www.rednova.com/news/health/172596/bitterpill/.

Linkowski, Paul. 1999. "EEG Sleep Pattern in Twins." *Journal of Sleep Research* 8, suppl. 1: S11–13.

Linkowski, Paul, et al. 1989. "EEG Sleep Patterns in Man: A Twin Study." *Electroencephalography and Clinical Neurophysiology* 73: 279–84.

———. 1991. "Genetic Determinants of EEG Sleep: A Study in Twins Living Apart." *Electroencephalography and Clinical Neurophysiology* 79: 114–18.

Linton, Simi. 1998. *Claiming Disability*. New York University Press.

Littner, Michael, et al. 2003. "Practice Parameters for Using Polysomnography to Evaluate Insomnia: An Update." *Sleep* 26, 6: 754–60.

Luce, Gay Gaer, and Julius Segal. 1969. *Insomnia: The Guide for Troubled Sleepers*. Doubleday.

Luhrmann, T.M. 2000. *Of Two Minds: The Growing Disorder in American Psychiatry*. Knopf.

Lupien, Sonia, et al. 1994. "Basal Cortisol Levels and Cognitive Deficits in Human Aging." *Journal of Neuroscience* 14, 5: 2893–903.

Maas, James, et al. 1999. *Power Sleep: The Revolutionary Program That Prepares Your Mind for Peak Performance*. Villard.

Mahowald, Mark, and Carlos Schenck. 2005. "Insights from Studying Human Sleep Disorders." *Nature* (October): 1279–85.

Manber, Rachel, and Roseanne Armitage. 1999. "Sex, Steroids, and Sleep: A Review." *Sleep* 22, 5: 540–55.

Manber, Rachel, and Tracy Kuo. 2002. "Cognitive-Behavioral Therapies for Insomnia." In *Sleep Medicine*, ed. Teofilo Lee-Chiong Jr. et al., pp. 177–85. Elsevier.

Mann, Charles. 1995. "Women's Health Research Blossoms." *Science* (August): 766–70.

Marchini, Evelyn, et al. 1983. "What Do Insomniacs Do, Think, and Feel during the Day?" *Sleep* 6, 2: 147–55.

Marsa, Linda. 2005. "Sleep for Sale." *Mother Jones* (January–February): 20–21.

Martin, Paul. 2002. *Counting Sheep: The Science and Pleasures of Sleep and Dreams*. HarperCollins.

Max, D.T. 2006. *The Family That Couldn't Sleep: A Medical Mystery*. Random House.

McEwen, Bruce. 2000. "The Neurobiology of Stress: From Serendipity to Clinical Relevance." *Brain Research* 886, 1–2 (December): 172–89.

McEwen, Bruce, with Elizabeth Lasley. 2001. *The End of Stress as We Know It*. Joseph Henry Press.

McEwen, Bruce, and Robert Sapolsky. 1995. "Stress and Cognitive Function." *Current Opinion in Neurobiology* 5: 205–16.

Medawar, Charles. 1992. *Power and Dependence: Social Audit on the Safety of Medicines*. Social Audit.

———. 1994. "Through the Doors of Deception?" *Nature* (March 24): 368, 369–70.

Medawar, Charles, and Anita Hardon. 2004. *Medicines Out of Control: Antidepressants and the Conspiracy of Goodwill*. Askant.

Meddis, Ray. 1977. *The Sleep Instinct*. University of Queensland Press.

Melbin, Murray. 1987. *Night as Frontier: Colonizing the World after Dark*. Free Press.

Mendelson, Wallace. 1990. "Do Studies of Sedative/Hypnotics Suggest the Nature of Chronic Insomnia?" In *Sleep and Biological Rhythms: Basic Mecha-*

nisms and Applications to Psychiatry, ed. Jacques Montplaisir and Roger Godbout, pp. 209–18. Oxford University Press.

———. 2000. "Hypnotics: Basic Mechanisms and Pharmacology." In *Principles and Practice of Sleep Medicine,* ed. Meir Kryger et al., pp. 407–13. Saunders.

Mendelson, Wallace, et al. 1984. "The Experience of Insomnia and Daytime and Nighttime Functioning." *Psychiatry Research* 12: 235–50.

———. 2004. "The Treatment of Chronic Insomnia: Drug Indications, Chronic Use, and Abuse Liability." *Sleep Medicine Reviews* 8: 7–17.

Mercia, Helli, et al. 1998. "Spectral Characteristics of Sleep EEG in Chronic Insomnia." *European Journal of Neuroscience* 10: 1826–34.

Mignot, Emmanuel. 2001. "A Commentary on the Neurobiology of the Hypocretin/Orexin System." *Neuropsychopharmacology* 25, suppl. 5: S5–13.

———. 2004. "Sleep, Sleep Disorders, and Hypocretin (Orexin)." *Sleep Medicine* 5, suppl. 1: S2–8.

Mignot, Emmanuel, et al. 2002. "Sleeping with the Hypothalamus: Emerging Therapeutic Targets for Sleep Disorders." *Nature Neuroscience* suppl 5: 10717–5.

Miles, Laughton, and William Dement. 1980. "Sleep and Aging." *Sleep* 3, 2: 119–220.

Moldofsky, Harvey, et al. 1975. "Musculoskeletal Symptoms and Non-REM Sleep Disturbance in Patients with 'Fibrositis Syndrome' and Healthy Subjects." *Psychosomatic Medicine* 37, 4: 341–51.

Moline, Margaret, et al. 2004. "Sleep Problems across the Life Cycle in Women." *Current Treatment Options in Neurology* 6: 319–30.

Monk, Timothy, ed. 1991. *Sleep, Sleepiness, and Performance.* John Wiley and Sons.

Monroe, Lawrence. 1967. "Psychological and Physiological Differences between Good and Poor Sleepers." *Journal of Abnormal Psychology* 72: 255–64.

Montplaisir, Jacques, and Roger Godbout, eds. 1990. *Sleep and Biological Rhythms: Basic Mechanisms and Applications to Psychiatry.* Oxford University Press.

Morin, Charles. 1996. *Relief from Insomnia.* Doubleday.

———. 2005. "Psychological and Behavioral Treatments for Primary Insomnia." In *Principles and Practice of Sleep Medicine,* ed. Meir Kryger et al., pp. 726–37. Saunders.

Morin, Charles, and Nathan Azrin. 1988. "Behavioral and Cognitive Treatments of Geriatric Insomnia." *Journal of Consulting and Clinical Psychology* 56, 5: 748–53.

Morin, Charles, and Virgil Wooten. 1996. "Psychological and Pharmacological Approaches to Treating Insomnia: Critical Issues in Assessing Their Separate and Combined Effects." *Clinical Psychology Review* 16, 6: 521–54.

Morin, Charles, et al. 1999a. "Nonpharmacologic Treatment of Chronic Insomnia." *Sleep* 22, 8: 1–23.

———. 1999b. "Behavioral and Pharmacological Therapies for Late-Life Insomnia: A Randomized Controlled Trial." *Journal of the American Medical Association* 281, 11: 991–99.

Morris, Bonnie. 2005. "Sleep Anxiety Leads Many to the Medicine Cabinet." *New York Times,* June 5.

Moynihan, Ray. 2003. "Sweetening the Pill." *Health Letter,* ed. Sidney Wolfe, 19 (September): 9.

Moynihan, Ray, and Alan Cassels. 2005. *Selling Sickness: How the World's Biggest Pharmaceutical Companies Are Turning Us All into Patients.* Nation Books.

Mueller, Rudolph. 2001. *As Sick as It Gets: The Shocking Reality of America's Healthcare: A Diagnosis and Treatment Plan.* Olin Frederick.

Murphy, Patricia, and Scott Campbell. 1997. "Nighttime Drop in Body Temperature: A Physiological Trigger for Sleep Onset?" *Sleep* 20, 7: 505–11.

Naiman, Rubin. 2006. *Healing Night: The Science and Spirit of Sleeping, Dreaming, and Awakening.* Syren Book Company.

"National Institutes of Health State of the Science Conference Statement: Manifestations and Management of Chronic Insomnia in Adults, June 13–15, 2005." 2005. *Sleep* 28, 9: 1049–57.

National Sleep Disorders Research Plan, sec. 4. "Sleep, Sex Differences, and Women's Health." National Center on Sleep Disorders Research. 2003. National Heart, Lung, and Blood Institute. www.nhlbi.nih.gov/health/prof/sleep/res_plan/section4/section4a.html.

Nofzinger, Eric. 2004a. "Advancing the Neurobiology of Insomnia, a Commentary on: 'Functional Imaging of the Sleeping Brain,' by Drummond et al." *Sleep Medicine Reviews* 8: 243–47.

———. 2004b. "What Can Neuroimaging Findings Tell Us about Sleep Disorders?" *Sleep Medicine* 5, suppl. 1: S16–22.

———. 2005. "Neuroimaging and Sleep Medicine: Theoretical Review." *Sleep Medicine Reviews* 9: 157–72.

O'Connor, Anahad. 2004. "Wakefulness Finds a Powerful Ally." *New York Times,* June 29.

Ohayon, Maurice. 2002. "Epidemiology of Insomnia: What We Know and What We Still Need to Know." *Sleep Medicine Reviews* 6, 2: 97–111.

Orr, William, et al. 1980. "Physician Education in Sleep Disorders." *Journal of Medical Education* 55, 4: 367–69.

Owens, Judith, et al. 2001. "Physician, Heal Thyself: Sleep, Fatigue, and Medical Education." *Sleep* 24, 5: 493–95.

Pack, Allan, and Miroslaw Mackiewitz. 2003. "Molecular Approaches to Understanding Insomnia." In *Insomnia: Principles and Management,* ed. Martin Szuba et al., pp. 195–212. Cambridge University Press.

Patrick, Regina. 2006. "Melatonin and Irritable Bowel Syndrome." *Focus: Journal for Respiratory Care and Sleep Medicine* 12 (January–February): 12, 66.

Paul, Annie Murphy. 2004. *The Cult of Personality: How Personality Tests Are Leading Us to Miseducate Our Children, Mismanage Our Companies, and Misunderstand Ourselves.* Free Press.

Perlis, Michael, et al. 1997. "Psychophysiological Insomnia: The Behavioral Model and a Neurocognitive Perspective." *Journal of Sleep Research* 6: 179–88.

———. 2001a. "The Mesograde Amnesia of Sleep May Be Attenuated in Subjects with Primary Insomnia." *Physiology and Behavior* 74: 71–76.

———. 2001b. "Beta/Gamma Activity in Patients with Insomnia and in Good Sleeper Controls." *Sleep* 24: 110–17.

Philip, Pierre, and Christian Guilleminault. 1996. "Adult Psychophysiologic Insomnia and Positive History of Childhood Insomnia." *Sleep* 19, 3, suppl. 1: S16–22.

Philipson, Ilene. 2002. *Married to the Job: Why We Live to Work and What We Can Do About It.* Free Press.

Preston, John. 2001. *Lift Your Mood Now.* New Harbinger Publications.

Prinz, Patricia, et al. 1990. "Sleep Disorders and Aging: Review Article." *New England Journal of Medicine* (August 23): 520–26.

Rechtschaffen, Allan. 1969. "Laboratory Studies of Insomnia." In *Sleep: Physiology and Pathology; A Symposium,* ed. Anthony Kales, 158–69. Lippincott.

———. 1979. "The Function of Sleep: Methodological Issues." In *The Functions of Sleep,* ed. Rene Drucker-Colin et al., pp. 1–19. Academic Press.

———. 1998. "Current Perspectives on the Function of Sleep." *Perspectives in Biology and Medicine* 41, 3: 359–90.

Rechtschaffen, Allan, et al. 1983. "Physiological Correlates of Prolonged Sleep Deprivation in Rats." *Science* 221: 182–84.

———. 1989. "Sleep Deprivation in the Rat. Part 10: Integration and Discussion of the Findings." *Sleep* 12: 68–87.

Regenstein, Quentin, and Peter Reich. 1983. "Incapacitating Childhood-Onset Insomnia." *Comprehensive Psychiatry* 24, 3: 244–48.

Relman, Arnold, and Marcia Angell. 2002. "America's Other Drug Problem." *The New Republic* (December 16): 27–41.

Reynolds, Charles, et al. 1986. "Sleep Deprivation in Healthy Elderly Men and Women: Effects on Mood and Sleep during Recovery." *Sleep* 9: 492–501.

Richardson, Gary. 2000. "Managing Insomnia in the Primary Care Setting: Raising the Issues." *Sleep* 23, suppl. 1: S9–15.

Richardson, Gary, and Thomas Roth. 2001. "Future Directions in the Management of Insomnia." *Journal of Clinical Psychiatry* 62, suppl. 10: S39–45.

Ridley, Matt. 2003. *Nature via Nurture: Genes, Experience, and What Makes Us Human.* HarperCollins.

Rodenbeck, Andrea, and Goran Hajak. 2001. "Neuroendocrine Dysregulation in Primary Insomnia." *Review of Neurology* (Paris), 157, 11, suppl. 5: S57–61.

Rodwin, Marc. 1993. *Medicine, Money, and Morals: Physicians' Conflicts of Interest.* Oxford University Press.

Roehrs, Timothy, and Thomas Roth. 2000. "Hypnotics: Efficacy and Adverse Effects." In *Principles and Practice of Sleep Medicine,* ed. Meir Kryger et al., pp. 441–18. Saunders.

Root-Bernstein, Robert, and Michele Root-Bernstein. 1995. *Honey, Mud, Maggots, and Other Medical Marvels.* Mariner Books.

Rosenteur, Phyllis. 1957. *Morpheus and Me: The Complete Book of Sleep.* Funk and Wagnalls.

Ross, Herbert, et al. 2000. *Sleep Disorders: An Alternative Medicine Definitive Guide.* Alternative Medicine.com Books.

Ross, Julia. 1999. *The Diet Cure.* Penguin.

———. 2002. *The Mood Cure.* Penguin.

Rubenstein, Hilary. 1974. *Insomniacs of the World, Goodnight.* Random House.

Rubinow, David, et al. 1998. "Estrogen-Serotonin Interactions: Implications for Affective Regulation." *Biological Psychiatry* 44, 9: 839–50.

Saper, Clifford, and Thomas Scammell. 2003. "Hypothalamic Pathways and Neurotransmitters Regulating Sleep." In *Insomnia: Principles and Management,* ed. Martin Szuba et al., pp. 239–47. Cambridge University Press.

Saper, Clifford, et al. 2001. "The Sleep Switch: Hypothalamic Control of Sleep and Wakefulness." *Trends in Neuroscience* 24: 726–31.

———. 2005. "Hypothalamic Regulation of Sleep and Circadian Rhythms." *Nature* 437: 1257–63.

Sapolsky, Robert. 1994. *Why Zebras Don't Get Ulcers.* Freeman.

Sapolsky, Robert, et al. 1986. "The Neuroendocrinology of Stress and Aging: The Glucocorticoid Cascade Hypothesis." *Endocrine Reviews* 7, 3: 284–301.

Sateia, Michael, et al. 2000. "Evaluation of Chronic Insomnia." *Sleep* 23, 2: 243–62.

Saul, Stephanie. 2006. "To Sleep, Perchance to Eat. Is It the Pill?" *New York Times,* March 14.

———. 2007. "U.S. Calls for Strong Warnings on Sleep Aids' Strange Effects." *New York Times,* March 15.

Schiller, Francis. 1982. "Semantics of Sleep." *Bulletin of the History of Medicine* 56: 377–97.

Schneider-Helmert, Dietrich. 1987. "Twenty-Four-Hour Sleep-Wake Function and Personality Patterns in Chronic Insomniacs and Healthy Controls." *Sleep* 10, 5: 452–62.

Schredl, Michael, et al. 1998. "Dreaming and Insomnia: Dream Recall and Dream Content of Patients with Insomnia." *Journal of Sleep Research* 7: 191–98.

Schur, Carolyn. 1994. *Birds of a Different Feather: Early Birds and Night Owls Talk about Their Characteristic Behaviors.* Schur Goode Associates.

Schwartz, Jeffrey, and Sharon Begley. 2002. *The Mind and the Brain: Neuroplasticity and the Power of Mental Force.* HarperCollins.

Schwartz, W. J., ed. 1997. *Sleep Science: Integrating Basic Research and Clinical Practice.* Basel.

Seeman, Teresa, and Richard Robbins. 1994. "Aging and Hypothalamic-Pituitary-Adrenal Response to Challenge in Humans." *Endocrine Reviews* 15, 2: 233–60.

Seeman, Teresa, et al. 1995. "Gender Differences in Patterns of HPA Axis Response to Challenge: Macarthur Studies of Successful Aging." *Psychoneuroendocrinology* 20, 7: 711–25.

Sewitch, Deborah. 1984. "The Perceptual Uncertainty of Having Slept: The Inability to Discriminate EEG Sleep from Wakefulness." *Psychophysiology* 21, 3: 243–59.

Shenk, David. 2001. *The Forgetting, Alzheimer's: Portrait of an Epidemic.* Doubleday.

Sherwin, Barbara. 1996. "Menopause, Early Aging, and Elderly Women." In *Psychopharmacology and Women: Sex, Gender, and Hormones,* ed. Margaret Jensvold et al., pp. 225–37. American Psychiatric Press.

Shipler, David. 2004. *The Working Poor: Invisible in America.* Knopf.

Shors, Tracey, and Benedetta Leuner. 2003. "Estrogen-Mediated Effects on Depression and Memory Formation in Females." *Journal of Affective Disorders* 74: 85–96.

Shorter, Edward. 1997. *A History of Psychiatry: From the Era of the Asylum to the Age of Prozac.* Wiley.

Siegel, Jerome. 2000. "Narcolepsy." *Scientific American* (January), www.sciam .com/2000/0100issue/0100siegel.html.

———. 2003. "Why We Sleep." *Scientific American* (November): 92–97.

———. 2004. "Brain Mechanisms That Control Sleep and Waking." *Naturwissenschaften* 91: 355–65.

"Sleep Centers—a Super Booming Industry." January 3, 2004. Pressrelease@ medicalnewstoday.com.

Sleep Disorders and Sleep Deprivation: An Unmet Public Health Problem; American Academy of Sleep Medicine Statement on Institute of Medicine Report. April 15, 2006. AASMnet.org/Articles.aspx?id=201.

Smith, Mickey. 1985. *A Social History of the Minor Tranquilizers: The Quest for Small Comfort in the Age of Anxiety.* Pharmaceutical Products Press.

Solomon, Andrew. 2001. *The Noonday Demon: An Atlas of Depression.* Scribner.

Spaar, Lisa, ed. 1999. *Acquainted with the Night: Insomnia Poems.* Columbia University Press.

Spiegel, Karine, et al. 1999. "Impact of Sleep Debt on Metabolic and Endocrine Function." *Lancet* 354: 1435–39.

———. 2004a. "Leptin Levels Are Dependent on Sleep Duration: Relationships with Sympathovagal Balance, Carbohydrate Regulation, Cortisol, and Thyrotropin." *Journal of Clinical Endocrinology and Metabolism* 89, 11: 5762–71.

———. 2004b. "Sleep Curtailment in Healthy Young Men Is Associated with Decreased Leptin Levels, Elevated Ghrelin Levels, and Increased Hunger and Appetite." *Annals of Internal Medicine* 141: 846–50.

Stepanski, Edward. 2000. "Behavioral Therapy for Insomnia." In *Principles and Practice of Sleep Medicine,* ed. Meir Kryger et al., pp. 647–56. Saunders.

———. 2002. "Etiology of Insomnia." In *Sleep Medicine,* ed. Teofilo Lee-Chiong et al., pp. 565–74. Elsevier.

Stepanski, Edward, and J. Wyatt. 2003. "Use of Sleep Hygiene in the Treatment of Insomnia." *Sleep Medicine Reviews* 7, 3: 215–25.

Stepanski, Edward, et al. 1988. "Daytime Alertness in Patients with Chronic Insomnia Compared with Asymptomatic Control Subjects." *Sleep* 11: 54–60.

Stickgold, Robert. 2005a. "Why We Dream." In *Principles and Practice of Sleep Medicine,* ed. Meir Kryger et al., pp. 579–87. Saunders.

———. 2005b. "Sleep-Dependent Memory Consolidation." *Nature* 437 (October 27): 1272–78.

Stickgold, Robert, et al. 2001. "Sleep, Learning, and Dreams: Off-Line Memory Reprocessing." *Science* 294 (November 2): 1052–57.

St. John, Warren, and Alex Williams. 2005. "The Crow of the Early Bird." *New York Times*, March 27.

Stoller, Melissa. 1994. "Economic Effects of Insomnia." *Clinical Therapeutics* 16, 4: 873–96.

Stores, Gregory, and Luci Wiggs, ed. 2001. *Sleep Disturbance in Children and Adolescents with Disorders and Development*. Mac Keith Press.

Styron, William, 1990. *Darkness Visible*. Vintage Books.

Szuba, Martin, et al., eds. 2003. *Insomnia: Principles and Management*. Cambridge University Press.

Tafti, M., et al. 2005. "Genes for Normal Sleep and Sleep Disorders." *Annals of Medicine* 37: 580–89.

Taheri, S., and Emmanuel Mignot. 2001. "The Genetics of Sleep Disorders." *Lancet Neurology* 1 (August): 242–50.

Taylor, Brian. 1993. "Unconsciousness and Society: The Sociology of Sleep." *International Journal of Politics, Culture, Society* 6, 3: 463–71.

Taylor, Daniel, et al. 2003. "Insomnia as Health Risk Factor." *Behavioral Sleep Medicine* 4: 227–47.

Thompson, E.P. 1966. *The Making of the English Working Class*. Vintage.

Turek, Fred, and Phyllis Zee, eds. 1999. *Regulation of Sleep and Circadian Rhythms*. Marcel Dekker.

U.S. Food and Drug Administration. 2001. *Peripheral and Central Nervous System Drugs*. Advisory Committee, Department of Health and Human Services, U.S. Food and Drug Administration, Center for Drug Evaluation and Research, June 6.

Utley, Marguerite Jones. 1995. *Narcolepsy: A Funny Disorder That's No Laughing Matter*. Self-published.

Van Cauter, Eve. 2005. "Endocrine Physiology." In *Principles and Practice of Sleep Medicine*, ed. Meir Kryger et al., pp. 266–82. Saunders.

Van Cauter, Eve, and Karine Spiegel. 1997. "Hormones and Metabolism during Sleep." In *Sleep Science: Integrating Basic Research and Clinical Practice*, ed. W.J. Schwartz, pp. 144–74. Basel.

Van Cauter, Eve, et al. 1996. "Effects of Gender and Age on the Levels and Circadian Rhythmicity of Plasma Cortisol." *Journal of Clinical Endocrinology and Metabolism* 81, 7: 2468–73.

———. 2000. "Age-Related Changes in SWS and REM Sleep and Relationship with GH and Cortisol Levels in Healthy Men." *Journal of the American Medical Association* 284, 7 (August 16): 861–81.

Van Coevorden, Anne, et al. 1991. "Neuroendocrine Rhythms and Sleep in Aging Men." *American Journal of Physiology* 260, 23: E651–61.

Van Dongen, Hans, et al. 2004. "Systematic Interindividual Differences in Neurobehavioral Impairment from Sleep Loss: Evidence of Trait-like Differential Vulnerability." *Sleep* 27, 3: 423–33.

———. 2005. "Individual Differences in Adult Human Sleep and Wakefulness: Leitmotif for a Research Agenda." *Sleep* 28, 4: 479–95.

Verdon, Jean. 2002. *Night in the Middle Ages*. University of Notre Dame Press.

Vgontzas, Alexandros, and G. P. Chrousos. 2002. "Sleep, the Hypothalamic-Pituitary-Adrenal Axis, and Cytokines: Multiple Interactions and Disturbances in Sleep Disorders." *Endocrinology and Metabolism Clinics of North America* 31: 15–36.

Vgontzas, Alexandros, et al. 1998. "Chronic Insomnia and Activity of the Stress System." *Journal of Psychosomatic Research* 45: 21–31.

———. 2001. "Chronic Insomnia Is Associated with Nyctohemeral Activation of the Hypothalamic-Pituitary-Adrenal Axis." *Journal of Clinical Endocrinology and Metabolism* 86: 3787–94.

Walker, Matthew, and Robert Stickgold. 2006. "Sleep, Memory, and Plasticity." *Annual Review of Psychology* 57: 139–66.

Walker, Sidney. 1996. *A Dose of Sanity: Mind, Medicine, and Misdiagnosis.* John Wiley and Sons.

Wallace, Robert, and Herbert Benson. 1972. "The Physiology of Meditation." *Scientific American* 226, 2 (February): 84–90.

Walsh, James. 1999. "Ten-Year Trends in the Pharmaceutical Treatment of Insomnia." *Sleep* 22, 3: 371–75.

———. 2004a. "Clinical and Socioeconomic Correlates of Insomnia." *Journal of Clinical Psychiatry* 65, suppl. 8: S13–19.

———. 2004b. "Drugs Used to Treat Insomnia in 2002: Regulatory-Based Rather Than Evidence-Based Medicine." *Sleep* 27, 8: 1441–42.

———. 2006. "Insights into the Public Health Burden of Insomnia." *Sleep* 29, 2: 179–84.

Wasleben, Joyce, and Rita Baron-Faust. 2000. *A Woman's Guide to Sleep.* Crown.

Webb, Wilse. 1975. *Sleep: The Gentle Tyrant.* Prentice Hall.

———. 1989. "Age-Related Changes in Sleep." *Clinics in Geriatric Medicine* 5, 2: 275–87.

Wehr, Thomas. 1992. "In Short Photoperiods, Human Sleep Is Biphasic." *Journal of Sleep Research* 1: 103–7.

———. 1996. "A 'Clock for All Seasons' in the Human Brain." In *Hypothalamic Integration of Circadian Rhythms: Progress in Brain Research*, ed. R. M. Buijs et al., pp. 321–42. Elsevier.

———. 1999. "The Impact of Changes in Nightlength (Scotoperiod) on Human Sleep." In *Regulation of Sleep and Circadian Rhythms*, ed. Fred Turek and Phyllis Zee, pp. 263–85. Marcel Dekker.

Wehr, Thomas, et al. 1993. "Conservation of Photoperiod-Responsive Mechanisms in Humans." *American Journal of Physiology* 265: R846–57.

Weil, Andrew. 1995. *Spontaneous Healing.* Ballantine.

Weitzman, Elliot, et al. 1981. "Delayed Sleep Phase Syndrome." *Archives of General Psychiatry* 38 (July): 737–46.

Wells, Melanie. 2006. "The Sleep Racket." *Forbes* (February 27): 81–88.

Whybrow, Peter. 2005. *American Mania: When More Is Not Enough.* Norton.

Wiedman, John. 1999. *Desperately Seeking Snoozin'.* Towering Pines Press.

Williams, Robert, and Ismet Karacan. 1978. *Sleep Disorders: Diagnosis and Treatment.* Wiley.

Wilson, Jennifer. 2005. "Is Sleep the New Vital Sign?" *Annals of Internal Medicine* 142, 10 (May 17): 877–80.

Wilson, Virginia, ed. 1996. *Sleep Thief: Restless Legs Syndrome.* Galaxy Books.

Worthman, Carol, and Melissa Melby. 2002. "Toward a Comparative Developmental Ecology of Human Sleep." In *Adolescent Sleep Patterns: Biological, Social, and Psychological Influences,* ed. Mary Carskadon, pp. 69–117, Cambridge University Press.

Wright, Lawrence. 1962. *Warm and Snug: The History of the Bed.* Routledge.

Yi, Daniel. 2006. "What Came First: Illness or the Ad?" *Los Angeles Times,* August 9.

Zarcone, Vincent. 2000. "Sleep Hygiene." In *Principles and Practice of Sleep Medicine,* ed. Meir Kryger et al., pp. 657–61. Saunders.

Index

Text: 10/13 Sabon
Display: Akzidenz Grotesk Condensed
Compositor: Binghamton Valley Composition, LLC
Printer and Binder: Maple-Vail Manufacturing Group